Medical Ethics
FOR
DUMMIES®

by Jane Runzheimer, MD, and Linda Johnson Larsen

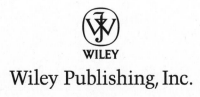

WILEY

Wiley Publishing, Inc.

Medical Ethics For Dummies®

Published by
Wiley Publishing, Inc.
111 River St.
Hoboken, NJ 07030-5774
www.wiley.com

Copyright © 2011 by Wiley Publishing, Inc., Indianapolis, Indiana

Published simultaneously in Canada

For general information on our other products and services, please contact our Customer Care Department within the U.S. at 877-762-2974, outside the U.S. at 317-572-3993, or fax 317-572-4002.

For technical support, please visit www.wiley.com/techsupport.

Wiley also publishes its books in a variety of electronic formats. Some content that appears in print may not be available in electronic books.

Library of Congress Control Number: 2010939506

ISBN: 978-0-470-87856-9

Manufactured in the United States of America

10 9 8 7 6 5 4 3 2 1

WILEY

About the Authors

Jane Runzheimer, MD, is a family physician who has been practicing primary care medicine for ten years. Her practice at Allina Medical Clinic in Northfield, Minnesota, includes pregnancy care, pediatrics, adult medicine, and geriatrics. She has a bachelor of science degree in molecular biology from the University of Wisconsin–Madison and is a graduate of the University of Minnesota Medical School. She is a member of the American Academy of Family Physicians and the Alpha Omega Alpha Medical Honor Society.

She has served on the Ethics Committee of Methodist Hospital in St. Louis Park, Minnesota, and Northfield Hospital. She has a special interest in medical ethics, especially in the areas of race and end-of-life care. She has also worked with the Indian Health Service in Zuni, New Mexico, and the Pine Ridge Indian Reservation in South Dakota.

Linda Johnson Larsen is an author and journalist who has written 24 books, many about food and nutrition. She earned a bachelor of arts degree in biology from St. Olaf College and a bachelor of science degree with high distinction in food science and nutrition from the University of Minnesota after she realized she didn't want to go to medical school after all.

She has been a patient advocate for her husband and several family members. She has spent thousands of hours in hospital and doctor's waiting rooms, learning the questions to ask when someone is sick, studying how doctors and nurses work together, and researching hospital standards. Linda understands that someone must be the voice for patients in the hospital. She has always been a student of ethics, and even made several life decisions (such as honoring a commitment to a college roommate when a semester studying abroad beckoned) depending on ethical issues such as nonmaleficence.

Linda is the Busy Cooks Guide for About.com and writes about food, recipes, and nutrition. Her books with an emphasis on health include recipes for *Detox Diet For Dummies, Knack Low-Salt Cooking, The Everything No Trans Fat Cookbook,* and *The Everything Low-Cholesterol Cookbook.*

Dedication

From Jane: First, I dedicate this book to my husband, Mark, the greatest gift in my life. I also dedicate this book to our three wonderful children — Jessica, Luke, and Marie Labenski. You four are deeply loved. I also would like to honor my parents, Kitty and Lee Runzheimer. They are two of the greatest examples of love, compassion for others, and ethical behavior that a person could ever have. And I can't forget my little brother, Kurt, who has been my best friend from the very beginning. Thank you all for the love and support you have given me. Finally, I dedicate this book back to God in gratitude for the many gifts He has given me — my loving family and friends, a profession that is my passion, my own (usually) good health, and the opportunity to spread a little light into places of darkness. Thank you, God, for your many gifts!

From Linda: I dedicate this book first and foremost to my husband, Doug. Throughout the last 29 years, we've had many ups and downs with medical issues and had the good fortune to be treated by excellent doctors and nurses. Through it all, he's been by my side and is my biggest cheerleader and confidant. I'd also like to dedicate the book to my parents, Duane and Marlene Johnson, for their support and encouragement. They always told me I could do anything I put my mind to!

Authors' Acknowledgments

From Jane: I would like to thank Linda Larsen for inviting me to work on this project with her. She has been an excellent coauthor — a gifted writer, a patient partner, and a great friend. I would also like to thank three of my fellow physicians — my husband, Dr. Mark Labenski, and my dear friends Dr. Amy Ripley and Dr. Laurel Gamm — for their professional input and their personal support.

I would like to thank all of my co-workers at Allina for putting up with a doctor who was more underslept than usual — I couldn't work with a better group of people. I send a special thanks to Linda Franek, LPN, my nurse of ten years, who is my dedicated friend and partner in our practice. I would also like to acknowledge Pastor Timothy McDermott and Lois Lindbloom for their spiritual input and support. And I would like to thank the two doctors who keep me healthy — Dr. Marty Freeman and Dr. Gretchen Ehresmann.

I should also say a special thanks to the man who first inspired my love of writing — my high school English teacher Roger Mahn. And also those professors who fueled my interest in medical ethics — Dr. Wayne Becker and Dr. Norm Fost (University of Wisconsin) and Dr. Arthur Caplan (University of Minnesota).

Finally, I would be remiss if I didn't mention my most important teachers and supporters — my many patients. Thank you all for the things that you have taught me, all the times that you have encouraged me, all the times you have forgiven me when I have failed you, and all the times we have worked together for a successful outcome.

From Linda: I'd like to thank my co-author, Jane, first of all, for being such a wonderful friend and guide while working on this book. We made a great team, and I'm grateful that we share the same sense of humor!

I'd also like to thank the biology department at St. Olaf College for giving me such a strong foundation in science, and for helping me realize I didn't want to become a doctor!

Thanks to our agent, Barb Doyen. She had such confidence in my ability to write this book and encouraged me every step of the way. Thanks to our wonderful editors for their support, suggestions, and guidance.

Special thanks to Amy Adams and Meg Schneider for their assistance and excellent logical reasoning skills. And thanks to my friends, especially my Facebook friends, and my faithful family for their support and love as I poured myself into this project.

Publisher's Acknowledgments

We're proud of this book; please send us your comments at http://dummies.custhelp.com. For other comments, please contact our Customer Care Department within the U.S. at 877-762-2974, outside the U.S. at 317-572-3993, or fax 317-572-4002.

Some of the people who helped bring this book to market include the following:

Acquisitions, Editorial, and Media Development

Project Editor: Victoria M. Adang

Acquisitions Editor: Michael Lewis

Senior Copy Editor: Danielle Voirol

Copy Editor: Susan Hobbs

Assistant Editor: David Lutton

Technical Editor: Karen Spears

Editorial Manager: Michelle Hacker

Editorial Assistants: Rachelle S. Amick, Jennette ElNaggar

Cover Photo: © Images.com/Corbis

Cartoons: Rich Tennant (www.the5thwave.com)

Composition Services

Project Coordinator: Sheree Montgomery

Layout and Graphics: Laura Westhuis

Proofreaders: Lindsay Littrell, Nancy L. Reinhardt

Indexer: Dakota Indexing

Publishing and Editorial for Consumer Dummies

Diane Graves Steele, Vice President and Publisher, Consumer Dummies

Kristin Ferguson-Wagstaffe, Product Development Director, Consumer Dummies

Ensley Eikenburg, Associate Publisher, Travel

Kelly Regan, Editorial Director, Travel

Publishing for Technology Dummies

Andy Cummings, Vice President and Publisher, Dummies Technology/General User

Composition Services

Debbie Stailey, Director of Composition Services

Contents at a Glance

Table of Contents

Introduction

While I (co-author Linda) was writing this book, my husband was admitted to the hospital and had to undergo a surgical procedure. Because I have studied medical ethics, it was interesting to see how the nurses, doctors, and other staff worked with us and each other, and how many of the issues in this book were addressed.

We had a very positive experience. Everyone was kind and helpful, and many of the topics I had researched were covered without a single glitch, down to asking about advance directives and telling us about the patient's bill of rights. But not every hospital or clinic visit is so smooth. Everyone who practices medicine takes a course or two on medical ethics, but applying what you've learned to real-life experiences takes effort. You gain knowledge from day-to-day experiences, and you learn from stories of other patients and providers. That's what *Medical Ethics For Dummies* is about.

For healthcare providers, Jane and I have provided many examples of real-life cases that require wrestling with ethical and philosophical problems. These examples cover many of the aspects you'll encounter as you build your practice. From the ethics of prenatal care, through family practice, medical research, and dealing with the last stages of life, the principles of medical ethics are examined and applied.

We don't always draw conclusions from the examples. Sometimes an issue can raise more questions than answers, and some of these issues are so personal they must be answered on a case-by-case basis.

About This Book

The practice of medicine is an art and a science. The art comes from dealing with human beings, who can be fragile and unpredictable when they are sick and need your help. The science comes from years of research and study. Medical ethics puts the art and science together in practical applications to tricky problems.

This book is arranged in a practical format. First, we examine the basics of medical ethics, its principles, and some controversies. Then we move on to putting morality in medicine. We look at the provider-patient relationship and how you can run a good, ethical practice. Everyone makes mistakes, but it's possible to learn from medical errors and design your practice so they are caught and fixed before they become serious problems or affect patients.

Then we follow patients through their lives, from prenatal care and dealing with the ethical issues of pregnancy, abortion, and reproductive technology, to treating children and working with parents. Then the discussion turns to death, both understanding when life ends and the ethics of end-of-life care. Finally, standards for medical research and the ethics of clinical trials using human beings are covered.

The great thing about *Medical Ethics For Dummies* is that providers and patients can both learn something relevant to their lives. Everyone is a patient at some point in their life, so understanding the philosophical side of medicine can only make the process smoother. And the more providers understand about the ethics of their profession, the more satisfying their work lives will be.

Conventions Used in This Book

The following conventions are used throughout the text to make things consistent and easy to understand:

- ✔ All Web addresses appear in `monofont`.
- ✔ Some new terms appear in *italic* and are closely followed by an easy-to-understand definition. We also italicize words that are often used in the medical field.
- ✔ **Bold** is used to highlight keywords in bulleted lists.

Co-author Jane has gleaned many stories relating to the ethics of practicing medicine from her practice and years of experience; we've placed those in sidebars throughout the text and marked them with an "A Note From the Doctor" icon. They are written in her voice and explain the issues she's faced in her work as a family practice physician and as a member of hospital medical ethics boards. Chapter 18, on ethical issues to address with your patients, is also written in her voice.

Because patients are both male and female, we've tried to alternate using male and female pronouns throughout the book — except of course in the chapters on pregnancy! Names and genders of the cases in the book have been changed, and actual information, although medically accurate, has been tweaked to protect privacy.

What You're Not to Read

We've written this book so you can find information easily and understand what you find. Each chapter covers one area of medicine and gives you the ethical basics you'll need to practice. But if you don't read every word, that's okay. Some text is set off from the main information, and it's interesting and relevant, but it's also stuff you can live without.

- ✔ **Text in sidebars:** Sidebars are the shaded boxes that give detailed examples or add interesting information that will help enhance your understanding of medical ethics.

- ✔ **The copyright and publisher's acknowledgments pages:** Unless you want to read legal jargon or are interested about all the people who put the book together (and they are important!), that's not the essential meat of the book.

Foolish Assumptions

This is what we've assumed about you because you're reading this book:

- ✔ You're a physician or medical student who wants to know more about medical ethics, either to enhance your practice or before you take licensing board exams.

- ✔ You're a nursing student who is curious about medical ethics. Nurses have their own code of medical ethics, which you've probably studied.

- ✔ You're in the medical field or a community member of a hospital ethics committee and have questions about ethical issues, or you need a refresher course on topics you may have studied in school.

- ✔ You're not in the medical field, but you want to know more about medical ethics from a patient's point of view. This knowledge will help make you a better patient because you can more actively participate in your health-care needs and decisions. We've tried to avoid using much medical jargon in this book so anyone can understand it. An interest in the topic is all you really need to learn more.

How This Book Is Organized

This book is divided into five parts. Each part deals with a certain aspect of medicine and discusses the relevant ethical issues. You don't have to read straight through the book; you can pick a chapter of interest and read that to find out all you need to know about that issue.

Part 1: Medical Ethics, or Doing the Right Thing

Medical ethics is based on essential principles. Those principles of autonomy, beneficence, nonmaleficence, and justice can be applied to difficult ethical situations. That's not as complicated as it sounds! When you decide which principle or principles apply, you can use them in a medical situation to reach an ethical decision on some pretty knotty subjects. You find out about codes of medical ethics and the importance of the doctor-patient relationship, especially the importance of confidentiality and informed consent. In this part, we also discuss how to set up an ethical medical practice and how to prevent medical mistakes, as well as learn from them.

Part II: A Patient's Right to Request, Receive, and Refuse Care

Should everyone have access to healthcare? If so, how are we going to make sure it's distributed fairly? We try to answer those questions and address the issues of religious and cultural differences. Finally, we include information about parental responsibilities and rights and the privacy rights of minor patients.

Part III: Ethics at the Beginning and End of Life

Personhood is the focus of this section. When does an embryo become a person? What are the ethical issues surrounding abortion? What about genetic testing and counseling for pregnant women? And because reproductive technology has exploded over the past years, we look at the ethics of in vitro fertilization (IVF), embryo storage, surrogacy, and sterilization. And at the other end of life, when does life end? What are the ethical standards regarding brain death? How can we help patients die with dignity and minimize suffering without violating ethical standards? We also look at some landmark ethical cases on the right to die and discuss physician-assisted suicide.

Part IV: Advancing Medical Knowledge with Ethical Clinical Research

Clinical research is the cornerstone of medicine. Just think how much the average lifespan has increased over the last 100 years. Much of that is due to modern medicine! Clinical research has given us more effective treatments for diseases, has found cures for some, discovered ways to diagnose problems earlier, and offers hope for the future. But there have been some dark times in medical research. Those need to be studied to avoid problems in the future. We look at the basics of ethical research trials, including the issue of informed consent and truth telling. We also take a look at some of the most controversial research projects: stem cell and genetic research.

Part V: The Part of Tens

Finally, we address some ethical issues you should talk about with your patients, look at some high profile medical ethics cases that set the current ethical standards (and even changed some laws), and try to gaze into a crystal ball at future ethics issues.

Icons Used in This Book

To make this book easier to read and simpler to use, we include some icons that can help you find and fathom key ideas and information.

We use this icon to highlight Jane's thoughts on the ethics of practicing medicine or to draw your attention to real-life situations she has encountered.

Whenever you see this icon, you know that the information that follows is so important that it's worth reading twice. Or three times!

This icon appears whenever an idea or information can help you in your medical practice or in your work with other providers.

When you see this icon, it's highlighting information that's important or that could be dangerous to you or your patient if not heeded.

Where to Go from Here

This book is organized so you can go wherever you want to find complete information. Want to know more about the ethical issues of abortion? Head to Chapter 11. If you're interested in the history of medical research and clinical trials, Chapter 14 is for you. If you want to know about the ethics of treating children and parental responsibilities, read Chapter 8. You can use the table of contents to find the broad categories of subjects, or use the index to look up specific information.

If you're not sure where to start, read Part I. It gives you all the basic information you need to understand the ethics of medicine and will tell you where to get the details.

Part I
Medical Ethics, or Doing the Right Thing

The 5th Wave   By Rich Tennant

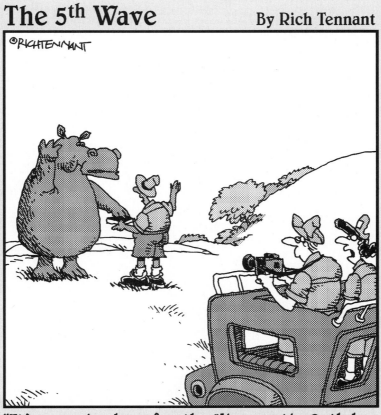

"It's amazing how far the Hippocratic Oath has evolved over the years."

In this part . . .

Medical ethics, also called bioethics, is the underpinning of any medical practice. To understand medical ethics, you need to look at the historical context and guideposts that have been developed over the years. "Doing the right thing" sounds simple, but can be difficult in practice. We define the four main principles of medical ethics, take a look at the basics of running an ethical practice, examine the doctor-patient relationship, and discover what to do when mistakes are made.

Chapter 1

What Are Medical Ethics?

Do the right thing. It sounds so easy, but it isn't. Every time a story is written about any medical issue, whether it's abortion, end-of-life care, or multiple births, everyone has an opinion about what's right and what's wrong. We're bombarded with two or more opposing viewpoints, and each one sound reasonable. But which one is right?

And that's medical ethics in a nutshell. What's the right thing to do? How do we structure clinics, hospitals, and government so the most people benefit and patients are treated with respect and compassion? What should you, as the provider, do in certain situations?

There are guidelines and principles in place to help us make decisions, but sometimes those come into direct conflict with each other. When that happens, we need to use logical reasoning skills, ethical theories, and some tools of philosophy to balance and weigh our options. Even after all of that is done, there are still questions. Medical ethics gets into the gray areas of life. As you look at these issues in more depth, you realize there aren't many that are truly black and white.

In this chapter, we define medical ethics, look at the differences between ethical and legal behaviors, and explain the difference between patient rights and provider responsibilities. We need to understand the guidelines and guideposts to follow while treating patients in all stages of life. We look at some of the common and hot-button controversies and take a peek at the ethics of medical research, which is on the forefront of medicine.

Defining Medical Ethics

Healthcare providers have always been respected and even revered. As societies were formed, ethical principles were developed by physicians and scholars from all walks of life. From Hippocrates to Muhammad ibn Zakariya ar-Razi to Thomas Aquinas, physicians and theologians have crafted guidelines to aid providers in their quest to help patients.

As a result, the American Medical Association has written a Code of Medical Ethics that covers most situations healthcare providers face in their careers. The Code is made up of guidelines and opinions written by ethical scholars and physicians. Whenever you have a question about an ethical issue, the Code will provide a good basis for your decisions. (See Chapter 2 for more on the AMA Code.)

In this section, we define the four principles of medical ethics. We also look at the differences between ethics and the law, and how you should reconcile patient care with ethical standards. One of the most important facts in medical ethics is that they are not static. Medical ethics have changed over the years and will continue to evolve as medicine advances.

What are ethics?

Ethics and morality mean the same thing to many people, and they are similar. Morals are used to describe personal character, whereas ethics defines behavior in different situations. Morality refers to personal character, beliefs, and behavior; ethics is about the reflection on morality and deciding how to act as a person or a professional. An ethical person and a moral person are usually one and the same. We use *medical ethics* to refer to those guidelines and behaviors that we expect a medical professional with moral integrity to exhibit.

Ethics has developed over the centuries as a code of conduct, especially for professionals. Healthcare providers have so much knowledge about the human body, so much potential power over patients, and the ability to change and save lives. Because of these factors, the ethical bar is set very high, and providers have moral obligations to their patients.

The field of medical ethics is really about reflection on how to behave as a medical professional as well as the morality of particular medical interventions. Medical ethics are simply some key ethical principles applied to the practice of medicine. These principles are the bedrock of good clinical practice, and they are autonomy, nonmaleficence, beneficence, and justice. But they often come in conflict with each other as they are applied to a case. By using these principles in each individual case, it can be easier to make difficult decisions with your patients as you guide them through their care.

The four principles of medical ethics

The four major principles of medical ethics are

- ✔ **Autonomy:** This principle is focused on the patient's independence or liberty. A competent adult has the right to make decisions about what happens to his body. The person must be capable of rational thought and not be manipulated or coerced into any decision. An adult can refuse medical care or treatment or accept treatment when his provider suggests it. That person then lives with the consequences of his decision.

- ✔ **Beneficence:** This principle states that a physician must act in the best interest of the patient. Providers are required to promote their patient's health and well-being. Most doctors agree that healing is the main purpose of modern medicine. Beneficence means providers must help their patients.

- ✔ **Nonmaleficence:** First, do no harm. Physicians must not harm a patient through carelessness, malice, vengeance, or dislike, or even through treatments intended to help the patient. This principle is balanced with beneficence in that any risks of a treatment or procedure to a patient must be outweighed by benefit. Some treatments always carry a risk of harm. But when the treatment is very risky, the benefit must be great, or the risk of not performing the procedure must be great.

  Double effect is an offshoot of nonmaleficence. A treatment that is normally used to help someone may have an unintended negative effect. For instance, a vaccine used to prevent disease can, in rare cases, actually cause the infection it is intended to prevent. This principle provides specific guidance when determining when unintended effects are justified and when they are not.

- ✔ **Justice:** Justice refers to fairness with respect to the distribution of medical resources. This principle draws upon ethics, the law, and public policy. Who should receive scarce medical resources, and how should we distribute them in order to realize the best outcomes? Making the system as a whole more fair is one of the goals of justice.

There are two other values of medical ethics: truthfulness (or honesty) and dignity. Although these are important qualities, they are more standards of conduct, not overarching ethical principles.

These ethical principles all have merit, but they are not absolute and they are often in conflict. You will also see some tools of philosophy applied to some of the difficult ethical situations addressed in the upcoming chapters. *Deontology* states that some actions are, in and of themselves, good or bad, no matter if the end result is good. *Universality* is the concept that what is right or wrong for a person is right or wrong for all people in all places and at all times. *Consequentialism* holds that the consequences of any action determine whether that action is just or right. And *utilitarianism* holds that the worth of any action is determined by the amount of good it produces.

Even with all of these principles and tools at our disposal, medical ethics can be complicated and messy. There will be times in your practice where you and your patient will simply not be able to decide on one course of action or agree about a treatment. Sometimes, all we can do is try to think clearly about what is ethical, then decide on a path, act, and hope for the best.

Differences between ethics and legality

What is ethical is not necessarily legal, and vice versa. For instance, doctors have a fiduciary and ethical duty to their patents to do no harm, tell the truth, and treat patients with respect. The law does not demand that patients receive respect or compassion; it simply demands good medicine applied according to current standards. Some have said that good ethics begins where the law ends. In fact, ethical obligations often exceed legal standards.

The law is expressed in our society through court rulings and legislation. A statute sets a conduct standard that must be met, and a court ruling is binding on all relevant parties. Ethics, on the other hand, are guidelines. And breaches of ethics are usually not legally enforceable, although providers can be sanctioned by different medical institutions or boards if a serious breach occurs. The law does have some bearing on medical ethics in several different areas. For instance, laws, legal opinions, and court rulings affect

- **Informed consent:** A consent form is a legal document, which states that the patient has been informed about his condition and treatments, and that he understands and agrees to them.

- **Advance directives:** Directions for end-of-life care or care when the patient is incapacitated are legally binding. Although the patient doesn't need a lawyer to create an advance directive, it should be notarized or witnessed.

- **Abortion and birth control:** Countries and states have different laws regarding access to abortion and birth control. Doctors and providers must follow these laws depending on where they live.

- **Euthanasia:** Two states in the United States (Oregon and Washington) and some countries allow physician-assisted suicide. Those laws state specifically what providers are and aren't allowed to do for a patient.

- **Privacy and confidentiality:** In the United States, confidentiality laws and regulations are strictly enforced to protect the privacy of the patient at all times.

- **Access to medical care:** State-sponsored medical care, including Medicare and Medicaid, are laws that provide access to people who usually couldn't afford the care. Universal healthcare is provided in most countries around the world.

Medical ethics standards do have an effect upon the law. Many laws are devised and written based on the ethical codes of doctors and nurses. It is important that you, as a provider, know the laws in your state as well as understand the ethics guidelines that apply in different situations.

Reconciling medical ethics and patient care

If you are in the medical profession, you do your best to become the kind of provider who is trusted by your patients. You want your patients to know that you have their best interests at heart, and you want to build relationships with your patients so you can give them the best care possible.

Medical ethics provide guidelines to becoming a better provider. Ethics can help you communicate better, be a better partner to your fellow doctors and nurses, reduce risk of errors, and increase job satisfaction. When you embrace ethics as simply doing the right thing, there will be few conflicts between medical ethics and good patient care.

In many cases, it may help to put yourself in your patient's shoes (or hospital slippers). What would you want if you were the patient? Would you want your doctor to be compassionate and caring? Would you want test results delivered to you quickly? Treating patients with a sense of courtesy comes first.

 The Golden Rule applies in medical ethics. If you treat your patients as you would want to be treated, or as you would want someone to treat a cherished family member, you will provide good medical care.

Turning to ethical guideposts and guidelines

If you have questions about a medical ethics issue, by all means turn to this book! But there are other sources for information, such as the Declaration of Geneva, an updated version of the Hippocratic Oath, or the AMA Code of Medical Ethics. If you work for a healthcare organization, your employer may have a code of ethics as well.

 It's a good idea to read over an ethics code every now and then, not just when you have questions about issues. These codes aren't perfect or even enforceable, but taking the time to learn their principles and following the basic rules will help you enjoy your practice more, will result in more satisfying patient relationships, and will help make you a more effective provider.

Looking at the Common Medical Ethics Issues

Medical ethics can be divided into five main areas of discussion: individual rights or privacy; beginning-of-life issues; end-of-life issues; access to health-care; and ethics in research are the main overarching areas that can generate the most need for medical ethics guidelines.

In this section, we look at each of the first four of these areas of ethics and talk a bit about how the four ethical principles can clash and intersect as people make decisions about their lives and providers make decisions about how to best help their patients. All four ethical principles apply to situations in these areas of ethics, and how a dilemma is resolved depends on which ethical principles you follow.

Privacy and confidentiality concerns

Privacy and confidentiality go hand in hand with the principle of autonomy. In fact, because privacy upholds all four medical principles, it can be considered the cornerstone of your practice. Patient autonomy rules this issue because competent, informed patients can legally and ethically make all decisions about their care. It can be frustrating when a patient refuses treatment you know will help, but respecting his decisions, whether those decisions are made on personal, religious, or cultural grounds, is paramount.

Complying with federal regulations and putting safeguards in place in your office and clinic are important. It's also important to train your staff about privacy and confidentiality, as we discuss in Chapter 3. Running an ethical practice means respecting patient privacy at all times.

If a patient doesn't trust that you will keep their information private, he will be less likely to confide in you about matters that may be important in making the correct diagnosis.

Patient confidentiality demonstrates all of the medical ethics principles. Confidentiality is crucial to respecting autonomy because patients need to know that their decisions about their health and any diagnoses are being kept in a personal space. Nonmaleficence is important because if that information falls into the wrong hands, the patient can be hurt. Doing the best for your patient, or beneficence, means honoring the trust he places in you. And justice demands that confidential information be kept private because when others can learn information about intimate matters, patients can feel violated.

In Chapter 4, we take a detailed look at how to manage paperwork, deal with managed care situations, and handle sharing information with third parties, particularly insurance companies. But complying with these standards is the bare minimum of keeping patient information confidential. It's important that you pay attention to what you are discussing with others and where, and what you communicate through the written and spoken word.

Most information about a patient, including test results, diagnoses, treatments, and vital statistics, can be shared only with others when the patient has given express permission for that release. That permission, when at all possible, should be in the written form.

When you have a system in place to comply with HIPAA (the Health Information Portability and Accountability Act), honoring confidentiality becomes second nature. Learning to not discuss patient information with anyone except other providers who are involved in the case or whom you are consulting is important. Practice it until it becomes second nature.

It's important to remember that in medical ethics, the law really is the lowest common denominator. Ethics goes above and beyond the law, from what is legal to what is right. So complying with the law is important, but to be the best healthcare provider, go beyond the law and add compassion, respect, and honesty to your practice. And speaking of honesty, medical errors do occur, and the best practice is to report them to your patient. We look at the best ways of disclosing medical errors in Chapter 5.

Reproduction and beginning-of-life issues

Reproduction includes access to birth control, abortion, the right of a woman to choose or refuse care, the rights of the fetus, reproductive technologies, and access to care. Autonomy often comes into conflict with the other principles in reproductive issues simply because these matters are so personal.

For instance, a pregnant woman is allowed to refuse healthcare for her and her fetus up until the moment of birth. Respecting the woman's autonomy means that she is allowed to decide for herself what happens to her body, even when pregnant. In Chapters 9 and 11 we look at how to weigh the rights of a mother versus the rights of her fetus and pro-choice and pro-life stances on abortion. The definition of personhood also is explored as it relates to the rights of the fetus.

Access to birth control becomes an issue when minors request it. Because the law has decided that mature minors can have access to prescribed birth control, how do we respect a minor's privacy and autonomy while not interfering with the parent-child relationship? In Chapter 8, we take a look at adolescent patient's rights, emancipated minors, mature minors, and how to balance privacy with your obligations to your patient and her parents.

Finally, assisted reproduction can raise many ethical issues. In Chapter 10, we look at the ethics of artificial insemination, in vitro fertilization, surrogacy, and sterilization. How do we balance risk and harm to the mother and fetus? Who should receive genetic screening, and how do you prepare your patient for the results? What are your responsibilities toward your patient as you try to provide the best care?

End-of-life issues

As at the beginning of life, the end of life raises many difficult ethical issues. With the advent of medical technology that is capable of supporting life far beyond what had once been possible, we need to understand anew when life ends. In Chapter 12, death is defined, and the rights of dying patients are discussed by looking at some landmark ethics cases. The physician's role in end-of-life cases is discussed, including the ethics of physician-assisted suicide.

We then look at honoring a patient's wishes at the time of death. Healthcare directives, or living wills, are addressed in Chapter 13 as vehicles for patient autonomy. How can we help patients die with dignity and as little suffering as possible? The rule of double effect (see the earlier section, "The four principles of medical ethics") is pertinent in this issue. Giving a patient drugs with the intent to make them comfortable can hasten death. Is that an ethical move?

Euthanasia and terminal sedation are hot-button topics. Who decides when it's someone's time to die? When it becomes obvious that life is ending, how much help should we offer someone who is suffering? One of medical science's advances is the ability to help relieve suffering. That's one of the greatest opportunities for beneficence. When someone is at the end of life, however, balancing beneficence and nonmaleficence can become tricky.

Access to care

In the United States, universal healthcare has been in the news. Passionate supporters of this concept and equally passionate opponents have made their voices heard. But what's the reality of the situation? And what does medical ethics have to say about access to care? The principle of justice takes center stage with this topic.

Congress passed, and President Obama signed into law, the Health Care Reform Act of 2009. Because this act will take years to implement, there are still millions of Americans who are uninsured and underinsured, and no real guarantee that provisions of the act will ever be put into place. Thousands of Americans die every year because they don't have access to medical care, and thousands more go bankrupt because of the prohibitive cost of medicine.

The principle of justice is most applicable to this issue. As we discuss in Chapter 6, providing the basic minimum of care to the most people possible, while not reducing the standard of care enjoyed by others, is the balancing act. This fulfills a utilitarian approach to ethics by maximizing benefit to the greatest number of people. As a provider, you can help your patients by volunteering at free clinics, by prescribing generic drugs and less invasive and expensive procedures first, and by encouraging people to live healthy lifestyles. Respecting patient autonomy, guarding against harm (including financial harm), trying to do the best for your patient, and treating all patients equally is challenging but necessary in the current healthcare climate.

In Chapter 7, we look at integrating your patient's spiritual and cultural beliefs into their care as a way of enhancing treatment as well.

Moving Medicine Forward: The Ethics of Research

Medical research has brought great advances in the 20th and 21st centuries. The life span for the average American has increased from 49 years at the beginning of the 20th century to 77 years at the beginning of the 21st century.

But with this progress has come some dark days. We look at the Tuskegee syphilis study and the abuses of medical research during the Holocaust. Patients have been abused, hurt, and killed in the name of medical research before standards were put into place, as documented in Chapter 14. Even now, some researchers fail to follow guidelines and end up harming patients.

For example, in July 2010, media sources revealed that the drug manufacturer SmithKline Beecham hid results that showed Avandia, their successful diabetes medication, was harmful to the heart. Patients in the clinical trial had serious heart issues, including a significant risk of increased myocardial infarction, that weren't recorded in the tally of adverse events. The FDA is now deciding whether the drug should be withdrawn from the market. Clearly, if SmithKline Beecham knew about adverse side effects from this drug, they should have been made public. If true, this was a clear violation of nonmaleficence.

In Chapter 15, we look at the important components in an ethical clinical trial. This is vital information, whether you are a researcher or a caregiver of patients in the trials. In Chapter 16, we look at research in some special populations, such as animals, children, and psychiatric patients. Special care needs to be given to protect research subjects who cannot give full informed consent. And finally in Chapter 17, we look at the ethics of stem cell research and the controversies around genetic testing and cloning.

Chapter 2

Morality in Medicine

*L*ife in today's society is complicated, and there aren't many professions as complicated or challenging as medicine. Furthermore, because doctors and healthcare providers have been so highly educated and the decisions they make may mean the difference between life and death, they're held to a higher standard of behavior and conduct. And because patients are so vulnerable when they're sick, the conduct of providers must be of the highest moral quality.

Doctors and healthcare professionals are usually regarded as upright and moral. But doctors, like anyone else, have the potential to be unethical. Throughout history, codes of ethics have been developed to help guide physicians. So where did morality in medicine come from? Who decides what is ethical and what isn't? And what about moral absolutes? Is there a time when lying to a patient or helping someone die is ethically acceptable?

In this chapter, we look at medical ethics and morality in medicine, including the Hippocratic Oath and how it has evolved. Humanitarian goals, culminating in the Declaration of Geneva, are also examined.

We also look at the American Medical Association and the American Nursing Association's Codes of Ethics and what you should know about them. Ethical behavior in the hospital is examined, and then we look at the influence of religion on ethical judgment. Finally, if you want to learn more about bioethics, we name some good places to get more information.

We have to decide how personal morals can affect clinical judgment, and when a conflict of interest is unethical. Doctors study life as a biological function, but the emotional, spiritual, and psychological parts of human beings must be considered as well. When we treat the whole person, morality and ethics become paramount.

Distinguishing among Ethics, Morality, and Law

Applying the principles of medical ethics and the theories of morality help healthcare providers decide what course of action to take. Basically, ethics is all about asking the question, "What is the right thing to do?"

What is *morality?* Most people define it as choosing the right beliefs or behavior in a difficult situation. *Ethics* is then reflecting on those moral standards and acting upon them. Ethics sets moral standards for behavior in many professions. With the four principles of medical ethics (see Chapter 1), providers often must weigh and balance one against another. When these principles seem to contradict, deciding which one has more moral weight, based on moral arguments, is the task of medical ethics.

At first, many scholars thought that ethics belonged solely to the study of religion or philosophy, but as medicine advanced, ethics became part of the practice of medicine through interdisciplinary studies.

Although many laws are derived from ethical or moral precepts, ethics and morality are not the same as the law. For instance:

- Some laws uphold ethical standards. For example, it's illegal for a doctor to have a sexual relationship with a young patient. And that behavior is highly unethical.

- Some ethical standards are stricter than the law. For instance, in Chapter 3 we discuss the case of the doctor who posted a sign on his door stating that anyone who voted for President Obama should seek care elsewhere. Although it was legal for this doctor to state this, the action wasn't ethical.

- Sometimes ethics partially conflict with laws. Some physicians are ethically opposed to abortions and will not perform them. The law in many states restricts abortion in the second and third trimesters. However, abortions are legal in the first trimester, and doctors are ethically required to tell this to their patients, even if they are morally opposed to abortion.

- And some laws are directly opposed to ethical standards. For instance, lethal injection is, in many countries, used as a means of capital punishment. But the AMA Code of Medical Ethics states that participating in this activity is a violation of ethical standards.

Some have said that good ethics take over where legal sanctions end. These ethical standards are not enforceable by law, but act as approved guidelines for healthcare provider behavior.

Every country in the world has a different code of medical ethics, although most have similar basic principles. For example, as discussed in Chapter 6, access to healthcare for all is an important ethical issue around the world. Patient autonomy, nonmaleficence, beneficence, and justice are usually embraced in most societies, but there are some exceptions. In some cultures, doctors don't tell the truth to terminally ill patients, as discussed in Chapter 7, because tradition states that doing so will undermine the patient's will to live.

Unfortunately, there have been times when ethical standards in medicine have been disregarded, both here and in other countries. As we discuss in Chapter 14, terrible and unethical experimentation on human beings prompted the Nuremberg Code, the Declaration of Helsinki, and the Belmont Report that guide modern medicine today. Institutional review boards and government agencies that oversee research are founded on these codes and declarations.

Looking at the Hippocratic Oath and Its Modern Descendents

The Hippocratic Oath is often invoked in discussion about medical ethics. But what is it? Is the Oath still the same as when it was first written? The Hippocratic Oath is a list of statutes, originating around 400 BCE in Ancient Greece. It governs the ethical behavior of the physician and addresses both physician behavior and the doctor-patient relationship.

Origins of medical ethics

The Hippocratic Oath may be the oldest and most well-known system of medical ethics, but it isn't alone. China and India began to incorporate ethics into medical practices about a hundred years after Hippocrates. They specified guidelines that encouraged humility of doctors, and concern and compassion for patients.

Early church teachings focused on medical ethics. Thomas Aquinas, the Roman Catholic scholar, wrote about issues in medicine and religion in the early 1200s. And doctors from all nations contributed to the field. For instance, the Muslim doctor Ishaq bin Ali Rahawi wrote *The Conduct of a Physician* in the ninth century, the first text dedicated to medical ethics.

Physician Thomas Percival wrote an expanded version of the Code of Medical Ethics in Britain in 1803 where he coined the expression *medical ethics*. (It was first published as a pamphlet in 1794.) Dr. Percival's code gave moral authority to doctors, along with independence and individual honor. At about the same time, Dr. Benjamin Rush at the University of Pennsylvania began teaching ethics to its medical students.

In this section, we look at the origins of medical ethics, the modern interpretation of the original Hippocratic Oath, and the Declaration of Geneva.

Noting why the Oath was updated

The Hippocratic Oath was written back in Ancient Greek times, when people worshipped gods and goddesses such as Aphrodite and Zeus. In fact, the first line of the original Oath states:

> *I swear by Apollo Physician and Asclepius and Hygeia and Panaceia and all the gods and goddesses, making them my witnesses, that I will fulfill according to my ability and judgment this oath and this covenant . . .*

There's some scholarly discussion about whether Hippocrates or Pythagoras first wrote the Hippocratic Oath. The phrase, "first, do no harm," wasn't in the Oath, but it appears in other writings by Hippocrates. Many people incorrectly assume that this phrase prompted the writing of the Hippocratic Oath.

Swearing an oath to Apollo and Asclepius isn't very relevant in today's society. And the original Oath had doctors promise loyalty and fidelity to their teachers, and to take care of their teacher's families. Whereas that may be an honorable thing to do, it's not in keeping with today's standards.

Several statements in the original Hippocratic Oath seem to be outdated or directly contradict current law and medical ethics in the United States. A few examples are:

- ✔ **I will not give a lethal drug to anyone if asked.** Legalized physician-assisted suicide, currently supported by state law in Oregon and Washington state as discussed in Chapter 13, directly contradicts this part of the Oath.

- ✔ **I will not give a woman a pessary to cause an abortion.** This statement directly contradicts the standard of legalized abortions in many countries around the world, as discussed in Chapter 11. And in modern medicine, a pessary is used to treat bladder or uterine prolapse and doesn't in any way lead to an abortion.

- ✔ **I will not use the knife, even on sufferers from stone.** This means that medical doctors would not perform surgery, which is no longer applicable.

These changing standards, laws, and morals prompted the rewriting of the Hippocratic Oath and the AMA Code of Medical Ethics. The modern Oath puts patients first and emphasizes strong shared values. The Oath has been rewritten many times in many countries. Some scholars think that it's time for the Oath to be updated again.

Taking a new oath at graduation

The Hippocratic Oath has been rewritten in modern language, and many medical schools require that graduating students recite the newer version of the Oath. In 1964, Louis Lasagna, the Dean of Tufts University School of Medicine, rewrote the Hippocratic Oath that is most commonly accepted. In part, it reads:

> I swear to fulfill, to the best of my ability and judgment, this covenant:

> I will respect the hard-won scientific gains of those physicians in whose steps I walk, and gladly share such knowledge as is mine with those who are to follow.

> I will apply, for the benefit of the sick, all measures [that] are required, avoiding those twin traps of overtreatment and therapeutic nihilism.

> I will remember that there is art to medicine as well as science, and that warmth, sympathy, and understanding may outweigh the surgeon's knife or the chemist's drug.

> I will not be ashamed to say "I know not," nor will I fail to call in my colleagues when the skills of another are needed for a patient's recovery.

> I will respect the privacy of my patients, for their problems are not disclosed to me that the world may know. Most especially must I tread with care in matters of life and death. If it is given me to save a life, all thanks. But it may also be within my power to take a life; this awesome responsibility must be faced with great humbleness and awareness of my own frailty. Above all, I must not play at God . . .

Understanding humanitarian goals: The Declaration of Geneva

The Declaration of Geneva is a revised version of the Hippocratic Oath, updated for the 20th and 21st centuries. The Declaration was written in 1948 in direct response to atrocities committed by Nazi doctors. It was approved during the second general assembly of the World Medical Association after World War II. It was updated in 1968, 1984, 1994, 2005, and 2006.

The basic message of the Declaration of Geneva is to "not use medical knowledge contrary to the laws of humanity." As currently approved, the Declaration of Geneva is:

> <u>At the time of being admitted as a member of the medical profession:</u>

> I solemnly pledge to consecrate my life to the service of humanity;

I will give to my teachers the respect and gratitude that is their due;

I will practice my profession with conscience and dignity;

The health of my patient will be my first consideration;

I will respect the secrets that are confided in me, even after the patient has died;

I will maintain by all the means in my power, the honor and the noble traditions of the medical profession;

My colleagues will be my sisters and brothers;

I will not permit considerations of age, disease or disability, creed, ethnic origin, gender, nationality, political affiliation, race, sexual orientation, social standing or any other factor to intervene between my duty and my patient;

I will maintain the utmost respect for human life;

I will not use my medical knowledge to violate human rights and civil liberties, even under threat;

I make these promises solemnly, freely and upon my honor.

Rules for Engagement: Today's Codes of Medical Ethics

Because humanitarian goals are the point of medical ethics, they were codified. Some speculate that the first medical ethics codes were written in response to behavior that many doctors thought was unacceptable and outrageous. The American Medical Association has a lengthy code of medical ethics, and the American Nursing Association has a code as well. In this section we look more closely at the basic standards set forth in these codes.

One of the AMA Code's purposes is to guide the doctor in his ability and authority to self-regulate. Most ethicists think that whenever you are in an ethically tricky situation, it helps to ask yourself some questions. These questions might include:

- ✔ Is there a published standard of behavior about this issue?

- ✔ Would I want a member of my family to be treated this way?

- ✔ How will this action or treatment affect the patient?

- ✔ How will my conscience feel after I take this action?

Ethical codes and standards are, of course, much more complicated than these simple questions. But stopping to think about an action or behavior before you do it is an important step in developing an internal ethical formula.

American Medical Association Code of Ethics

The American Medical Association established a code of medical ethics in 1847 because there were no overarching government regulations or ethical standards. The code has been modified through the years; the first version of the code specified physician behavior and manners.

The AMA Code of Medical Ethics is not enforceable, but still serves as the standard of behavior for medical professionals with moral integrity. You can find a complete copy of the Code of Medical Ethics at www.ama-assn.org/ama/pub/physician-resources/medical-ethics/code-medical-ethics.shtml.

Knowing what's in the code

The AMA Code of Medical Ethics has eight basic principles:

- ✔ Provide competent and compassionate medical care
- ✔ Maintain the highest professional standards
- ✔ Respect the law
- ✔ Keep the confidence of patients and colleagues
- ✔ Advance scientific and medical education
- ✔ Do not discriminate among peers and patients
- ✔ Improve public health
- ✔ Honor responsibilities to patients and support access to care

The Code publishes opinions and reports on specific aspects of physician behavior that explain the principles in more detail.

The AMA has established the Ethical Force Program (EForce) to promote and measure high ethical standards and expectations for healthcare providers. It creates, tests, and publicizes ethical issues and standards. The EForce panel will create questions that doctors and patients can ask themselves and develop criteria for performance and policies.

Dealing with violations

Only about 30 percent of all American doctors are members of the AMA. The AMA itself doesn't investigate doctors who violate the Code, but refers complaints to local medical societies. If the doctor is an AMA member, the local society or board informs the AMA's Council on Ethical and Judicial Affairs about its findings. The Council holds hearings, and can then

- ✔ Acquit the doctor
- ✔ Admonish or censure the doctor
- ✔ Place the doctor on probation
- ✔ Expel or suspend the doctor from the AMA

The AMA doesn't have the power to remove a doctor's license to practice medicine. Local medical boards or specialty boards can sanction doctors based on ethical violations.

American Nursing Association Code of Ethics

The American Nursing Association (ANA) revised its Code of Ethics in 1995. The original Code was written in 1950. It is meant to guide nurses through their practice of medicine and help them make ethical decisions in their everyday work environment.

The nine provisions in the Code deal with:

- ✔ Respect for human dignity as expressed through autonomy
- ✔ Commitment to the patient by setting boundaries and collaborating with other professionals
- ✔ Protection of the health, safety, and rights of the patient, especially through respect for privacy and confidentiality
- ✔ Accountability and responsibility of the profession
- ✔ Self-respect and integrity, using the same standards of respect and dignity they assign to their patients
- ✔ Maintenance and improvement in the healthcare environment
- ✔ Advancement of the profession through education and practice, to meet professional obligations
- ✔ Collaboration with others to meet society's health needs, focusing on issues such as hunger and violations of justice
- ✔ Assertion of values; upholds intraprofessional integrity, and shapes social policy through professional associations and social reform

The basic duty of nurses is to assist the patient and their families however they can, with dignity, respect, care, and compassion. The Code places the patient as the center of a nurse's responsibility, but acknowledges that as a professional, the nurse has an obligation to act with responsibility and dignity in society.

Bedside Manners: Ethics inside the Hospital

Healthcare providers are constantly trying to balance the social and scientific parts of their brains. Emotion and compassion have to be balanced with medical knowledge and the ability to reason and diagnose. The bedside manner is where these two parts come together in an ethical dance.

In this section, we look at ethics inside the hospital, including what a hospital ethics panel does. Most hospitals have a patient bill of rights; we look at what purpose these documents serve. And we look at ethics in the emergency room, where different rules prevail.

We've all heard stories about doctors who lack good bedside manner. Although it's true that doctors and providers must be at least somewhat removed from emotion while treating a patient, there is a balance between diagnostic excellence and caring for the whole patient.

Understanding the hospital ethics panel

Most hospitals have ethics panels, composed of doctors, nurses, and other providers, administrators, social workers, lawyers, chaplains and other clergy, and some laypersons. All of these members are volunteers.

Dolores's case: Consulting the ethics committee

Dolores was a 69-year-old woman who sustained a heart attack that severely damaged her heart. Her ejection fraction, or pumping function of her heart, was reduced to 5 to 10 percent, which is life-threatening. She was kept alive in the ICU with continuous IV drip medications and a ventricular assist device that helps the damaged heart pump. Her husband of 40 years was very devoted, and they had no other family. Even though doctors had discussed with him that further treatment was futile, he refused to let them withdraw treatment.

The care providers and the husband were at a standoff, and the hospital ethics committee was consulted. The husband and lead cardiologist met with the committee, and each person presented their side of the case. The different committee members, including doctors, nurses, an administrator, a lawyer, and a chaplain, all gave compassionate commentary on the situation. After a long discussion, the committee gave a recommendation. Over the next three days, medications and machines would be slowly withdrawn. Doctors would also try to get Dolores on the heart transplant list in case she survived this incident. After further discussion, both the husband and cardiologist agreed to this plan with the support of the ethics committee.

These panels convene to discuss ethics situations, advise providers and patients about making healthcare choices, review hospital policies, and help educate hospital staff about ethical issues.

The ethics panel can be convened at the request of a provider or patient or a patient's family when there is some disagreement about the course of treatment. The panel can also convene at the request of other hospital staff, such as nurses or administrators, if there are conflicts in care. What is best for the patient is at the center of every discussion, and the patient's family values play a big role in the decisions made by the ethics panel.

Some of these topics addressed by ethics panels include:

✔ Disagreements between providers and patients, within families, or within hospital staff about the best course of treatment for a patient

✔ Clarification of ethical issues in a particular situation for providers and families

✔ Review of criteria for waiting lists for treatments or transplants

✔ Appropriate course of action when medical errors are committed

✔ Whether or not to continue life-sustaining treatment

✔ The need for informed consent and how this is best communicated with the patient

✔ Proxies and decision-making, such as living wills and advance directives

✔ Equity of care for minorities, the poor, or those with different religious beliefs

✔ Review of hospital policies involving ethical issues such as end-of-life care or abortion

When discussing and deciding on these dilemmas, the ethics panel will consider:

✔ What the patient really wants for the best outcome

✔ What the proxy, or designated representative, thinks the patient would want

✔ What doctors and other providers believe is the best course of treatment

✔ What to do when care is futile

✔ When lifesaving treatments should be withdrawn

✔ Whether to approve or deny cutting-edge medical treatments

✔ How cultural or religious beliefs factor into healthcare

Ethics panels and new procedures

In 2006, a London hospital's ethics panel approved the world's first full-face transplant. The panel was brought in to make sure that this new procedure followed ethical protocols, that risk is minimized, and to set standards. Because the procedure is so new, it was considered research, not treatment. The go-ahead for this new and controversial procedure was given because all other medical treatments had been exhausted. The panel recommended that the patient receiving the transplant undergo extensive counseling and education so informed consent could be achieved, and to make sure that the patient was psychologically stable enough to undergo the surgery and extensive after care, including lifetime immunosuppressant drugs.

Hospital ethics committees facilitate an open discussion and bring out the ethical issues involved in a case. They may or may not make a recommendation, but it remains the role of the provider and patient or patient's family to make the final decisions about the care given to the patient.

Hospital ethics panels do not

✔ Sanction or discipline doctors or other providers

✔ Publicize their decisions

✔ Issue binding legal judgments

It's important to remember that using a hospital ethics panel to help decide course of treatment is often a last resort. When a conflict about care can't be resolved, this panel is a great and underutilized resource. Some of the panel's additional responsibilities are to guide hospital administrators on policies involving ethical issues, and to educate staff about medical ethics and decision-making.

Patient bill of rights

Most hospitals and clinics publish a patient's bill of rights. These documents set forth the type of treatment and care a patient and his family can expect to receive in that hospital or clinic. In 1990, the Association of American Physicians and Surgeons published a list of patient freedoms, which was formally adopted as a Patient Bill of Rights in 1995.

Any patient's bill of rights for different hospitals will be slightly different, but all have the same basic principles:

✔ To choose a physician freely

✔ To agree on terms with their provider

✔ To be treated with respect and consideration

✔ To have an advance directive on their chart

✔ To expect confidentiality and privacy

✔ To be fully informed about their condition and any treatments or drugs

✔ To receive responses to questions or requests in a reasonable time frame

✔ To be informed about business relationships among providers, the hospital, payers, and other entities

✔ To make choices about their care

✔ To refuse medical treatment

✔ To full disclosure of their condition, insurance plans, and treatment plans

✔ To expect continuity of care

Along with rights, patients also have responsibilities, which are discussed in Chapter 3. Patients must fully disclose information about their condition, and should ask questions if they don't fully understand their diagnoses or course of treatment.

Emergency room ethics

Emergency medicine has special ethical rules. The patients and providers usually do not have a longstanding relationship, and decisions about life and death can sometimes be made in seconds. So what are the ethical standards that should exist in emergency rooms? Doctors must quickly evaluate a situation, think about available options and treatments, and then take action.

When considering decision-making in the ER, providers should first look for a policy or precedent that may apply to the situation, then look for an option that can be found while the patient is stabilized, and use logical reasoning skills to reach a decision. Providers should also consider these questions: What would you want, if you were the patient? Could you defend this action to others? And would this decision work in other situations?

Some of the unique situations in emergency room ethics include:

✔ **Triage:** Doctors and providers must make quick decisions about who to treat first, who can wait for treatment, and who is so severely injured or sick that treatment is futile. This is one of the first considerations in an ER, especially when there is a community-wide emergency.

✔ **Quick action:** In an emergency situation, providers have to make split-second decisions about treatment and care, sometimes with little or no information about patient history.

✔ **Implied informed consent:** In an emergency situation, informed consent is implied when a patient is unable to provide consent. That is, providers assume that the patient would want treatment to save his life, even if he is unable to consent. Aggressive care is expected until the situation is futile.

✔ **Staff teamwork:** Patients are often very sick with life-threatening conditions. A team of staff with defined roles must work quickly and efficiently to care for the patient. Because medical treatment may sometimes be given with little or no discussion and under unpredictable conditions, ER providers must be ready to help each other at a moment's notice.

✔ **Respect for the law:** From domestic violence issues to child abuse to attempted murder, emergency room providers can face many situations where law enforcement is involved.

✔ **Impartiality:** Because many patients present to the emergency room from poor socioeconomic conditions, they must all be treated with respect no matter what their living situation is. Even those charged with violent crimes must be treated fairly and with the same standards as every other patient.

✔ **Resilience:** The emergency room can often be chaotic with many very sick patients being managed at the same time, and providers must remain as calm and flexible as possible in the face of trauma. Adaptability is an important virtue for emergency room staff.

All of the other ethical considerations in medicine, such as beneficence, respect for autonomy, nonmaleficence, and justice apply to the emergency room, of course, but these additional values and skills are important additions to the provider's toolbox.

Bioethics as a Field of Study

Medical ethicists commonly work at colleges and universities, teaching and publishing papers. Some hospitals and clinics have medical ethicists as consultants to help them navigate the often difficult maze of ethical situations. They often serve on hospital ethics committees. These professionals can help providers by rendering decisions about ending life-sustaining treatments or judging the capacity of patients. Medical ethicists help providers keep the ethics of every situation in mind as they do their jobs.

Bioethics has existed only since the 1960s, prompted by advances in traditional medicine that included dialysis, intensive care units (ICUs), transplants, and respirators. These advances forced doctors to address complicated moral issues such as when to remove life-sustaining treatment, or when to admit or remove someone from an ICU. Medical advances continue to drive new ethical issues, such as advances in genetics that may raise questions about genetic testing.

The Institute of Society, Ethics, and Life Sciences, now called the Hastings Center, was founded in 1970 in New York. The Institute began as a way to bring together scholars in religion, philosophy, law, science, and medicine to tackle the issue of bioethics. And the Kennedy Institute of Ethics was founded at Georgetown University in 1971. Now there are more than 50 universities in the United States alone that have departments in medical ethics. Several publications focus on this field, including the Journal of Clinical Ethics, the Hastings Center Report, the Cambridge Quarterly of Healthcare Ethics, and the American Society for Bioethics and Humanities.

The American Society for Bioethics and Humanities has tried to codify core competencies and critical areas of knowledge for medical ethicists. They stated that medical ethicists should be familiar with healthcare, moral reasoning, laws affecting healthcare, and be able to listen and communicate well when asked to participate in ethics consultations.

Chapter 3

The Provider-Patient Relationship

· ·

In This Chapter

▶ Protecting patient privacy

▶ Understanding full disclosure and referrals

▶ Choosing whom to serve

▶ Understanding patient rights and obligations

· ·

octors and patients must have a good relationship for the best care. This relationship is based on clear communication, mutual trust and respect, and shared goals. This standard of care goes back to Hippocrates. Important aspects of this relationship include patient privacy, confidentiality, and respect for autonomy.

Patients have many rights, including a right to receive complete information from their doctors, to discuss benefits, risks, and costs of treatments, and to make informed decisions about their healthcare. Doctors have rights, too. They have the right to be treated with respect, to choose their patients as long as laws against discrimination aren't broken, and to refuse patients in some situations. And they have a right to honest information from their patients.

But a doctor's responsibility for his patient goes beyond establishing a casual relationship. Doctors have a *fiduciary duty* toward their patients. This means that there is a legal relationship between the doctor and patient and that the doctor must establish trust and confidentiality at every step during his relationship with the patient. The doctor must

✔ Provide the best care possible.

✔ Deal with the patient in good faith.

✔ Respect confidentiality about patient information.

✔ Show loyalty and honesty toward the patient.

✔ Serve the patient's best interests at all times.

✔ Avoid any conflict of interest.

In this chapter, we look at the matter of confidentiality between a doctor and patient: how to build and maintain it, and how legal requirements affect the relationship. We also examine who makes the decision about medical records access, especially genetic information, and how that information can be shared. And we explore the concept of full disclosure and when and how to refer a patient to another health practitioner.

Hippocrates' standard of "do no harm" is at risk as we go through the digital age. If private medical information can be easily accessed by others, the patient's confidence in providers, future insurability, or even employment could be threatened. Technological and economic factors can muddy the waters, so we look at new methods to ensure privacy, respect, and confidentiality.

Most ethicists think that good doctor-patient communication helps patients adhere to treatment plans, reduces doctor and patient stress, and reduces the risk of malpractice lawsuits. Best-practice communication skills need to take a more prominent role in the doctor-patient relationship.

Protecting Patient Privacy

Patient privacy is central to medical care. Without it, the provider-patient relationship will break down, the patient may not receive the best treatment, and the doctor may end up in court. A patient is more likely to follow advice and instructions if the provider-patient relationship is strong and healthy. Be sure to look at each patient as a partner, not as the lesser part of a paternalistic relationship.

In this section, we define confidentiality, explain the tricky act of balancing privacy with the public good, and address how to balance a patient's privacy with the need to collect data in research studies.

Understanding confidentiality

Confidentiality is an ethical principle that stipulates communication between a patient and a provider must remain private. Anything a patient says in a doctor's visit or over the phone to a nurse cannot be discussed with a third party without express written permission from the patient.

A breach of confidentiality occurs when a doctor shares patient information with a third party, but does so without the patient's consent or a court order. The disclosure can happen in conversation or in writing, whether by fax, e-mail, or another form of electronic means.

The case of President Clinton: A high profile breach of confidentiality

In 2004, 17 hospital workers at New York Presbyterian Hospital (including doctors, supervisors, and lab techs) were suspended for improperly accessing the medical record of former President Bill Clinton who was hospitalized there. This occurred despite stern warnings to hospital employees at the time of his admission. At this time, many clinics and hospitals have a *zero tolerance policy* when it comes to looking into a patient's chart for reasons other than patient care. This means employees are immediately terminated without further warning for these breaches in confidentiality.

administrative work is completed, the patient may or may not be told. In some cases, disciplinary action may be needed. For more about admitting mistakes, please see Chapter 5.

Confidentiality comes from two ethics principles: beneficence and autonomy. This means you must use information about current medical status, treatments, and discussion of further treatment only for its intended purpose. This respects the patient's right to privacy (autonomy) and helps ensure that every action is working toward a good outcome (beneficence).

Patients won't feel free to talk to you about their health and symptoms unless they trust that you'll keep their information private. Just imagine; if you knew your doctor was discussing your case with a friend, would you feel comfortable telling him intimate details of your life? Outcomes can be compromised if patients withhold information about symptoms because they don't trust you.

The doctor's discretion plays a big part when setting confidentiality limits. In most cases, the only way you can share medical information about a patient with another party is with written consent. In Chapter 4, we discuss the Health Insurance Portability and Accountability Act (HIPAA) and the legal limits placed on communication. HIPAA has specific regulations about confidentiality and controlling patient health information and all providers need to be familiar with its statutes. Risk assessments and security programs must be in place in any office, hospital, or clinic to guard privacy.

Maintaining confidentiality can be tricky. Considerations include:

✔ The need to share information with other providers, including nurses, office management, and lab technicians. There is no breach of confidentiality when doctors share information with other doctors and providers who are involved in the patient's care.

✔ How treatments and care are paid for, because insurance companies and third-party payers can look at patient records. The information must be encrypted or encoded when your office is transmitting to these parties.

✔ The security of computers and electronic medical records. Because hackers can break into almost every computer system no matter how advanced the protection (even the Defense Department), many advocates say patients should be told that absolute privacy does not exist.

✔ The public good when communicable diseases such as tuberculosis and H1N1 can affect the public health.

✔ The safety of a third party or the patient himself in some mental health cases and domestic abuse situations. If a patient threatens another person or persons in an explicit way, the doctor has a duty to inform that person and the authorities.

✔ If a patient in incapable of making a decision about care because of impairment, or if disclosure would be in the patient's best interest.

In all of these cases, the doctor should try to get consent from the patient before patient information is shared. But in some cases, if another person's safety is threatened or the patient is incapable of consenting to the release of information, this is not practical or possible.

Balancing privacy with public good

When balancing privacy with the public good, doctors must balance autonomy, beneficence, and nonmaleficence. Patient autonomy is key. Patients must keep the right to decide who has access to their personal information.

Blogging doctors

Social Internet media sites, such as Facebook, Twitter, and personal and professional blogs, are treading on confidentiality. Many doctors blog about their experiences. If a patient is able to identify himself in a blog even if names are not disclosed, there could be legal consequences.

Many ethicists think that healthcare providers should not be broadcasting troubles with patients or discussing issues in their practices on the Internet. If you feel a need to write about your experiences, keep a personal journal instead.

The classic ethics dilemma involves patient privacy and the *public good,* or the best interests of the community in terms of safety and health. To ethically breach confidentiality, these standards must be met:

- There must be an immediate, apparent, and well-documented threat to public safety or health, such as when a psychiatric patient threatens to kill or harm another person during a counseling session.

- The public should be protected without personally identifying the patient or his medical records, such as a patient with tuberculosis being reported to the Department of Health so their compliance with treatment can be tracked. Any methods used to protect the public must be kept as confidential as possible.

- The methods for releasing information must cover only the relevant material and not disclose any other private information. For example, a patient likely does not need to release their mental health records to the surgeon who is going to perform their gall bladder operation.

Confidentiality in research

The public good includes advances made in medical research. To develop safe and effective clinical trials, private information about genetics and any reaction to drugs must be disclosed to researchers to improve treatments and reduce side effects. But as science advances, many patients fear discrimination from employers or insurance companies if their genetic information is released. Privacy must be balanced with accuracy in any database used for research.

Accountability comes into play here. Expensive new treatments and drugs must be evaluated for efficacy and cost. Insurance companies and researchers have the right to know if a treatment leads to good outcomes and then decide if it is worth the cost, both in time and money.

One way to balance the need for privacy with the need for research material is for you, the provider, to stress future benefit to the patient. As we state in Chapter 14, patients need to understand that future benefit is not treatment. If more people participate in research databases and offer their private information to medical researchers, more successful treatments will be developed. And that will help everyone, including the patient herself, down the road.

Clear and Ethical Communications

Clear communication and understanding is the best predictor of a good outcome. When doctors understand what patients are saying to them, they can diagnose and prescribe treatment. And when patients understand what the doctor says, they are more likely to continue with treatment and follow advice. Almost 80 percent of the information for an accurate diagnosis comes from what the patient says to her doctor!

Communicating clearly and fairly to the patient respects the patient's autonomy and ties into beneficence. Listen carefully, think before you speak, and pay attention to nonverbal cues for better outcomes. Poor communication is not only a predictor of poor outcome; it can be costly to the provider. Many doctors who face malpractice cases didn't communicate clearly and dismissed the patient's concerns and opinions.

It is important to remember that even though you, as a provider, are comfortable spending every day in a clinic or hospital, this is often an anxiety-provoking experience for patients. I have seen many people who have come to see me after avoiding doctors for years. They are visibly anxious, and their blood pressure is often elevated due to *white coat hypertension*. They may have a serious diagnosis that I need to convey to them.

I acknowledge their anxiety, and I try to encourage them to bring a friend to family member in as a "second set of ears" as we discuss important issues. I give them a written summary of our visit and encourage them to call me back with any questions that come up. Good communication can definitely be impacted by a patient's emotional state, and this should be recognized and acknowledged.

In this section, we discuss how to best communicate with the patient and how to make sure the patient understands the diagnosis and treatment protocol.

Communicating with the patient

Time is a valuable and scarce commodity in the doctor-patient relationship. An average visit in a managed-care setting lasts only 15 minutes. In the short time you have together, you must make sure you understand the patient's symptoms and concerns so you can make a correct diagnosis, and you also must make sure that the patient understands her diagnosis and the treatment.

Healthcare providers need to ask the right questions and then let the patient speak without interrupting. Doctors can learn communication skills and take the time to implement them. In an office visit, you should

- ✔ Keep track of body language and nonverbal communication.
- ✔ Use open-ended questions rather than questions requiring yes or no answers.
- ✔ Develop trust and pay attention to emotional issues.
- ✔ Be as specific as possible with a diagnosis and treatment and make sure patients understand them.
- ✔ Let the patient know the protocol for delivering test results.
- ✔ Offer choices and treatment alternatives.
- ✔ Prioritize directions and the order of treatment.
- ✔ Treat patients as respected partners in their care.

Body language is important in any type of communication. If you sit down when talking with a patient instead of standing, the patient perceives that you are taking more time to talk. Don't answer a pager or cell phone during the visit. Make eye contact with your patient and allow silence in the conversation.

Getting information from the patient

Unless you're psychic, you need to find out the reason for the patient's visit. Open-ended questions usually bring the best results. Ask a question like: "What brings you here today, and how can I help you?" Be sure that you understand what the patient has told you; then reassure the patient that you understand their concerns.

You can use the mirroring technique to show the patient that you understand what he's said. Repeat back to the patient his concerns and symptoms, using slightly different language. The mirroring technique

- ✔ Increases patient autonomy
- ✔ Helps a doctor make an accurate diagnosis
- ✔ Lets the patient know that you are listening closely

Patients often bring up symptoms or concerns at the very end of the visit. These factors can be key to an accurate diagnosis. Don't be in a hurry to leave the examination room.

Also take time to ask about the patient's home and work life. Often, the source of problems occur at those venues. Listen carefully if your patient wants to talk about his personal life or difficulties at work.

You must also listen for clues about the patient's emotional health. A 1997 study by Suchman et al found that doctors often ignore a patient's statements about their emotional health and steer the conversation back to technical terms and treatments. This can lead to missed clues that may be important to the patient's health and best outcomes.

It is also important to remember that the patient is not just looking for someone to give him a diagnosis. Often an important role is to offer support and compassion during a time of suffering, serious illness, or family discord. These situations are so much easier for patients to face if they know they are not going through a difficult experience alone.

Making sure the patient understands

The patient must understand the diagnosis and treatment. But because healthcare providers are trained in medical terminology and patients are often a bit anxious, it can be difficult to communicate in language a patient understands. Translating from medical jargon to lay terms takes skill and practice. You must never just assume that the patient understands a diagnosis or treatment.

Allow time for the patient to ask questions. Don't assume that because no questions are asked the patient understands what you have said. It may help to use a mirroring technique by asking the patient to repeat the treatment protocol as they understand it. If the patient can't explain to you what they've heard, ask if they would be more comfortable reading the information, or if they need to hear it again. Be careful to avoid medical jargon, and when you repeat information, use simpler language.

Ask if the patient understands. If a diagnosis is bad, the patient may be in emotional distress and unable to fully comprehend the diagnosis, let alone treatment options. An illness itself, or other medications, may affect the patient's ability to understand a diagnosis. Feedback is critical to patient care.

The interrupting doctor

Studies in the Journal of American Medical Association found that, on average, doctors let a patient describe symptoms and problems for 18 to 23 seconds before interrupting. The study found that patients need only six more seconds to complete their story. Only 2 percent of patients complete their tale before diagnosis. In addition, most doctors think they take eight to nine minutes explaining treatment, when they really only spoke for one minute. More than half of all doctors thought it was important to let patients know test results were normal, but only about one-fourth actually did so. Also, only 30 percent of doctors ask if the patient has any questions at the end of a visit.

Informed consent

Informed consent, or patient agreement to treatment based upon a clear understanding of the situation and all potential ramifications, is central to the doctor-patient relationship. You, the provider, must tell the patient about alternatives to his care and the pros and cons of those treatments and then respect the patient's decision. The ethical dilemma here is between beneficence and autonomy. Although a doctor may see the best outcome for his patient with one treatment, the patient may choose another drug or no treatment at all.

When a patient understands the treatment and its risks and benefits, she can make an informed decision about her care, including the risks of choosing no care at all. But what alternatives are best for the patient? When is a risk too great, or benefit too small? The legal standard states that a doctor must use common sense and tell the patient what a reasonable physician would do in her case.

These are the standards for informed consent:

✔ The doctor has to tell the patient about medically viable options. This means treatment, which is the medically accepted standard of care, must be offered to the patient, as well as other options with the potential to help the patient more than harm him.

✔ A patient can be told of nonmainstream medical approaches when a respectable minority of physicians endorse it.

✔ If a doctor knows of more experienced doctors who can perform the treatment the patient requests, the doctor should tell the patient about those other experts.

There are two major exceptions to the informed consent rule. You don't need informed consent before performing a simple and common procedure that has little risk, such as a blood test; however, the patient still needs to agree to the procedure. And you do not need patient consent to treat in an emergency life-threatening situation.

And there are even more exceptions to those exceptions. You must make an attempt to contact a family member for informed consent in an emergency, and can't treat the patient if you know the patient has a previously filed legal notice to refuse lifesaving treatment. If the patient has an advance directive, living will, or Do Not Resuscitate (DNR) order, as discussed in Chapter 13, those instructions must be followed if you are aware of them. Prior to treatment it's always a good idea to ask a patient or a family member if the patient has a living will.

Understanding Full Disclosure: Telling the Patient What Matters

The doctor must be as honest with the patient as possible. But the selection of information to disclose is an ethical issue. Healthcare practitioners should disclose any conflict of interest they have when dealing with patients. People have the right to know all of the risks and benefits of their treatment.

So the patient can make an informed decision, the doctor must tell the patient

- ✔ About his condition
- ✔ What may happen if the condition is not treated
- ✔ About all possible and medically reasonable treatments, including drugs and surgery
- ✔ All the risks and the benefits of these treatments

In this section we look at the definition of conflict of interest and what and when to disclose in financial and clinical matters. We also discuss the benefits and harm of *therapeutic privilege,* or withholding information that may do more harm to the patient than good.

Decoding conflicts of interest

A conflict of interest occurs when a healthcare practitioner or any member of his family has a financial interest in pharmaceutical sales, medical equipment, medical research, patient care, or administration.

Good medical practices rely on minimizing bias or conflicts of interest. Any interest or involvement of a medical provider which interferes with his ability to make decisions solely based on the patient's best interest is problematic. For example, an orthopedist who orders MRI scans on patients and then receives a kickback payment for every MRI scan ordered brings bias into his medical decision-making. There are two types of bias: intentional and unintentional. Bias can be real or perceived. The Association for Medical Ethics has created the Ethical Rules of Disclosure. These rules try to guarantee full and honest disclosure to ensure the best patient care. They are

- ✔ Try to limit bias and conflict of interest. Instead, rely on facts and evidence-based medicine. Always keep the patient's best interest as the first priority.
- ✔ Financial ties and incentives may result in bias.
- ✔ Healthcare providers should disclose the financial interest of more than $500 per year that might result in perceived or real bias.

Pharmaceutical detailing

Pharmaceutical detailing occurs when representatives from drug companies go to doctor's offices to pitch a specific drug. These visits can keep doctors up to date on new drugs and help providers choose newer, more effective treatments, but you must be aware of the conflicts of interest these visits can create. A problematic aspect of these visits is that the drug samples are new and expensive. Patients get started on these free drug samples that are given in the clinic, but soon have to pay for them when the sample runs out. Sometimes a less expensive and equally effective drug is available. Some clinics are now prohibiting visits from pharmaceutical reps due to the conflict of interest this creates. Electronic detailing, or e-detailing, is now becoming more common because physicians have less time for face-to-face meetings.

TIP

Self-referral, or ordering a test on a machine the doctor's practice owns, can be ethically tricky and can be a potential financial conflict of interest. The healthcare practitioner must be honest when prescribing any form of care. The tests must be medically necessary. A new machine, drug, surgery, or other treatment should not be used unless it is the best choice for that patient. And the patient should be told about the doctor's self-interest so he can decide if that test or drug is best for him.

Deciding who has access to medical information

The Health Information Portability and Accountability Act (HIPAA), as discussed in Chapter 4, has guidelines about patient and family member access to medical records. *Access* means the right to look at and copy medical records. Doctors must balance beneficence, patient autonomy, and justice when granting access to medical records.

Granting and denying access to medical records

According to the law, these persons and groups can have limited or full access to a patient's medical records:

- ✔ Family, depending on state law and the competency of the patient
- ✔ Guardians for minors and dependents
- ✔ Insurance companies
- ✔ Government agencies such as Medicare Workers Compensation, and Social Security Disability Insurance (SSDI)
- ✔ Employers when they self-insure

✔ Health researchers and the Center for Disease Control (CDC)

✔ Officers of the court when medical records are relevant to a legal case

Patients are advised to ask for medical records on a fairly routine basis. A small fee can be charged, but it must be reasonable and cover only the cost of producing the report. The records must be released within 30 days.

Drug manufacturers often buy patient lists to expand their market. In this practice, called *prescription data-mining,* pharmacy information companies buy prescription data from pharmacies and sell it to drug companies. Baby product companies use birth records to advertise cribs, strollers, and nursing aids to new parents. Privacy must be guarded in these situations and you, as the provider, must be careful to release only that information the patient agrees to release. The patient must always give express permission for information release.

In some cases, requests for medical records can be denied. A request for medical records can be denied

✔ If information on the record can endanger the patient's health. For instance, if the medical record reveals a serious diagnosis in a mentally ill patient, the record can be withheld for fear that the patient might harm himself if he sees the record.

✔ If information on the record can endanger someone else's health.

✔ If the request is frivolous or vexatious, such as asking to see the same records over and over again for no meaningful reason.

Considering personal versus joint information

The genetic component of personal information is rapidly increasing. As more genetic testing becomes available, doctors and patients must decide who has access to results. Some of the most damaging diseases are purely genetic; that is, unless you have the gene responsible for the disease, you won't get it. If one person in a family tests positive for a disease such as Huntington's Chorea, do you think the rest of the family members deserve access to that information?

Many doctors and researchers are dividing private information into two categories: personal and joint. Members of a family do have a right to some personal information that directly affects their health, just as they would have information about a jointly held bank account.

If information that could affect other family members is uncovered during tests or an exam, you should discuss this situation with your patient. If she doesn't want to pass on the diagnosis, and you know that withholding that information could cause harm to another person, you can ethically break confidentiality and disclose it.

As we discuss in Chapter 9, discussing the possible ramifications of any test, especially genetic tests, is an important first step before the tests are performed. For instance, if tests reveal that a pregnant patient is a carrier for a disease like Fragile X Syndrome, and you know that her sister is also pregnant but doesn't know she may be a carrier, first encourage your patient to tell her sister. This is not a breach of confidence of the patient.

Choosing not to disclose information to a patient

Healthcare providers have long discussed the issue of *therapeutic privilege*, or the withholding of medical information from a patient because it might harm them. This is an exception to the principle of informed consent. Many ethicists feel this practice fails to respect patient autonomy and undermines trust in the relationship.

The old definition of therapeutic privilege came from the paternalistic version of the doctor-patient relationship. Not telling a patient that he has a serious disease because he would be upset isn't a good reason for nondisclosure. You must have a valid and compelling concern that information could cause your patient to harm himself or even end his life.

The courts have limited the use of therapeutic privilege as a justification for physicians to withhold information from a patient. It cannot be invoked if the doctor thinks the patient will refuse the therapy; the condition must be serious psychological harm to the patient.

Understanding Appropriate Referrals

An implied contract exists between a doctor and patient starting at the first visit. A referral brings a third person into this contract. Whether you are referring a patient to another doctor or seeing a patient referred to you, there are rules to follow.

Respecting patient autonomy and ensuring beneficence are the primary ethics guidelines in these situations. The patient always has a right to choose his doctor. And all doctors who are consulted must consider the best outcomes for the patient.

In this section, we discuss the rings of uncertainty, an ethical principle that can help determine when a referral should be made. We also talk about giving and getting second opinions, whether requested by the doctor or the patient.

Considering second opinions

In the doctor-patient relationship, both the patient and the provider can ask for a second opinion about a patient's health condition. You shouldn't hesitate to remind a patient that he has this option, and you shouldn't be embarrassed to tell a patient that you want to seek another doctor's counsel about his condition.

All patients have the right to ask for a second opinion. This can be difficult for some patients because they may be afraid of alienating or insulting you.

When a patient asks for a second opinion:

- ✔ Agree to this decision.
- ✔ Offer names of other physicians to contact.
- ✔ Do not pressure the patient to make an immediate decision.
- ✔ Make all of the patient's records available for the other doctors.
- ✔ Don't make it difficult for the patient to get another opinion.

There are some situations when a healthcare provider should bring in another doctor for consultation. The *rings of uncertainty* is an ethical model that describes how certain a doctor is that he can perform a surgery or diagnose a condition. Any doctor needs to be very certain that his level of competence is high enough to undertake a treatment or surgery alone. If the doctor is not completely confident of his competency in this area, a second physician should be brought in to assess the situation.

You should ask for a second opinion when

- ✔ You have had poor results with patients with this diagnosis. It's responsible and ethical to admit you have had problems with some treatments. Recommending the patient see another doctor in certain situations ensures the best outcomes.

- ✔ If you think that patient won't follow through with recommended treatment. In this case, the doctor-patient relationship has broken down and another doctor might be able to gain the patient's trust.

- ✔ If the patient has a problem you can't adequately treat. Some patients need several courses of treatment or levels of care before the treatment you recommend can occur.

Discovering the need for specialist referrals

No doctor can be a specialist in all areas. A family practitioner wouldn't feel comfortable performing kidney surgery, and an obstetrician wouldn't be qualified to perform cardiac bypass surgery. Specialists in medicine are highly trained in a specific area. The trick is knowing when to refer a patient to a specialist.

A specialist is brought in for two reasons: to consult or to administer care. In a consultation, the primary care doctor is fully responsible for the patient. If the specialist needs to treat the patient, the primary care doctor must relinquish control of the patient to the specialist. When referring a patient, keep these guidelines in mind:

- ✔ The doctor must be sure that the referral is relevant to the diagnosis and based on objective, not subjective, reasons.

- ✔ The doctor must keep in mind that the welfare of the patient comes first, before any monetary or business interests.

- ✔ Referral fees are unethical. Federal laws called Stark Regulations prevent doctors from offering or accepting referral fees in most, if not all, cases.

- ✔ Be ready to make alternative arrangements if a referral fails because your patient doesn't establish a good relationship with the new doctor.

Refer the patient to a specialist who you are confident can treat the patient competently and with the best outcomes. Experience will teach you the best providers to whom you should send referrals. Make sure you receive good communication back from the specialist as well.

Choosing Whom to Serve

As citizens of the United States, doctors have choices in whom they want to serve and treat. But doctors must treat patients they may personally dislike, or patients whose politics they disagree with. Doctors must treat smokers, obese patients, and others who may be careless with their lives and health. In this section, we discuss a doctor's choice of patients, when and how to sever a relationship, and when to offer medical advice to non-patients.

Dr. O'Riley's case: Applying conscience laws

Dr. O'Riley is an internist who is also a devout Catholic. He is morally opposed to abortion and prescribing birth control because of his faith. He chose internal medicine as a specialty because he rarely encounters conflicts to his personal beliefs in his patient population, which is primarily geriatric. Occasionally, a woman may see him for an exam and request birth control pills. When this occurs, he notifies the patient that due to his personal beliefs he is unable to prescribe them. He sends her to one of his partners in the office to obtain the requested prescription.

Conscience laws, or refusing to perform certain procedures or prescribe treatment against a doctor's moral or religious beliefs, exist so a healthcare provider can't be forced to prescribe a treatment to which he is morally opposed. These laws are amended in certain ways. For instance, the patient must be able to obtain a specific treatment or surgery elsewhere, as long as it is legal.

Refusing to treat a patient

Doctors do have the right to refuse a patient, based on certain guidelines. There are exceptions to this rule.

- ✔ In an emergency a doctor must respond to the best of his ability.
- ✔ A doctor cannot refuse to treat a patient with an infectious disease, according to the Americans with Disabilities Act of 1990.
- ✔ A doctor cannot stop caring for a patient in the middle of treatment or when that patient needs medical care.
- ✔ A doctor cannot decline a patient based on "race, color, religion, national origin, sexual orientation, or any other basis that would constitute invidious discrimination." — AMA Code of Medical Ethics

The *public square,* or the broad society that includes all members, comes into play here. In any group of people or any country there are going to be others with different beliefs. The principle of justice demands that all people deserve access to all aspects of healthcare. A doctor's personal views are less importance than the patient's autonomy or best outcome.

Doctors can also refuse to add new patients if their practice has become too large. Never take on more patients than you can treat well. They can also leave patients if they move away and take their practice elsewhere.

Ending a doctor-patient relationship

When a doctor decides to no longer treat a patient, certain conditions must be met to legally end the relationship. Notice to the patient must be in writing. These are the rules:

- ✔ Doctors must support continuity of care. Before ending a relationship with a patient, you must give advance notice so the patient can find another doctor.

- ✔ When a relationship exists, a patient's treatment cannot be discontinued unless the doctor has assisted the patient in finding a new doctor and making arrangements for treatment.

- ✔ A doctor can end a patient relationship if the patient has committed fraud (for example, falsifying prescriptions under the doctor's name) , the patient exhibits inappropriate behavior (threatening or sexually inappropriate behavior), or repeatedly refuses the recommended treatment.

- ✔ A doctor can end a relationship if the patient wants a treatment that is not scientifically valid or interferes with a doctor's personal or moral beliefs.

- ✔ A clinic can end a relationship with a patient if they have repeatedly refused to pay their bills and have refused to set up even a minimum payment plan. If the patient's doctor confirms that they do not have a life-threatening medical illness, the clinic will notify the patient in writing that he is "terminated." The clinic should give the patient a reasonable amount of time, usually about 30 days, to find a new doctor.

Patient dumping, or abandonment, is unethical and constitutes malpractice. When the patient requires care, it is unethical to refuse treatment. The patient must be assisted in finding another provider before you can end the relationship.

Politics and medicine make strange bedfellows

In 2010, a urologist in Florida put a sign on the front door of his office stating, "If you voted for Obama . . . Seek urologic care elsewhere." Is this ethical? According to the AMA Code of Ethics, politics has no place in the doctor-patient relationship. The Code states, "Under no circumstances should physicians allow their differences with patients or families about political matters to interfere with the delivery of high-quality professional care." This doctor's actions may be legal because he wasn't asking patients directly about their political choices, but they are not ethical.

Hector's story: An abrupt good-bye

Hector was a 95-year-old man who lived in a nursing home. His daughter brought him to the doctor for care. Because Hector was in a wheelchair, this took a lot of effort. Hector had several physical problems and was often agitated, sometimes disturbing other nursing home residents in the middle of the night. At one visit, Hector's doctor told the daughter that he would no longer treat Hector as a patient. The doctor did not give notice in writing, did not offer any help finding a new doctor, and immediately severed the relationship, leaving the daughter to return Hector to the nursing home without a checkup. These actions were unethical.

Ending a relationship for nonpayment when the patient is undergoing necessary or lifesaving treatment is unethical. If a patient refuses to pay or cannot pay, the doctor must arrange for treatment elsewhere and give the patient sufficient notice to arrange for care elsewhere.

The reasons for ending relationships with a patient must be applied uniformly across all patients. The policy must be applied equally to all patients in all situations without discrimination or prejudice.

Giving medical advice to non-patients

Imagine that you are a small-town family physician at your daughter's soccer game. An acquaintance comes up to you and asks your opinion about a lump on her arm. What do you do? Do you diagnose a condition, encourage her to make an office visit with you, or refer her to another physician?

An actual doctor-patient relationship doesn't exist in this situation, but one can be implied. You can offer a disclaimer that you are only imparting information and not medical advice, but that may not be a legal defense in the event you're sued.

It's not wise to diagnose any condition based on casual conversation. Without a medical history and thorough workup, offering advice can be unethical and even harmful to the patient. It's too easy to make serious errors when not in a clinical setting and without the proper diagnostic tools. And you could be held legally liable for any advice you give in a casual conversation. It's also hard to know how to document these encounters in the patient's medical record.

All you can do is encourage your acquaintance to seek medical attention from her primary care doctor. Tell her that it could be harmful and unethical for you to offer a specific opinion or advice.

Patient Rights and Obligations

The doctor-patient relationship used to be seen as paternalistic. Doctors knew what was best for patients, and patients obeyed. Period! That has changed in the past 50 years. The new relationship has evolved into a partnership, with the doctor and patient both taking active roles. Doctors still have more power in the relationship because they have been highly trained and educated. Both the doctor and patient must follow guidelines and take responsibility for the patient's health.

In this section, we take a closer look at patient autonomy and the patient's right to make decisions and steer his care. We discuss how encouraging honesty is the best way to facilitate a healthy doctor-patient relationship. And we show how balancing treatment and cost is necessary in these days of skyrocketing healthcare costs.

Patient autonomy: Patient as decision-maker

Autonomy refers to freedom of will and freedom of action. Doctors must respect the patient's decisions as long as they are made with a sound mind and with all available information. You must create the environment necessary for your patient to make an informed choice.

Before a patient can be considered autonomous, certain conditions must be met. The patient must have the ability to reason, have power and legal control over her life, and the ability to understand the benefits of treatment. She must also understand the risks of refusing treatment or choosing not to follow the doctor's advice.

Geraldine's case: A patient's right to refuse treatment

Geraldine is an 80-year-old woman who was recently diagnosed with breast cancer. A small lump was found at her annual physical. Even though Geraldine is otherwise in good health and lives independently, she is refusing further treatment such as a simple lumpectomy, which may stop the cancer's spread. "I'm 80 years old and I'm ready to go any time. I don't want to prolong my life and don't want to find out if the cancer has spread. Just let me live my life and keep me comfortable." Even though her doctor wishes she would pursue further evaluation and treatment, he must go along with her decision.

There are times when the principles of autonomy and beneficence come into conflict. If a patient refuses treatment that the doctor knows will help her and improve her health, the doctor must respect that decision.

Many offices, clinics, and hospitals post a Patient Bill of Rights, often found on the wall near the entrance or patient admitting area. Hospitalized patients are often given a written copy of the Patient Bill of Rights at the time of their admission. Make sure that your patients are informed about these rights and understand them. In most cases, patients have a right to

- Be treated with respect
- Receive care in spite of age, religions, race, disability, or nationality
- Confidentiality within the law
- An accurate diagnosis and explanation
- Their medical records
- Informed consent
- A second opinion
- Refuse information about diagnosis, treatment, and prognosis
- Receive information and diagnoses in a timely manner
- Make decisions about end-of-life care
- Refuse treatment

Some patient responsibilities come along with those rights, and it's important that patients understand them. Patients have a duty to

- Be truthful and express their symptoms, questions, and concerns
- Provide a complete and accurate medical history, including all drugs and supplements they're currently taking
- Ask questions and seek more information when they don't understand
- Make decisions in a responsible manner
- Cooperate with treatment, keep their appointments, and question a treatment plan
- To meet their financial responsibilities or tell their doctor
- Treat their bodies with respect
- Act properly and with respect toward healthcare providers and other patients

Patients should be able to make their own decisions regarding their healthcare as long as they are intellectually and emotionally able. Doctors help by providing honest and complete information and respecting the patient's ability to shape their own life.

Encouraging honesty

One of the important ethical principles is truth telling. Patients should be as honest as possible, both in their description of symptoms and as they help decide their treatment. When patients are dishonest or withhold information, their treatment and even their life can be compromised or put in danger.

Everyone lies at one time or another. Some patients lie because

- ✔ They are afraid of being judged.
- ✔ The examination room and clinic setting scares them.
- ✔ They are afraid of the diagnosis.
- ✔ They want to please the doctor.

It's important to tell the patient you are not going to judge their lifestyle or actions, and that you must know their complete medical history to make the correct diagnosis. It's also important to give positive feedback when patients do tell the truth. A physician is not a teacher who disciplines a student. You are a partner in your patient's care.

How something is asked or stated is critical to getting an honest answer. Instead of saying, "Why didn't you take the pills?" say "Some of my patients don't like taking these pills. Are you having that problem?" This less judgmental and accusing question will probably elicit more answers. When the patient is honest, even if they reveal something embarrassing, you can help them change. If an exercise routine or swallowing a pill is too difficult, there may be other options you can recommend that will help.

Take the time to ask questions, especially open-ended questions. This can seem like a lot of trouble in the middle of a busy day. But if the patient lives a better life because you take a bit more time in the exam room, it's worth it.

To tell the truth

A study from Johns Hopkins found that what patients say they did and what they actually did are two different things. The study looked at patients using an inhaler to help with breathing problems. The inhaler recorded the time and date of each use. The researchers found that 73 percent of patients said they used the inhaler three times a day, but only 15 percent of them actually did. Even worse, 14 percent of patients emptied their inhalers before their doctor's visits so it would look like they were using the device. This concerning study points out that many patients are more interested in pleasing their doctor (or avoiding reprimand!) than they are in telling the truth. Patients also may not accurately remember their treatment protocol when reporting it to the provider.

Balancing treatment and cost

As discussed in Chapter 6, healthcare costs are spiraling out of control. Fewer people have access to healthcare in the United States, yet costs continue to increase beyond the rate of inflation.

Countries with universal healthcare have set many standards balancing treatment, outcomes, and cost. These standards are not widely used in the United States. It's not possible to offer all the care a patient wants to every person in the world. Choices must be made and treatment and costs weighed for each patient. There is no consensus on how to limit cost in this country.

Doctors are often being asked to play a role of *restricted advocacy*. This means they must consider the cost of treatment when recommending the best care to their patients. In health maintenance organizations (HMOs) and managed care operations, this benefits the patient because the patient has an interest in the financial health of the operation.

One of the best ways to manage healthcare costs is to make sure that the patient is following the course of treatment. When the provider-patient relationship is strong, the patient will be most likely to follow the doctor's advice and will get the best result for less cost.

Chapter 4

Outside the Examining Room: Running an Ethical Practice

A few old television sitcoms like *The Bob Newhart Show* and *Becker* featured doctor's offices as the setting. Although losing a patient's records or mixing up appointments may be a funny plot line in a TV show, those situations should not happen in your medical practice. Running a medical practice today is very different from 20 or even 10 years ago. Today, ethical issues include safety and confidentiality when communicating with third parties, keeping medical information private, and navigating the issues, demands, and problems of managed care.

In this chapter, we look at complying with the Health Insurance Portability and Accountability Act (HIPAA), how you should train your staff to handle medical records, and the issue of medical releases. We also examine how to set good administrative policies in the age of managed care, and take a look at third-party issues such as dealing with insurance companies and pharmaceutical representatives.

Above all, your responsibility is to your patients and ensuring that they get the best care possible, while respecting their rights to privacy and autonomy.

A study conducted by Physicians Practice Inc. and the University of Pennsylvania's Wharton School of Business found that doctors with better medical practices spend more money and time on support staff. Their practices make more money and have more satisfied patients. A well-trained and complete support staff lets you focus more time on your patients, leading to a higher quality of care.

Good professional and ethical conduct, both inside the examining room and in clinics and hospitals, results in better care for patients and a more satisfying career for you and your coworkers.

Propriety in the Paperwork: Medical Records

The practice of medicine is based on accurate and complete medical records. And running an efficient office is essential to an ethical practice. The golden rule in running a practice is this: Treat your patients as you would want yourself and your family to be treated. Running a good practice means you attempt to follow all four principles of medical ethics (see Chapter 1), and know how to balance them.

In this section, we look at the details of complying with government regulations regarding medical information. We also look at ways to train staff to handle medical records and releases. And we look at the best ways to safeguard patient anonymity.

Before you train your staff, you must first hire ethical and qualified employees. Encourage continuing education and training, including the areas of ethics and HIPAA regulations. Your support staff is a valuable part of your team, and you all must work together.

Complying with the Health Insurance Portability and Accountability Act (HIPAA)

The Health Insurance Portability and Accountability Act (HIPAA) is a federal law designed to regulate and define healthcare information and its use in the United States. It sets security policies and procedures, defines what information — also called Protected Health Information (PHI) — should be kept private, and determines how the information should be handled in this age of electronic communication.

All doctors' offices and clinics must have comprehensive security programs in place to protect patient information. The office must make a reasonable effort to comply with the law. The government defines this as a prudent and professional effort to use established transmission methods like encrypted e-mail, and follow HIPAA guidelines.

The leaky elevator

A study in Philadelphia by the Annals of Internal Medicine found that in 7 percent of elevator rides, staff, nurses, and doctors breached confidentiality about patients during normal conversation. All healthcare providers must be trained to avoid mentioning any potentially private information in casual conversation in the work place and out in public. In fact, it's best not to gossip while you're at the office . . . for many other reasons, too!

The ultimate goal is to protect private data and keep it secure. If you establish procedures and policies to reduce the risk of accidental disclosure, your office will be secure. The steps to become HIPAA compliant are

- ✔ Conduct a *risk assessment,* or review of information management and all procedures.

- ✔ Develop a policy to protect and secure private data.

- ✔ Develop a plan to implement your clinic's policy and reduce risk, including identifying a privacy officer, who can be any staff member trained to oversee the plan.

- ✔ Fund the implementation plan and put it into practice.

- ✔ Train staff and employees on all procedures, policies, and workstation use, and have frequent refresher training sessions. Ensure privacy during staff workstation use.

- ✔ Make sure that computer systems and information technologies are encrypted and that fax, e-mail, telephone, and transcription services are secure.

- ✔ Set up a plan to routinely monitor and enforce the program, and develop a contingency plan for system emergencies.

Many states have enacted stricter guidelines than HIPAA mandates, but states can't relax HIPAA standards. It's always wise to check your state's mandates when evaluating HIPAA compliance.

Training staff to handle records

When you train your staff to handle patient's medical records, confidentiality needs to be stressed above all else. Information contained in medical records should be kept private by law. Many offices are eliminating paper records and turning to electronic records management (ERM). This requires more staff training. Electronic medical records make it easier for breaches of confidentiality to occur. All patients' medical records are available at the touch of a button. On the other hand, it's much easier to detect these breaches because there is a computer record of every person who accesses a patient's chart.

It's very important that staff keep up with medical records, keeping the information current and accurate. Notes, orders, laboratory results, and patient summaries should be updated as soon as possible, preferably the same day the information is received. In the case of an abnormal lab result or stress test, for example, this could mean the difference between life and death.

Chart delinquency is a serious problem and should be avoided at all costs. Doctors and nurses must give patient information to staff in a timely manner. Some clinics or practice groups give doctors delinquent medical record notices if this becomes a problem.

Standards for handling medical records should be written and taught to each member of your staff. These considerations can include

- ✔ Location of the records
- ✔ Security procedures, including who has access to records
- ✔ The person or persons responsible for passing on information in patient files
- ✔ Who is in charge of compliance with federal laws

Processes must be standardized, and all staff must be trained according to your system. In larger practices it may be helpful to have one member of the staff focus mostly on compliance training so there is consistency in your office.

Preventing identity theft

Identity theft is a worldwide problem. Thieves can literally steal someone's identity and impersonate that person to commit fraud or theft. A patient who uses a fake identity or stolen medical insurance card does not have to pay the doctor or hospital bill unless they get caught. Also, doctors' offices and hospitals have been targeted by identity thieves; these offices must enact special policies and procedures to protect their patients. Medical records contain lots of personal information that can be used for fraud.

In 2010, the FTC issued regulations called the Red Flags Rule to help prevent identity theft. The Rule cover businesses that act as creditors. As mandated by federal law, doctor's offices and hospitals must have a written program to spot the "red flags" of identity theft. Your practice is covered under this rule if you are a creditor or hold covered accounts with your patients. In other words, if you accept deferred payments for your services, you are considered a creditor. The FTC has delayed compliance of the Rule until December 31, 2010 because the AMA has objected to doctor's offices being listed as creditors, but likely it will be implemented after that.

You need to establish red flags for your particular practice. Some red flags include

- Fake IDs or altered IDs
- A patient listed under multiple names
- Suspicious documents, such as a Social Security number that doesn't match information from another source
- Suspicious activities, such as mail returned as undeliverable
- Alerts from other businesses, such as a credit report
- Inconsistency between exam results and medical histories
- Notices about identify theft from another source, such as an insurer or pharmacy

After you've identified the red flags, you need to take steps to implement your policy. If a member of your staff sees a red flag, you may need to ask for more information from the patient or contact a third party to ask more questions.

Keep your red flag program updated with the latest information from government and law enforcement because identity thieves are always changing their tactics and improvising new techniques.

Releasing medical records

Medical releases are forms that let a provider give confidential patient information and medical records to others, such as insurance companies, other providers, or designated family members. Each state has a different type of medical release form, so make sure you are in compliance with the laws and rules in your state.

Medical release forms are mainly intended to give other providers the medical records they need to understand the complete history and status of a patient for whom they are caring. There are different parts of the medical record which can be designated on the form depending what information is needed. These include

- Provider notes on the patient's care, dating back to the start of the relationship or another specified date
- Other communication about the patient, including telephone calls and nurse encounters

✔ Lab and radiology reports

✔ Actual radiology films such as X-rays

✔ Mental health records, which should be approved by the patient, separate from other records

✔ Consultation reports from other physicians

✔ Insurance information

✔ Summaries of admission, discharge, and procedures from hospital facilities

Accuracy in medical releases is paramount because a misunderstanding or miscommunication can harm a patient. Make sure all abbreviations and terminology are correct. And the release should be typed, not hand-written, to avoid confusion or misunderstanding.

It is essential to keep medical release forms in good order. Forms must be complete, signed and dated, with all necessary information kept up to date. The medical release form should be scanned or filed on the patient's chart. Records are released when a patient is transferred to another doctor or clinic, when a referral is made, for a legal claim, to a government agency for a worker's compensation claim, or to the patient herself. Information should never be released over the phone or in an e-mail. A patient can revoke a medical release authorization in writing at any time.

You can release medical records without a patient's consent if he is physically unable to consent and if his needs relate directly to his condition. In these situations, you're practicing the ethical principle of beneficence. For example, Jim was a patient who collapsed while jogging. An onlooker called 911 and Jim was brought to the ER, unconscious at the time of presentation. Jim's wife arrived and said that he had recently being seeing his doctor for some tests. Even though Jim couldn't sign a medical release form, it was legal for the ER to get his clinic records as quickly as possible because they were likely related to his current condition. The records verified that Jim was undergoing evaluation for a heart condition, so his collapse was likely cardiac-related.

There are special laws and rules that relate to medical release forms in HIV cases. There are limits to a patient's right to privacy in these cases. Medical information about those at risk for HIV can be released to other parties without a patient's consent when

✔ In an emergency situation to medical personnel.

✔ A public health authority requests the information.

✔ For the purpose of public health research and statistics.

✔ A court order is granted.

✔ The doctor knows of the patient's sexual partners and the patient has not told them of his diagnosis. The doctor must make an effort to counsel the patient, and but then disclosure is needed to protect the partners' health.

Most states have laws that require mandated reporting of certain conditions, such as bullet wounds, communicable diseases, and conditions that render people unfit for some occupations (such as driving a large commercial truck or flying an airplane). These decisions must be reported with or without patient consent.

Safeguarding anonymity

Anonymity is a stricter standard than confidentiality, with more guarantee of privacy. With more and more medical records becoming electronic, medical practices should add de-identification of patient data to their systems. This statistical practice removes 18 identifiers from patient data, including names, telephone numbers, social security numbers, zip codes, and account numbers.

Health researchers have found that when they must get consent for clinical studies, participation rates go down. It's possible to use some information on medical records for secondary research, such as surveys, without consent if it is de-identified. The problem is that it can be easy to identify a patient even when the information is de-identified. Information such as a disease, birth date, marital status, gender, and zip codes can be combined to identify patients. In fact, just the date of birth, gender, and zip code can identify more than 80 percent of United States citizens in public databases.

Just because data looks anonymous doesn't mean it is anonymous. It's important that medical information is not just encrypted when transmitted, but that *noise,* such as nonsense words or meaningless symbols, should be added to the data, and some values should be scrambled and exchanged. This process is called *k-anonymity,* an algorithm developed by Sweeny et al that changes medical codes and suppresses or generalizes attributes so a patient can't be identified with linked data.

There are quite a few other entities that have access to some parts of patient's medical records. In fact, some data-sharing is quite common. They include

- Insurance companies
- Government agencies, such as Social Security and Medicare
- The Medical Information Bureau
- Prescription drug databases
- Employers, for a background check or if a company is self-insured, with patient consent
- Records subpoenaed in court
- Medical records used for research and given to agencies such as the National Institutes of Health
- Direct marketers if a patient uses free health screenings

Modern Managed Care and Today's Office Practice

The Health Maintenance Organization Act of 1973 was the start of managed care. Health maintenance organizations (HMOs) were the first entities to emerge from that legislation. Managed care is meant to improve the quality of medical care and reduce the cost at the same time. They work through various incentives, including cost sharing, controls on hospital admissions and length of stay, contracting with providers, and managing high cost cases. At this time, more than 90 percent of all Americans with health insurance are enrolled in managed care plans.

Unfortunately, managed care hasn't reined in healthcare costs. One of the big problems of this type of system is that the plans are managed by for-profit companies, and some companies put profit above patient care. Doctors are forced to spend less time with patients and the companies make it more difficult for patients to see specialists, all without saving significant amounts of money. Many states have enacted laws that mandate managed-care standards, which have increased costs.

In this section we look at the ethical issues surrounding managed care, especially when support staff rather than doctors treat patients and how to supervise this trend. We also look at the balance between taking good care of patients and earning money.

Managed care has produced a lot of dissatisfaction from providers and patients. Having a gatekeeper approve medically indicated treatments can be frustrating, and patients have died waiting for appeals of denied treatment.

Some critics have stated that managed care reduces costs simply by making it too difficult for some patients to get treatment, so they just give up. This is an unethical practice because it violates the principles of beneficence, nonmaleficence, and justice.

Ethical concerns of managed care

Managed care works in several ways, using many different methods. Incentives are offered so providers are encouraged to become more efficient, or provide care while minimizing cost. Incentives can include bonuses for those who see the most patients with the least overall cost, peer pressure on those who do not reduce costs, and penalizing providers by withholding income or bonuses if goals are not met. Managed care methods include

✔ Emphasizing preventive care

✔ Restricting enrollees to a specific set of providers

✔ Paying doctors a fixed amount for each patient no matter how much care that patient needs (capitation)

✔ Offering incentives for wellness programs and efficient care

✔ Restricting access to specialists, tests, and some medicines

✔ Using case managers to organize care for each patient

✔ Emphasizing patient education

Ethicists are concerned that some incentives, whether monetary or not, will lead providers to compromise care. You should have your patients' best interests as your primary responsibility. When you also have to consider time spent with a patient and are forced into cost-cutting measures, patient care can be pushed down on the priority list.

Many providers are also concerned about the doctor-patient relationship in managed care. Because doctors are forced to spend less time with patients, there is less opportunity to develop a good relationship, which can reduce trust and compromise care. And because managed care organizations (MCOs) can terminate relationships with doctors, a patient may lose their doctor when a health plan changes.

Doctors can choose which organizations to join. As an ethical principle, you should carefully evaluate the contracts you sign with these companies. You have a responsibility to examine the standards of the organization. Before you sign with an MCO, be sure to look for:

✔ Guidelines that set a reasonable time frame for seeing patients. A ten-minute visit usually isn't enough time to adequately assess a patient's needs.

✔ Reasonable fee structures, so you can spend enough time with each patient. Doctors are paid either by the amount of time they spend with patients or by the level of complexity of the medical care given or procedure performed. Be sure that you get adequate reimbursement for both the time spent with the patient and the level of complexity of the care given.

✔ Clauses that may restrict patient referrals and discussions about their care, also known as *gag clauses*. These can prevent a doctor from telling a patient about a beneficial treatment because the MCO doesn't authorize its use.

✔ Adequate pathways to appeal denied services. When a manager at an insurance company denies treatment, patients can get sicker and die. It's important that there are methods set up to adequately address this problem.

You can try to negotiate with the company to remove terms that you find unacceptable, especially if they compromise your ethical integrity or medical judgment. Incentives that hurt patients are unethical.

Teamwork results in better care

In our clinics I am blessed to work with excellent NPs and PAs. We have set up a system so each midlevel provider has a supervising physician to work with, especially when they are new to the practice. That physician is available to answer questions and help out if a patient situation is more critical or complex. The provider then becomes a support to the physician's practice and is available to see a patient if the doctor is gone or busy. The doctor/midlevel provider team provides improved care and access for patients.

And remember that you should frequently evaluate your relationship with an MCO, and consider whether your patients are getting the best care in that particular system. If you find yourself cutting patient visits short, routinely appealing denied care, or feeling too much financial pressure, look for another organization.

There's something new on the horizon: Accountable Care Organizations, or ACOs. These systems use *global capitation* as a payment system. An entire team of providers is paid a set fee for disease treatment, and the payment is divided among the providers. This system helps ensure efficiency because repetition of services won't be paid for, and the team works to prevent readmissions. One of the problems with ACOs is that they will not work with doctors in private, independent practices.

Working with midlevel providers

Support staff is critical to a good practice. The patient's first contact is with a receptionist. She then sees a nurse, and then perhaps a nurse practitioner or physician assistant, rather than a doctor. All of these people must be trained to be compassionate, caring, and responsible, and they all must understand medical ethics.

Support staff has assumed a greater role in managed care. Not every visit or every illness demands you see a doctor. In many cases, a nurse practitioner (NP) or physician's assistant (PA), also called *midlevel providers*, can deliver quality care with less cost. Nurse practitioners are also called *clinical nurse specialists*.

Every state has different rules about what support staff can do. Some nurse practitioners have a doctorate degree (called a Doctor of Nursing Practice, or DNP), and most have a master's degree. In some states the practitioner must be under the direct supervision of an MD.

As the doctor, you should set clear guidelines and standards for support staff. Work and practice methods must be continuously reviewed to make sure that patients are receiving the best care and that staff isn't ordering or giving inappropriate treatment. When supervising staff, remember to

- Make sure communication is always open throughout the day
- Develop specific protocols for staff, including nurse practitioners and physician assistants
- Review staff function regularly
- Review charts on a regular basis
- Have a plan in place for emergencies, including back-up assistance by on-call physicians
- Have a review plan for prescriptions, especially controlled substances

The important thing to remember is that nurses and other support staff should be considered part of a team that has healthy patients as its goal. Your staff are equal partners in your healthcare team and are there to help you do the best job you can.

It's important to let patients know that when they see a nurse practitioner, even if that person has a doctorate, they are not seeing a medical doctor. A DNP is a respected doctorate, but it is not the same as a medical degree. To keep patients fully apprised of their care, to keep them informed, and to keep the relationship open and trusting, midlevel providers need to be identified as such. Some patients will have a strong preference about seeing a physician, and others are happy to see all types of providers. Many patients will come to identify with an NP or PA as their primary provider.

A new trend in medicine is the establishment of retail health clinics, or *minute clinics*. These clinics in pharmacies or big-box stores are staffed by a nurse or midlevel provider. Patients are seen for a few simple medical problems, such as sore throat, pink eye, or colds. Visits cost less and are quicker, but there are concerns about quality of care. There is also loss of continuity of care with a patient's primary provider, who knows the patient's health and risk factors for more serious problems.

Prescribing good care while still getting paid

Today's doctors have to deal with a lot of paperwork. There's paperwork for insurance companies, paperwork for HMOs and MCOs, paperwork for government policies and regulations, paperwork for patients, and paperwork for running a practice. More regulations mean more paperwork. And doctors also have to meet the financial goals of managed care plans and their own practices.

But it's possible to have satisfied patients and a good career even in the midst of all these regulations and restrictions. If you remember to keep your focus on the patient, work on creating and maintaining good doctor-patient relationships, and treat staff with respect and trust, your practice will thrive.

For the best medical practice, there are some rules to follow:

- ✔ **Focus on the patient.** Make all decisions in their best interests.

- ✔ **Communicate, communicate, communicate.** Always explain risk versus benefit of treatments, and make patients partners in their health care.

- ✔ **Choose your tests and medications carefully.** Make sure that you order tests and treatments that are absolutely necessary, but don't go overboard with diagnostic tests or prescribe drugs that might not be best for the patient. And keep the patient's economic standing in mind when prescribing drugs.

- ✔ **Keep your priorities straight.** Your job is to rule out any serious problems, treat the problem the patient comes to you to fix, and make them feel better.

- ✔ **Be an advocate for your patients.** Intervene for them when there are problems with insurance companies or MCOs. And try to move the process along because delay can mean serious consequences for the patient. Delayed treatment because of insurance payment issues can seriously affect patient outcomes.

- ✔ **Remember to be compassionate and caring.** People who come to your office are often scared and upset. Part of your job is to reassure them when you can and be present with them in difficult circumstances. Being compassionate and caring does not have to take extra time, and often leads to more effective and efficient care.

Third-Party Issues

There are often conflicts of interest between doctors and third parties, including insurance companies, HMOs, MCOs, the government, drug companies, and researchers. Balancing these conflicts is an important part of your medical practice.

In this section, we look at how to handle third parties while keeping the patient at the center of your practice. Unfortunately, third parties do not have the same objectives or ethical responsibilities that you do. Insurance companies and drug companies need to show a profit to their shareholders.

And what about perks, freebies, and advertising? When can a provider cross the line accepting gifts, and how much and what kind of advertising is ethical? We look at these issues, too.

Felicia's case: Arguing the necessity of medical procedures

Felicia was a 24-year-old pregnant patient who came in for an 18-week OB visit including an ultrasound. She and her partner wanted to know the baby's sex. She had had an early OB ultrasound at nine weeks to determine the pregnancy due date because she was uncertain about her last period. Felicia was a heavy smoker and at her visit, the baby seemed to be small. Felicia had only gained one pound during the pregnancy. An OB ultrasound was ordered and the baby was found to be a boy, but also experiencing intrauterine growth retardation (IUGR). Felicia's insurance company wouldn't pay for the ultrasound because the policy covered just one unless there was a substantial medical indication for a second. Felicia's doctor wrote a letter to the insurance company stating that the ultrasound was ordered not to determine the baby's sex, but to check fetal growth based on indications from the OB visit. The company accepted the appeal and paid for the ultrasound.

Dealing with insurance companies and HMOs

Insurance companies, whether traditional groups, HMOs, or MCOs, have profit in mind. Everyone has heard stories of insurance companies refusing to pay for treatment that a patient needs. So what's your role in this issue?

Doctors and other providers should stand up for their patients. Lay persons should not be second-guessing medical decisions because they do not have the patient's best interests in mind. Your responsibility is to your patients.

Sometimes insurance companies may ask you to do something that is unethical. For instance, in 2008, Blue Cross of California sent out a letter telling doctors that new patients who do not submit a complete medical history with an insurance application will be dropped unless the doctor fills in the blanks. In other words, the insurance company was asking the doctor to violate confidentiality for a business decision. Pitting doctors against their patients for monetary gain is unethical.

Pay-for-performance (PFP or P4P), is an emerging trend in health insurance, whereby providers are rewarded for the quality of their services and for meeting goals for quality and efficiency. Physicians are rewarded financially for meeting pre-established care goals. For example, a patient is hospitalized with new congestive heart failure. There is a checklist of what insurers will be looking for when the hospital admission is reviewed: Did the patient have an echocardiogram? Were they instructed in a low salt diet? Were they started on an ACE inhibitor (heart failure medication)? All these are shown to reduce re-hospitalization and improve care. Providers who do all these will be paid better than those who forget certain components of the care. When reviewing whether to participate in pay-for-performance with certain insurers, look for

- ✔ Incentives that are broad and applied across large groups of doctors, which can help lessen the impact on each doctor's individual reimbursement

- ✔ A large-as-possible patient pool, which allows you to care for a diversity of patients without taking a hit for seeing only a specific underserved group

- ✔ Annually evaluated incentives, not monthly because the longer time frame allows for more variation and more time to improve outcomes

- ✔ Efficiency-promoting incentives based on quality care, not on money-saving cuts

- ✔ Access to care that is supported for all patients, no matter how sick or healthy they are

Patients should be informed about financial incentives that affect their care. If you are uncomfortable telling a patient about a particular incentive, that's a good clue it isn't ethical.

What are the ethical issues about P4P? Some studies have shown that it does lead to improved care of patients, or beneficence. Some MCOs want to link payment to negative outcomes, such as medical errors, which would support nonmaleficence. But there's an unintended consequence of P4P that has a negative effect on justice. Doctors are more likely to avoid high-risk, sicker patients and noncompliant patients because they will lower their performance numbers. These patients will have a more difficult time finding a doctor, and this is unjust.

Working toward optimal care for diabetic patients

In our state, insurers will soon be moving from paying physicians per patient visit to paying for performance based on meeting certain optimal care goals. At our clinic, we are continually working toward optimal diabetes care. My nurse and I work together to help every one of our diabetic patients meet the following guidelines: Glycosylated hemoglobin (HgA1C or 3 month blood sugar test) less than 8.0, LDL cholesterol below 100, blood pressure below 130/80, smoking cessation, and taking an aspirin daily. All these goals reduce morbidity and mortality in diabetes. Patients who have not reached these goals are seen regularly to adjust medication and encourage lifestyle changes. Our patient goal and clinic goal is to have 40 percent of patients meeting all five goals of optimal care. As of now we are not paid on whether we achieve these goals, but it is addressed in our annual employment reviews. In the future, insurers will look at rates of success at various healthcare provider groups and reimburse physicians more highly for better care.

Should doctors lie to insurance companies?

A 2000 survey by the American Family Physician found that most doctors would deceive an insurance company for some procedures. More than 57 percent of respondents said they would lie to get authorization for coronary bypass surgery, even though this violates the AMA Code of Medical Ethics. More than 30 percent would lie to get a mammogram covered. It seems that doctors are more willing to deceive insurance companies when their patients have severe medical issues because only 2 percent of doctors would lie to get approval for cosmetic surgery. These doctors stated that their first responsibility was as an advocate for their patients. This highlights the conflict and tension between patient advocacy and the ethics of controlling medical costs. Although the rules of third parties were important, they became less important when they compromise the patient's best interests.

Many ethicists think that appeals processes should be expanded so doctors don't feel they have to lie to care for their patients. If the appeals process for denial of claims is complicated and cumbersome, which could cause unacceptable delays in treatment, doctors are more likely to use deception. And the public supports this practice. In fact, the public is more than twice as likely to sanction deception as healthcare providers are. One of the problems with this practice is that exaggerated symptoms, for instance, become part of the patient's medical chart. Doctors could use support staff to spend more time on appeals for denied services.

Insurance companies and HMOs are shifting from fee-for-service and capitation systems to something called diagnosis-related groups (DRGs), in which the doctor is paid based on standard treatment for a diagnosis. For example, there is a set rate paid for a patient who is hospitalized with pneumonia or a hip replacement. If you can treat a patient for less money, you get to keep the difference. If your patient costs more than the DRG, you are penalized and must absorb the loss.

Trying to save money on a patient should be low on your list of priorities. Moving patients through your practice quickly to offset high expenses on a few patients where you lose money could lead to missed diagnoses and is unethical. And what about patients who do cost more? Will patients who need more than standard treatment be turned away?

The point is that the pull and tug of money concerns, insurance company rules and demands, and hospital administrator's concern over cost tends to overshadow patient care. Ethically, your commitment to your patients should come first.

Perks and freebies

Most industries offer some type of perks and freebies to their employees. Company picnics, bonuses when goals are met, and complementary vacations to boost morale are all common in business. Pharmacy reps and outside parties try to influence healthcare provider behavior, such as prescribing a new drug or ordering a new treatment. But they often do this by giving physicians free gifts. These can be as simple as pens with a drug name on it, a luncheon where you listen to a drug rep talk, or more expensive, such as paying for physician travel. It's hard to prescribe an $11 generic drug for hypertension when you know the company that makes a new expensive drug is sending you to Colorado on a ski trip. And the information presented by drug reps to doctors is often based on biased market research. You must remember that your patient's needs come first (beneficence) and you should resist outside influences as much as possible.

The American Medical Association has guidelines for accepting gifts and perks from companies. Remember that any gift that could be construed as a conflict of interest should be declined. The guidelines include the following:

- ✔ Gifts should show some benefit to patients, such as books or supplies.
- ✔ Cash is not acceptable.
- ✔ The gifts should not have a lot of value. Value is determined by how much the item would cost if you bought it, not the cost of the gift to the company offering it.
- ✔ Conferences and trips should be focused primarily on education and medical goals, not on recreation.
- ✔ Subsidies for continuing education are permitted, but should be paid to the sponsor of the educational organization who will use that money to reduce costs and fees.
- ✔ Subsidies for medical-education-related travel aren't ethical, although honoraria or reimbursement for travel expenses, as long as they are reasonable, are permitted.
- ✔ No gift or freebie should ever have strings attached, and no subsidy should be accepted with the understanding that reciprocity is implied.

Sales reps visit doctors who are influential. They offer samples and gifts more often to specialists than to primary care doctors. Although visits from reps can keep you up to date on the latest medical advances, you should not let these visits influence your medical judgment or prescribing patterns.

Doctors can give patients health-related products without fear of conflict of interest. But selling health products from your office is trickier. Make sure any product you offer is based on peer-reviewed evidence-based medicine. And only offer or sell something that offers a direct benefit to your patient. You must disclose your financial interest in the product when it is sold.

Targeted advertising and ethics

Physicians advertising their services is a relatively new phenomenon. Twenty-five years ago, doctors didn't advertise. Now advertisements for hospitals, clinics, and individual doctors are all over the place. So how do you advertise while still respecting patient privacy and the truth? Above all, all advertising should be truthful and accurate. Can you honestly say you are the "best doctor" in a certain area? Never misrepresent your qualifications or specialty. Medical consumers are especially vulnerable, so advertising a particular specialty or service can raise false hopes.

There are no restrictions on advertising, according to the AMA Code of Medical Ethics. However, the ads should be specifically designed so the average layperson can understand them. Medical jargon can be confusing to the public, so make sure that any of your ads are clear and representative of your practice. Also, never imply that you can guarantee results or that you are more successful treating certain kinds of illnesses than other doctors. Creating unrealistic expectations in your potential patient base is unethical. Any ad placed by a doctor or other healthcare provider must be true both explicitly and implicitly, with a reasonable basis of the truth.

Targeted advertising, or focusing on one or two particular medical conditions, can be ethically tricky. Some clinics advertise to attract the attention of patients with good insurance policies or who need expensive surgery. Some ethicists call this *targeting to DRGs* (diagnosis-related groups). Aggressive and high-pressure advertising is not ethical. And patient testimonials, although they can be effective, can violate confidentiality and misrepresent your practice. Testimonials about patient satisfaction can be used, but only if they are true of most of your patients.

Chapter 5

Learning from Mistakes: Disclosing Medical Errors

*T*o err may be human, but many patients see their doctors as infallible. Unfortunately, that just isn't the case. No one is perfect. Medical errors happen every day. In fact, the AMA estimates that in the United States, up to 98,000 patients die every year because of medical errors. This is similar to the number of deaths caused by car accidents, breast cancer, and AIDS combined. These errors also cost our country billions of dollars each year.

In this chapter, we look at the different types of medical errors, and how to tell the patient when a mistake has been made. We look at the relationship between ethics of disclosure and legal protection, how to tell if another provider has become impaired, and how to handle this situation by helping a colleague and protecting patients. And we examine how reporting errors can actually help the medical profession as a whole.

First, do no harm. Medical errors primarily violate the ethical principle of non-maleficence, but also of beneficence, and justice. Even though providers do their best to care for patients, medical errors that cause suffering and even death do occur. It must also be stressed that errors do not automatically equal negligence. A physician may be giving medically appropriate care, and an error still may occur. It is critical that as a provider, you implement any tools you can to try to reduce all medical errors, whether due to negligence or simple human error.

Medical practice is an uncertain business with ambiguous problems. Every person is different, and many diseases can be difficult to diagnose. Errors have been made in every medical specialty and at every level of care. All healthcare providers must strive to reduce medical errors, whether they result from a mistake in surgery, an error in medication, or an error in recording information on a patient's chart.

Types of Medical Errors and Ways to Prevent Them

Medical errors occur when an incomplete or incorrect diagnosis or treatment leads to a negative outcome. Errors are defined as preventable events in medicine that harm patients. These are errors of *commission* (what is done to a patient) and errors of *omission* (what should have been done but is not).

Errors are usually not caused by a single event, but happen because of a chain of events that create multiple mistakes. Medical errors represent a breakdown of the medical system. And the more people who are involved with a patient, the greater the possibility an error will occur.

Errors happen because there is a failure in one or more areas:

- ✔ The design of the system
- ✔ Equipment failures
- ✔ Procedural mistakes
- ✔ Mistakes made by providers
- ✔ Defects in supplies and materials
- ✔ Errors in creating the hospital or clinic environment, including organizational design

The healthcare provider's part in these system failures occurs in equipment malfunction, procedural mistakes, oversight by providers, and mistakes in the environment. These include diagnostic, treatment, medication, communication, administrative, laboratory, and equipment errors. These are all errors of execution.

In this section, we look at these different types of errors, how they occur, and how they can be minimized or prevented. It's true that the more complex any system is, the more likely that errors and accidents can occur. Although it's not unethical to make an error, the issue of ethics comes into play when you decide what to do about the error. We address this in later sections in this chapter.

When you hit a nail with a hammer, there are only a certain number of things that can go wrong. But when you're operating on a human being, errors can occur in many areas: the patient could have a reaction to the anesthesia, become disabled, have a heart attack or stroke, or could die. The human body is a complex system. When something goes wrong in one part of the body, a cascading effect can take hold with catastrophic results.

Understanding diagnostic errors

Diagnostic errors are failures to diagnose a condition or disease correctly. Incorrect treatments and medications can be prescribed when a diagnostic error is made. They are usually an error of omission. An illness can be missed completely, a patient can be diagnosed with a condition they don't have, or a healthcare provider can fail to act when test results are abnormal.

Studies have found that diagnostic errors happen under certain conditions:

- Getting an inaccurate medical history from the patient
- Misinterpreting test results
- Becoming stressed, distracted, or fatigued
- Failing to ask advice from other doctors
- Avoiding intervention because a patient isn't of typical age for a particular disease or symptoms are unusual
- Failing to put together all the clues presented by the patient

There is no central agency that collects data on diagnostic errors. Because it's difficult to quantify diagnostic errors, it's also difficult to find a solution.

Studies have shown that many doctors are actually overconfident and don't want to rely on other sources for diagnostic help. There are computerized decision-support systems and diagnosis-reminder systems that can help a doctor correctly diagnose a patient. No one doctor can know everything about medicine because the amount of information has become so complicated and expansive. When doctors are asked if they have made diagnostic errors, only about 1 percent will even admit to having made a mistake. Yet studies have found that diagnostic errors are made 5 to 15 percent of the time.

A study in the American Medical Journal found that doctors who are overconfident in their knowledge and skill can develop *confirmation bias,* or jumping to a conclusion or diagnosis before all the facts have been examined. It's human to think that you can solve problems on your own, but learning something new and rethinking opinions is difficult.

The problem is that doctors must be confident in their ability to practice medicine, or they won't be able to do their jobs. The trick is to find a balance. Understand that you are well trained and able to do your job, but be willing to take advice and ask for help when necessary.

Don't be too quick to focus on a particular diagnosis, especially when the case seems complex or the patient has many symptoms. Narrowing down to a diagnosis too quickly is called *premature closure.* Considering the whole body in any diagnosis is important. Also, don't be too confident about the accuracy of sophisticated diagnostic testing results. Just as it's easy to be overconfident, you can become complacent. Little errors can add up to big problems. A 2004 study in the Annals of Family Medicine used cascade analysis to look at the chain of events that lead to an error. The study showed that the first errors in a chain almost always led to more errors.

Many primary care doctors never know when they misdiagnosed a case. If a patient isn't satisfied or doesn't feel better, she may just leave her doctor and seek medical treatment elsewhere. A patient treated in an emergency room may go to another hospital the next time he is sick, and the ER doctors will never know what happened. And sometimes people just get better on their own despite a misdiagnosis: nature is a good healer.

The best way to reduce diagnostic errors is for doctors and healthcare providers to seek another opinion of a colleague or specialist if things don't seem to add up. Close, regular follow-up of the patient is important because new symptoms may eventually lead to the correct diagnosis. By calling patients who don't keep their follow-up appointments, you may receive critical feedback on what happened to the patient. It is also important to stay up to date with continuing medical education so you are current with diagnostic tools and skills.

Understanding treatment errors

Treatment errors occur when patients are given the wrong medication or treatment. Errors may result from a diagnostic error, from the result of a mistake at the lab or pharmacy, or from a surgical mistake. Sometimes an outdated treatment is given to a patient. Treatment errors include:

Preventing diagnostic errors with aggressive follow-up

As a family physician, I am aware that the most common diagnostic error made by primary care providers leading to a lawsuit is missing a breast lump on physical exam that later turns out to be cancer. A breast exam is difficult, and a lump can be missed even with the help of an ultrasound and mammogram. These tests can come back as normal even in the case of a palpable breast cancer.

If I have a patient with a breast lump, even if the imaging is normal, I always see the patient again in one month for a recheck. If the lump is still present or growing, I refer the patient for biopsy. If I'm not sure, I send the patient to a local surgeon for a second opinion.

The most important point to stress to the patient is if they have a breast lump that is persisting or growing, they need follow-up. This conversation should be documented on the chart as well. This is an example of how early follow-up, referral for a second opinion, and patient education can help prevent a critical diagnostic error.

Edward's story: Recognizing the benefits of a second opinion

Edward was a 25-year-old male who developed pain in his abdomen. He went to see his doctor, who at first thought Edward had appendicitis. Those tests came back negative. The doctor, who was in his 70s, then proceeded to test Edward for tapeworm, lactose intolerance, and food allergies. The doctor eventually diagnosed him with irritable bowel syndrome, even though the patient had a significant weight loss of 40 pounds over five months. Edward then developed an infection in his right testicle. Another doctor in the practice diagnosed testicular cancer, which had metastasized to a large tumor in the abdomen. This was the cause of the pain. The first doctor had never done a check on his testicles, which had a large lump. Surgery, chemotherapy, and radiation followed. If Edward's doctor had discussed this case with his partners, or referred him to a specialist when the symptoms didn't add up, the correct diagnosis could have been made much earlier, leading to earlier treatment and better care for Edward.

✔ Mistakes made in surgery, including accidentally injuring adjacent structures or operating on the wrong body part or the wrong patient

✔ Mistakes made in doses of radiation given to cancer patients

✔ Improper use of medical equipment

✔ Mistakes in dosing or administering medication, either in the hospital or on outpatient prescriptions written in the clinic

✔ Mistakes made because of misinterpretation or mishandling lab results

Systems analysis for treatment errors should be implemented in hospitals and clinics. These programs can identify areas of highest risk and put procedures in place to reduce those risks. This can prevent errors before they happen.

An example of systems analysis is the process many hospitals have put in place to prevent surgeons from operating on the wrong limb. A patient is asked in the pre-operative area which limb is to be operated on. This is confirmed by looking at the surgeon's note and the primary doctor's pre-operative not. The limb is then marked, usually by a bright colored band or marking pen. Then in the operating room, the correct limb is reconfirmed again.

Medication errors

Medication errors are the most common type of treatment error. They occur when a patient is given the wrong prescription, the wrong dose of a prescription, or not given a prescribed medication. There are five types of medication errors:

- ✔ Administration errors, when the provider gives the wrong medicine to the patient

- ✔ Pharmacy fulfillment errors, when the pharmacist fills the prescription with the wrong drug

- ✔ Transcription errors, when the pharmacist misreads the prescription or it is written into the chart incorrectly

- ✔ Prescription errors, when the prescription is written incorrectly; a patient may be given the wrong dose of medicine, or receive unauthorized medication

- ✔ Drug interaction errors, when a provider prescribes a drug that has a serious interaction with a medication the patient is already taking

Nationwide, adverse drug events (ADEs) affect 6 percent of patients. Studies have found that mistakes made when writing prescription orders cause most of the errors.

When you're writing a prescription, avoid abbreviations. A misplaced decimal point or microgram being read as milligram can mean the difference between a patient getting better and a patient being hospitalized. The Institute for Safe Medication Practices (ISMP) has a list of common abbreviations that are misinterpreted. The ISMP List of Error-Prone Abbreviations can be found at `http://www.ismp.org/Tools/errorproneabbreviations.pdf`.

Always ask the patient about any medication or supplement they are currently taking. And tell the patient the name of the drug, the dosage, the purpose of the drug, what the medication looks like, and any special instructions. Remember — she is your partner in her care, so she should be educated about medications.

Electronic systems are better than hand-written prescriptions. The electronic medical record (EMR) is a great improvement for preventing medication errors. The EMR calculates pediatric doses based on weight. It allows only safe doses of adult medication to be prescribed, and automatically checks the new prescription with the patient's other medication to look for adverse drug interactions. It also removes the doctor's handwriting, which, because it can be illegible, can lead to errors.

Distractions and interruptions are a huge problem that can cause medication errors. It's best not to talk to a patient while writing or typing their prescription. If a pharmacist is interrupted when she is counting out pills or entering an order into the system, mistakes happen easily. Some hospitals have instituted quiet zones for prescription fulfillment. To ward off distractions and interruptions, some pharmacists and technicians wear vests that literally say "Do Not Interrupt" on them in large letters.

Communication errors

Communication among doctors, nurses, administrators, office staff, pharmacists, and lab technicians is crucial to a good patient outcome. According to a study by the Joint Commission on Accreditation of Healthcare Organizations, communication errors caused 60 percent of all medical errors in the United States in 2005. Communication errors can range from a nurse not understanding how a doctor wants a patient treated, to a staff member seeing a problem but not telling anyone about it.

A website www.silencekills.com reports on problems in communication between healthcare workers. Studies show that more than 70 percent of medical errors are caused by poor communication.

Clear, effective, and continuous communication is key to running a successful practice that benefits patients. To help improve communication, healthcare providers can

- ✔ Improve written communication by typing instead of writing and avoiding abbreviations
- ✔ Improve verbal and telephone orders by repeating the order back to the provider giving it
- ✔ Use Failure Mode and Effects Analysis or other systems to track errors and improvements and make changes
- ✔ Offer training in communication and disclosure, including developing teamwork and initiating a culture of safety
- ✔ Improve handoff communications by using electronic medical records and taking time to talk about a patient during a handoff

Communication between the patient and doctor can also result in medical errors. In Chapter 3, we discussed more effective ways to communicate with patients. Differences in culture, education, gender, and personality can hinder communication with patients. Use the methods described in that chapter to improve communication with your patients.

Administrative errors

Administrative errors can range from the wrong diagnostic codes entered into a patient's medical records to failure to accurately monitor status or not provide adequate staffing to meet patient needs. In 2009, the California Department of Public Health fined 11 hospitals for administrative errors that constituted an immediate jeopardy to the health and safety of patients.

Case study: Lab error

Monica was a 26-year-old who came in for her annual check-up. It had been a few years since her last pap smear, and she had had a few new sexual partners. Her pap smear was performed and somehow, the paper report was filed on her chart without the physician seeing it. Unfortunately, the report showed severe cervical dysplasia (precancerous change). Her clinic had no way of making sure abnormal labs were followed up, and Monica assumed her pap smear was normal because she didn't get a phone call saying otherwise. When she returned a few years later for another pap smear, results showed a lesion on her cervix. This was biopsied and diagnosed as cervical cancer. When the physician looked back over Monica's records, it was not clear how the previous abnormal result was put into her chart without being addressed.

Errors can also occur in filing systems or recording laboratory and other test results. Most of these errors are preventable. Installing safety systems can be expensive and take time, but are worth the investment because they can reduce or eliminate errors.

One cause of administrative errors is understaffed offices and hospitals. Assistants, receptionists, and secretaries who have a large workload and are under stress are more likely to make mistakes. Hospital nurses who have too many patients cannot give compassionate and error-free care. And doctors who have been awake on call for too many hours are at risk of making serious errors as well. It's important to stress to staff that taking the time to do the job correctly is crucial to achieving the best outcomes and for administration to support appropriate staffing. Understaffed clinics and hospitals are a serious threat to patient health and safety. Management should make sure that, as an ethical responsibility, staffing levels are adequate.

The crucial point is to identify errors before they actually affect patients. An error reporting system is an important tool that can help identify problem areas and find areas for improvement. These systems can also identify clusters or issues and errors that occur repeatedly. We take a look at error reporting systems later in this chapter.

Lab errors

A lab error is an error made while performing a test, interpreting test results, or recording the results incorrectly. Errors in the laboratory can range from a malfunction of lab equipment, failing to notify a patient of results, incorrectly identifying a biopsy, misplacing tissue or blood samples, or allowing cross-contamination in samples. A certain number of errors occur due to chance or test variability, including false positives and false negatives.

Lab errors can cause significant harm to patients, which obviously violates the principles of nonmaleficence and beneficence. A false negative on a cancer test can lead to an early death, whereas a false positive can force a patient to undergo surgery and treatments she doesn't need. And repeating a test adds to the overall cost of healthcare.

A system of checks and balances can help reduce the number of errors in the lab. To reduce the number of laboratory errors, doctors should

- ✔ Be sure that the lab used is accredited and approved by the College of American Pathologists.
- ✔ Double-check that names are written correctly on slides and pathology vials.
- ✔ Consider having a slide or test reviewed by another pathologist for serious diagnoses.
- ✔ If a diagnosis is for a disease or condition that has a high false negative or positive rate, consider redoing the test.
- ✔ Institute quality assurance programs, electronic transmission of results into the physician's inbox on his computer so they cant' be misplaced, electronic error-reporting systems, and specimen processing systems.

Quality assurance programs can improve morale, increase patient safety and satisfaction, and ensure confidence in patients and providers. These systems should incorporate training, lab test and error tracking, proficiency testing, and stress competence. Many government agencies already require continuing education and compliance courses and testing. These quality assurance systems will enhance and complement compliance.

Equipment failures

Equipment failures can range from heart defibrillators with dead batteries to defective IV pumps that administer an overdose of medication. Equipment can also be used improperly by healthcare providers. Machines that administer anesthetic can be misused, ventilator or bipap settings can be inappropriate, and x-ray equipment can be set to deliver a dose that's too high.

To reduce equipment failures, healthcare providers should

- ✔ Select medical equipment only from reputable manufacturers.
- ✔ Regularly test, inspect, and maintain medical equipment.
- ✔ Keep a detailed history of maintenance and failures about each piece of equipment.

> ✔ Identify maintenance, inspection, and testing procedures for all hospital equipment.
>
> ✔ Monitor any equipment failures, and report them as described in the Safe Medical Devices Act of 1990.

Admitting Your Mistakes

The hardest part about making a medical error is telling the patient. In another job, an error might mean incorrect paperwork, an ineffective product, or loss of money. In medicine, an error can severely affect a patient's life. Making a mistake that harms a patient or even leads to death can be devastating for the patient, the family, and the provider.

In this section we examine the patient's right to know when mistakes have been made, and look at truth telling — to the patient, to colleagues, and to management. We also try to understand balancing the ethics of telling the truth with legal protection.

Not disclosing errors undermines patient trust and violates the provider's responsibility to act in the patient's best interest. Telling a patient about an error respects their autonomy as well. Recent court decisions have highlighted the fact that providers have a legal duty to tell the patient about errors. A doctor's fiduciary duty demands that he is honest with his patients at all times. Making an error may not be unethical, but lying about it is.

Providers don't always agree that patients should be told about minor mistakes that don't cause harm. This acknowledgment may cause the patient to lose trust in the doctor, but that loss may become more serious if a patient discovers they have been lied to. All organizations should have a consistent standard for deciding which type of errors to disclose.

Understanding truth telling

Telling the truth is important in any discipline. Truth telling is not only crucial to the doctor-patient relationship; it can also be a learning opportunity for providers. Even when a mistake is made but caught before it caused harm, the event can be shared with colleagues in a confidential manner as a learning experience. Some ethicists believe that truth is a medical ethical principle.

In the past, traditional medical ethics favored a different principle than truthfulness in doctor-patient relationships: *beneficent deception*. In beneficent deception, a doctor may choose not to disclose the whole truth to the patient if they felt it was in the patient's best interest not to know. For instance, a doctor may not have told a patient about a new diagnosis of cancer to prevent undue anguish. Beneficent deception is still practiced in some cultures. In our country in recent years, there has been a strong move toward full truthfulness as the most ethical form of communication.

Withholding information alters the power in the relationship, creating a paternalistic scenario that diminishes the patient. If a healthcare provider loses his reputation for truth telling, it can mean the end of his career. And there's a difference between less than full disclosure and an outright lie. If a patient is irrational or depressed, providers must consider exactly what to tell that patient. In Chapters 3 and 7 we discuss what patients from some cultures and religious beliefs expect in a diagnosis and when it's better to withhold some information. It's also important to consider a patient's mental state. For someone who is very anxious, for example, it may make sense to slowly inform them of a serious diagnosis over a couple of visits to allow time for them to digest the information. The patient's autonomy and nonmaleficence need to be balanced and weighed in these situations. It's important to tell the truth in a compassionate manner, and to spend time with the patient when they need it.

There are also questions about uncertainty. There are degrees of certainty and uncertainty in medicine. When you are telling the patient "the whole truth," is it really the truth? Should you talk about every possible diagnosis or every step of a prognosis? Using the *reasonable person standard* is important in many cases. Tell the patient what a reasonable person would want to know in order to make decisions about his care. You can also treat your patients as you would like to be treated. How much information would you want to be given in the same situation?

Disclosing an error to a patient

Telling a patient about a mistake reaches beyond telling the truth (see Chapter 3 for more on truth telling). When you tell a patient the truth, you show that you respect his autonomy. Even if news is bad, it is your duty as a provider to tell the patient the truth.

When an error is made, healthcare providers should

- First make sure that the patient is stabilized, and take action to prevent further injury or harm. Immediately eliminate the source of the error.

- Make sure that records, medications, and equipment are secured so they can be examined for the cause of the error. And report the event to management. Never tamper with the medical record.

- Tell the patient that an error has been made. Don't try to explain how or why the error happened until the situation has been investigated. Do not speculate.

✔ Take responsibility for the error. The patient trusts you, and you must assume responsibility for their care. In the event of a serious error, management should also accept responsibility for the event. Accepting responsibility does not mean you accept blame for the event, but that you are in control of the situation.

✔ Apologize for the mistake. Apologizing is crucial for beginning the healing process. The act of apologizing also expresses compassion and humanity. And apologies are part of telling the truth.

✔ Tell the patient what will be done to prevent this error in the future. This is an important part of the response that is sometimes overlooked. This step can help give a positive meaning to patient suffering.

✔ Analyze the error and investigate. Uncover the factors and issues that led to the error and develop changes to prevent that error in the future. Talk to your employer's medical-legal department or malpractice insurance carrier about the error. Document all evidence and results. However, never change prior documentation or destroy part of a medical record. That is illegal.

Sometimes patients will ask you to withhold some information from them. You must use your professional clinical judgment to decide if you abide by their wishes. If a patient has an incurable disease, he may not want to know all of the stages his body will go through before death.

And remember that the truth is often a relief to patients. They may have been struggling with symptoms for weeks or months before a diagnosis is made, or have even realized that an error was made. The truth can confirm their suspicions and reassure them that they were correct to suspect something was wrong.

Standing by a patient through a poor outcome

Discussing an error or poor outcome with a patient is the hardest thing to do. I remember a case early in my practice where I removed a small skin lesion from a patient's face. Unfortunately, he had more than the expected scarring at the site of excision due to a reaction to the suture material. He was very angry about the outcome. I did not want to take his phone calls and certainly didn't want to see him in the office again. In fact, I wanted to take a permanent vacation from my medical practice.

I did agree to see him and let him express his anger. It was hard to look at the ugly scar. I referred him to a plastic surgeon and continued to call him to check on his progress. I struggled with anxiety the next few times I excised skin lesions. I thought this patient would leave my practice, but he decided to stay with me and our relationship survived. He has become one of my most trusting and endearing patients. Although my reaction was to run away from a poor outcome, I realized the most important thing is to let a patient express their hurt and frustration, and never abandon them in their time of need.

Truth telling can also be cathartic to the providers who made the mistake. Other providers can give emotional support to someone who inadvertently harmed a patient, but only if they told that a mistake was made.

Balancing ethics with legal protection

All healthcare providers worry about malpractice lawsuits, but ethical principles demand that you do the right thing. Taking responsibility for mistakes is the right thing to do. It may be a hokey, old-fashioned statement, but it's true: honesty is the best policy. Some research has shown that one reason that patients contact an attorney is because they feel they have been lied to. In fact, lawsuits can be the only way a patient may feel they can get the truth about what happened to them. Studies have shown that when healthcare providers are honest with their patients, those patients are less likely to sue.

Just because you as a provider make an error doesn't mean that you have committed medical malpractice. Malpractice occurs when a provider commits an error (either by act or omission) that deviates from accepted standards of medical practice due to negligence. This act must then be shown to cause significant injury or death to the patient. In a medical malpractice case, the plaintiff or patient must show that the provider failed to conform to the accepted standard of care (negligence and that this was the cause of substantial damages, either physical or emotional. Without damages, there is no basis for a claim. Likewise, damages without negligence are no basis for a claim. It's interesting to note that 60 percent of liability claims against doctors are dropped, withdrawn, or dismissed without payment.

Some malpractice policies actually have *cooperation clauses* that state an insured healthcare provider shouldn't admit any liability. Arguments against this stance are

- ✔ This clause might be unenforceable because the doctor is telling the truth.
- ✔ Hiding a mistake might end up costing the insurance company more than revealing the error would.
- ✔ The U.S. Supreme Court has ruled that insurers cannot force doctors to violate their moral obligation under the Medical Code of Ethics.
- ✔ There is a negative correlation between concealing mistakes and containing malpractice costs.
- ✔ When insurance companies try to deny coverage when a doctor was following his ethical code of conduct, they have lost in court.

Malpractice cases are not just hard on the patient. They can be devastating for the physician as well. For doctors, a malpractice lawsuit is a very personal attack on their sense of integrity and ability, and often leads to significant guilt and self-doubt. There are resources available to help doctors experiencing litigation, usually through larger healthcare organizations and online.

Telling a higher-up that you've made an error

When an error has been made and you must tell a supervisor or manager, there's a logical progression of steps to take. Most clinics and hospitals have action plans that detail what kinds of errors should be reported and the chain of command. Don't try to hide or cover up the error because those actions can make the situation worse. When you tell a supervisor about an error:

✔ Tell her as soon as possible. It's better to own up to the mistake yourself rather than wait and have her learn about it from someone else.

✔ Ask to speak to her in private and talk about the problem openly and honestly. Take responsibility for the error and be honest about what happened.

✔ Propose steps and actions to take that can alleviate the error.

✔ When the problem has been solved, make plans with your supervisor or manager the team can implement to ensure this mistake will not happen again.

When Colleagues Don't Disclose: Your Ethical Obligations

As a physician, you will mostly likely come across a number of situations where you become aware of an error committed by one of your partners. It is also likely that one of your partners will become aware of an error committed by you. It is important that a climate exists within your practice group where these errors can be addressed. Partners should be able to discuss mistakes with each other and a system for dealing with errors should be in place.

You will also find that hospitals and healthcare organizations have anonymous ways of reporting and addressing errors. Patient safety is of utmost importance. If an error is not addressed, it may be repeated. This can have an adverse effect on patient care. Although making mistakes is forgivable, not taking some type of action to prevent a repeat of the mistake is not.

The ethical principles that apply here are nonmaleficence and beneficence. Where the patient is involved, truthfulness and justice can be positive for both the patient and the provider.

We're trained from a very young age to dislike tattletales. Now that we're grown up, we've learned that *whistleblowers* (the grownup word for tattletale) can be an important resource that can actually help improve medicine. There's also a difference in intent. Most children who tattle do so to get another child in trouble. Whistleblowers, on the other hand, have the patient's and the public's best interest in mind.

When confronting a colleague about a situation, be gentle and do this in private. Never disparage another physician or provider in front of the patient. This is inappropriate and creates a loss of trust by the patient. In fact, this type of action can set up another provider for a malpractice lawsuit.

Encourage the provider to address the error directly with the patient. However, if you meet resistance, you may need to report the provider to the supervising doctor or medical committee. This person or entity can review a case and talk to a physician about inappropriate care.

Most doctors are perfectionists; that's why many of them got into the business in the first place. But nobody is perfect. Everyone has made a mistake, and has a visceral memory of the fear and shame that accompanies mistakes, so it's natural to think about looking the other way. We encourage you to do the right thing and talk to your colleague when you're aware of an error he has made.

You have *dual loyalty* to your patients and to your colleagues. To be a respected member of the healthcare community, use compassion and confidentiality, and keep truth in your pocket as your ultimate defense.

Healthcare Provider Impairment

Like all people, healthcare providers can become impaired in different ways. They may have a condition that interferes with their ability to practice medicine. This includes physical and mental problems, as well as substance abuse. Or they may actually be incompetent.

There are several ways a provider can become incompetent. Examples of physical and mental problems include:

- A progressive neurological disease such as Parkinson's disease or multiple sclerosis
- Progressive dementia
- Loss of vision or hearing
- Mental impairment
- Profound depression or anxiety
- Untreated bipolar disorder
- A problem with addiction, such as a sexual addiction
- Substance abuse, most commonly alcoholism or the abuse of prescription drugs

The case of provider impairment

Dr. Thomas was a new emergency room physician at a small hospital. He started seeing a local doctor, Dr. Jones, who prescribed Vicodin (a narcotic) for Dr. Thomas' back pain.

Soon, Dr. Thomas started showing up late for his shifts at the hospital. His patients noticed he seemed a bit groggy at times. When he completely missed one of his shifts, his supervising doctor looked into his past and found that Dr. Thomas had been disciplined by the state board of medical practice a few years ago for abuse of prescription narcotics. Further investigation revealed he was forging prescriptions from Dr. Jones to get larger amounts of Vicodin. Dr. Thomas was confronted by the supervising doctor and admitted to the problem. With the help of the board of medical practice, his license was suspended until he completed treatment. He had to submit to random drug testing and outpatient treatment through Narcotics Anonymous to be able to return to work.

The AMA says an impaired provider is "unable to practice medicine with reasonable skill and safety to patients because of physical or mental illness, including deterioration through the aging process or loss of motor skill, or excessive use or abuse of drugs including alcohol." An impaired provider can easily harm a patient, violating the principles of nonmaleficence and beneficence. And because of the power and respect granted to providers, justice demands that they approach their practice with respect and honor.

In this section we look at the warning signs of impairment, when you should intervene in another provider's case, and how to handle facing a medical ethics board.

Knowing the warning signs of impairment

A study in the Annals of Internal Medicine concluded that at least 30 percent of all doctors will experience periods of impairment, which can include alcohol or drug abuse or mental health issues. There are both subtle and clear signs and situations that indicate that a provider may be impaired. They include

✔ Personal signs, including personality changes, poor hygiene, and signs of drug or alcohol abuse like slurred speech or use of mouthwash or fragrance.

✔ Changes in family life, including an increase in outbursts, changes in a child's behavior, divorce, or withdrawal from family or patients.

✔ Comments from friends and colleagues, remarking about embarrassing behavior, like suddenly becoming unpredictable, or sudden isolation.

✔ Comments from nurses and other staff. Nurses may be the first to notice a problem when a doctor becomes impaired.

✔ Changes in professional manner, including taking frequent breaks, decreased productivity, complaints about behavior problems from coworkers and patients, or a sudden change in work hours.

There are also clues that can appear before an impaired provider is hired. If letters of reference are vague or very brief, or if a job history is quite erratic, look closer before hiring.

Similar to the rest of the population, about 10 percent of healthcare providers can have a problem with drugs or alcohol. But prescription drug abuse is higher among providers simply because they have more access to these substances.

You need to use your best judgment to decide if a fellow provider is impaired. In some cases, just one sign, such as slurred speech or trouble walking, would be enough to intervene. In other situations, such as a pattern of unpredictable behavior, you may need to see a pattern over a period of days or weeks before deciding there's a problem. If you see any compromise in good patient care, or if a patient raises concerns, that's the time to intervene immediately before further harm is done.

Addressing a colleague's impairment

Doctors are an independent bunch. Judging a colleague is difficult, especially when that person may also be a friend. But being a friend means not just accepting that person, but helping when they need help. Providers have an actual duty, as opposed to a prima facie duty, to report impaired or incompetent colleagues. Actual duties are morally binding, whereas prima facie duties are guidelines for behavior.

If you feel that a provider poses a threat to patients and the public through his medical practice, you must act in some way. A study conducted by the American Association of Critical-Care Nurses found that that almost 90 percent of doctors and 50 percent of nurses observed a colleague showing poor judgment. More than 80 percent of doctors and 50 percent of nurses also had concerns about the competency of some of their co-workers. But less than 10 percent of those providers with concerns actually told their coworker about their concerns.

This poses a danger not only to patients but to the medical profession as a whole. That study in The Annals of Internal Medicine found that whereas almost 100 percent of surveyed doctors said that impaired providers should be reported, 45 percent of them knew of an impaired colleague but did not report him.

When you must speak up about an impaired colleague

- ✔ Talk to the colleague first. That person may very well own up to the situation and take responsibility. It may help if more than one colleague is present in this conversation to help stress the seriousness of your concern and your support.

- ✔ If talking directly to your colleague doesn't produce any results, tell someone else in the organization. Go to the direct supervisor of the colleague, not further up the chain.

- ✔ Follow up on the situation and try to make sure that something is being done to address the problem.

If nothing is being done about the colleague, you need to go further up the chain to a higher supervisor or report them directly to the state board of medical practice. And keep a private record of your actions and any response, so you have a written record of the situation as it develops. However, if the problem is substance abuse, it may be better to report the provider in addition to confronting them directly, especially if patient care is being compromised. Anyone addicted to a substance is usually in denial and may rebuff any attempt to intervene.

And some states have hotlines any provider can call, anonymously, to discuss a situation to see if it warrants further investigation. Unless the situation is critical and deemed an emergency, a report usually isn't acted upon until some corroboration is obtained.

Sometimes a provider wants to self-report. This should be encouraged and the person should not face sanctions for being honest and addressing problems.

Testifying before a medical board

All states have licensing and disciplines boards. These organizations act to protect the public and to ensure that healthcare providers meet high professional standards. They can order remedial programs to help impaired providers. And most states have Medical Practice Act laws that give anyone who makes a report about an impaired colleague immunity from liability.

If you report an impaired colleague and the case gets to a medical board, you may be required to testify about what you've witnessed and how you made your report. Documentation, as we discussed in a previous section, is critical to the case. Presenting the facts as you have observed them, with supporting documents or evidence, is the best way to approach this situation.

A board can take several steps to help an impaired provider. It's important to remember that this process stays confidential until a board takes some type of final action. The board will hear all of the facts of the case, then begin an investigation. Subpoenas may be issued, and many colleagues will be interviewed. A medical board can

- ✔ Reprimand or suspend a provider.
- ✔ Revoke a medical license.
- ✔ Order mandatory participation in an education program, random drug or alcohol screening, counseling, or treatment.

Most medical boards use the laws in their state along with the AMA Code of Medical Ethics as their guide and standard.

How Reporting Errors Helps Medicine as a Whole

No one likes to admit they have made a mistake. In some occupations, making a mistake can mean just giving someone the wrong sandwich. But in medicine, mistakes can be lethal. Reporting errors helps improve the practice of medicine. From an ethical standpoint, reporting errors leads to changes in systems, which then prevents errors from occurring. This is best for both providers and patients, leading to both nonmaleficence and beneficence.

In 1999, the Institute of Medicine released its report "To Err is Human." That report found that most medical errors are a result of problems in the medical system, not incompetent doctors. Many medical systems can be modified to anticipate errors and stop them before someone gets hurt.

In this section, we look at how reporting medical errors makes the practice of medicine a better profession. Fixing errors doesn't have to be an arduous process that ruins careers.

Creating a no-blame system for reporting errors

One way to improve the system of reporting errors is to create a *no-blame status* for errors. Many hospitals and clinics have a shame-and-blame system that creates fear and trepidation among the staff. Because most errors result from a failure somewhere in the system, blaming a specific person or persons for a mistake is counterproductive.

When healthcare providers are not ridiculed for mistakes, reporting rates increase and the system improves. There are several ways to create a more proactive system:

- ✔ Make sure that protocols and procedures are constantly evaluated to identify weak points in the system.

- ✔ Hospital leaders should create a system that encourages error reporting and takes steps to avoid repeated errors. Be proactive about the design of high-risk procedures and activities.

- ✔ Make sure the emphasis is on guiding and improving, not shaming and blaming.

Understanding how to reduce errors

The Institute of Medicine recommends that hospitals and clinics use two kinds of error-reporting systems: errors that cause no harm would be reported voluntarily, and reports on errors that cause death or permanent serious injury would be mandatory.

Because minor errors can lead to bigger mistakes, it's important that they be reported. Most hospitals and clinics have error reports which are to be filed even for simple errors, such as giving a patient the wrong, but harmless, dose of medication. Then administrators and providers can identify weaknesses in the overall system and start measures to improve things.

A proactive approach is important. Simply reacting to errors and mistakes means you're playing catch-up and will never get ahead of the curve. There should be

- ✔ Uniform standards for education about preventing and reporting errors

- ✔ Good communication, including shared information

- ✔ Emphasis on individual accountability and responsibility

- ✔ Safety for providers when reporting errors

- ✔ Database programs that run spot checks on prescriptions and diagnoses

Always involve the patient in his or her care. The patient is his own best advocate and can be a great help in identifying and thereby preventing medical errors. When prescribing medicine, tell patients to read their prescriptions. Have them repeat advice back to you. Remind them to ask the pharmacist if the medication they pick up is the same as the one you prescribed. And always ask if they have questions about their treatment or care. This can reveal errors in your treatment plan. Finally, give patients easy ways to provide feedback and report errors that have occurred, such as comment cards in the lobby and easy access to the appropriate administrators.

Part II

A Patient's Right to Request, Receive, and Refuse Care

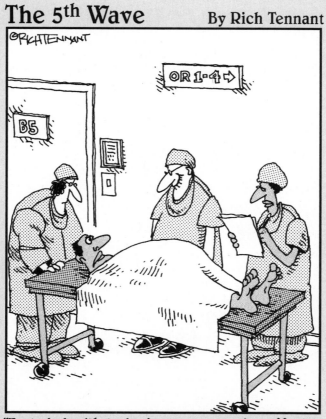

The 5th Wave — By Rich Tennant

"Included with today's surgery, we're offering a manicure, pedicure, haircut, and ear wax flush for just $49.95."

In this part . . .

Respecting patient autonomy, no matter what the outcome, can be difficult for many providers, but it's necessary to medical ethics. When can patients refuse care? And how much care can patients demand? How do we allocate scarce medical resources in a just and fair manner? In this part, we also examine how cultural and religious beliefs affect care. And what about the rights of minor children? What should a provider do when parental rights and responsibilities conflict with what their children want?

Chapter 6

The Ethical Challenges in Distributing Basic Healthcare

. . . .

In This Chapter

▶ Looking at the ethics of distributing healthcare

▶ Decoding the ethics of healthcare rationing

▶ Looking at healthcare in the United States

▶ Understanding pros and cons of universal healthcare

. . . .

*H*ealthcare is an inflammatory issue in America. The fourth principle in medical ethics, justice, more specifically distributive justice, comes into play as we consider the fairest ways to distribute healthcare as a limited resource. Justice demands all citizens receive the *decent minimum*, or basic care that ensures they have the best chance at living a normal life. The goal is to limit total suffering (satisfy nonmaleficence), maximize outcomes (satisfy beneficence), fairly allocate resources (satisfy justice), while allowing citizens the healthcare treatments they want and need (satisfy autonomy).

In this chapter, we look at some of the basic ethical concepts and questions about healthcare distribution. We explore balancing the costs and distribution of healthcare with each person's desire for good health. *Egalitarian ethics,* or the fair and equal distribution of goods and services, and *utilitarian ethics,* or the effort to maximize positive outcomes, are the important standards in this debate. *Rationing,* or placing limits on the types and amounts of medical tests and treatments, is examined next. We look at rationing based on different factors, such as cost, time, access to service, severity of illness, and citizenship. How do we ensure that basic care is offered to all without reducing the benefits well-off groups currently enjoy?

Finally, we look at the current, proposed, and future distribution of healthcare in the United States and the ethical implications of each method. We examine universal healthcare in more detail and take a brief look at healthcare in other countries.

Ethics of Healthcare Distribution

We first look at a few basic ethical questions and principles that are unique to the area of healthcare distribution. First, is healthcare a right? And how should healthcare resources be ethically distributed? We look at the principle of distributive justice and apply philosopher John Rawls' theory of justice to help us answer these questions. We then explore rationing with these principles in mind.

Is healthcare a right? And what is a human right? Human rights are protections and benefits possessed by all human beings. In 1948, modern human rights were defined by the United Nations in the Universal Declaration of Human Rights as "societal preconditions for physical, mental, and social well-being." Based on this definition, it seems that healthcare should be a right. Healthcare upholds all four principles of medical ethics by preventing harm (nonmaleficence), helps people (beneficence), and lets people act freely when they are in good health (autonomy). And if healthcare is a right, it should be available equally to all people to satisfy the principle of justice.

But some people feel that health care is a privilege rather than a right. One argument on this side states that there is no set definition of basic healthcare like there is for other human rights. The definition of basic healthcare changes as technology advances. In the 1960s, kidney dialysis was considered extraordinary care, but now it's ordinary care. And if the definition of basic healthcare is always changing, how do we decide how much healthcare is a human right? This discussion touches on a couple of the many aspects of this difficult ethical debate.

So how should healthcare be ethically distributed? The concept of *distributive justice* is helpful. Distributive justice refers to what society owes individuals in proportion to

- ✔ That individual's needs and responsibilities
- ✔ Resources available in society
- ✔ Society's responsibilities to the common good

Egalitarian ethics argue for fair and equal distribution of limited resources. And utilitarian ethics argue for the best outcomes for the most people. We try to maximize patient health (beneficence) while distributing healthcare to the most people (justice). This is the dilemma.

John Rawls was an American philosopher who developed the theory of *justice as fairness* that applies to healthcare distribution. He said that human beings are rational and reasonable, so they can decide ways to fairly distribute limited resources. Rawls argues that to set up the fairest system, we should decide the rules of society and distribution of assets from behind a *veil of ignorance*. This means that no one who is deciding societal rules will know what place in society they will occupy. Because no one knows if they will be rich or poor, black or white, man or woman, they will strive to make society as fair as possible.

When rules are set, Rawls moves on to the *difference principle*. This principle argues that people with similar skills should have equal chances to a good life, and that any inequalities in society should be set up to help those who are less fortunate.

If we use Rawls' arguments, and put ourselves in the position of someone who is underserved in society, we should strive to make the distribution of healthcare as equal as possible to satisfy the principles of medical ethics.

Exploring Healthcare Rationing

Healthcare must be and is rationed, just like every other good and service in the world. Very few people around the world receive every treatment they need or want. Most people agree that it's not moral or ethical to deny healthcare treatments based on income. But we need some type of system to distribute healthcare. Which system is the most fair?

The goal of rationing combines the utilitarian benefit of maximizing outcomes for the greatest number of people with the egalitarian benefit of ensuring that the care of better-off groups is maintained. In other words, it ensures that as more people receive basic healthcare, those who currently enjoy good care will not lose those benefits.

In the United States, privately funded healthcare is rationed by cost. If you can afford it, you can receive as much care as you want, including experimental treatments and private nursing care. If you can't afford it, you may not receive primary or preventative healthcare. In countries with universal healthcare, that is, a health care system (often government administered) that provides for universal coverage for all members of that society, treatments and care are rationed by longer wait times and limits on the use of expensive treatments, especially for the terminally ill, and experimental care.

In the following sections, we examine the reality of healthcare rationing and the medical ethics principle of justice as it appears under the different methods of rationing. We also look at how countries place a monetary value on life, and how countries handle the healthcare needs of immigrants and noncitizens.

How services are rationed

Every single service in the world is rationed in some way. Rationing takes place in many ways, depending on the service being rationed, how valuable it is, and how critical the service is to a person's life. Healthcare is rationed by the following methods:

- ✔ Cost
- ✔ Time
- ✔ Personnel/access to services/scarcity of drugs
- ✔ Severity of illness and likelihood of recovery
- ✔ Citizenship
- ✔ Triage during emergencies/pandemics

The free market naturally results in many of these methods of rationing. When governments get involved in healthcare, they force rationing on the healthcare system based on need and create objective systems that decide how much a life is worth and how care should be distributed. Americans may hate the thought of rationing healthcare in such a calculated manner, but we also need to face reality. Rationing in some form other than cost is an ethical mandate for the sake of achieving justice in access to healthcare.

The ethics of rationing

In an ideal world, every patient would receive the care and treatment they need to live a healthy life. But this world is far from ideal. So we need to work with what we have and figure out a way to help all citizens reach the decent minimum of health, while letting patients with means get the best healthcare available.

Every method of rationing satisfies ethical principles, especially for certain populations. Most forms of rationing try to satisfy the principle of justice, but each method of rationing is unjust in certain ways.

Rationing by cost

Healthcare is rationed in the United States by cost. This type of rationing leads to inequality in healthcare access between those who have money or insurance and those who don't. For the well-off, their autonomy is optimized because they can choose their doctors and the treatments they want and need without limitation. Because many people must forego care, there are more doctors available to treat patients, more operating rooms open for surgery, and more appointment slots open in doctor's clinics.

But rationing by cost forces many people to forgo care altogether. This has a very negative impact on their health, which violates the principles of benefi-cence and nonmaleficence. Because health insurance is most often tied to employment in the United States, losing a job means not only losing an income, but access to healthcare. If you can't afford healthcare, your choices are very limited. For these "have not" patients, financial concerns severely limits their autonomy, or ability to make choices about their healthcare. This is clearly unjust.

Every person who goes to an emergency room in the United States will receive treatment. But the difference between patients who have insurance and those who don't is revealed in the uninsured patient's health.

According to studies from Harvard University, Harvard Medical school researchers, and the Henry J. Kaiser Family Foundation, uninsured patients who are denied access to healthcare because of cost rationing are

- ✔ Twice as likely to die in the emergency room
- ✔ More likely to die from traumatic injuries and accidents
- ✔ More likely to die younger
- ✔ Twice as likely to visit emergency rooms for primary care

Surveys of adults with chronic illnesses show that many Americans give up recommended treatments and drugs because of cost, violating the principle of autonomy. For more about patient autonomy, see Chapter 3. More than 50 percent of Americans state they don't fill prescriptions, don't visit the doctor, and refuse care because of cost. In countries with universal healthcare, such as Britain and Canada, only about 7 to 10 percent of patients put off recom-mended treatment because of cost.

In the United States healthcare system where we ration by cost, bankrupt-cies are rampant. According to the *American Journal of Medicine*, 62 percent of all bankruptcies in the United States in 2004 were caused by medical bills. Three-quarters of those people were middle-class and well-educated and had private health insurance.

Going back to John Rawls' arguments about justice as fairness, and that people with similar skills should have equal access to a good life, we can see that rationing by cost is unjust.

Rationing by time

In many countries with universal healthcare, care is rationed by time because there are more people to receive care and proportionally fewer providers. In Canada, for instance, there are longer wait times for hip transplants because more people can afford that particular treatment, and because it is not a life-threatening illness, that surgery has a lower priority in the overall system. In any society, the law of supply and demand rules up to a point. If there are more people who want or need a service, wait times for that particular service increase. It makes sense that wait times for care will increase when there are more patients in the system.

Countries with universal healthcare try to solve this problem by ranking illness or injury in order of severity. Someone with a life-threatening illness who has only a few weeks or months to live will get care before someone who needs a treatment for an illness that, although still important, will not take their life any time soon. This helps balance the scales and satisfies the principles of beneficence and nonmaleficence to a higher degree.

So is it ethical to ration healthcare by time? Well, more, if not all, people have access to healthcare, satisfying the principle of justice. Patient autonomy is reduced somewhat because patients can't have everything they want exactly when they want it. If you are disadvantaged or poor, universal healthcare reduces nonmaleficence. Those who are seriously ill aren't affected by longer wait times, but those waiting for elective procedures may experience some harm while waiting for treatment.

Rationing by personnel/access to services/scarcity of drugs

With more patients in the system, there will probably, at least at first, be rationing because of the number of medical personnel available to treat patients. There is a shortage of primary care doctors in the United States. If 45 million Americans who are currently without healthcare enter the system, there will be rationing based on provider shortage, which will lead to rationing by time. This may also lead to rationing by cost because certain providers may only accept self-pay patients or those with favorable insurance.

How can we address this shortage of providers? We can put a priority on recruiting more providers and stressing job stability, good income, and opportunities for advancement in the healthcare field. This is a job for government and current providers. Becoming a mentor to future providers is something that you can do, and will help satisfy the ethical principle of justice and may help ease strain on the healthcare system in the future.

What about scarcity of drugs or treatments? The United States has already faced that issue in the past few years with the shortage of flu vaccines. We need to have better systems in place to anticipate shortages and increase production before medications become scarce. Companies can be mandated to increase production of needed drugs or medical products, and the government is already in the business of paying researchers to develop and distribute drugs such as seasonal flu vaccines.

The hurry-up-and-wait aspect of universal healthcare

A Commonwealth Fund report compared U.S. healthcare wait times versus wait times in countries with universal healthcare.

✔ Canada reported 30 percent of patients waited six or more days for a general doctor's appointment in 2007, compared to 20 percent in Germany and the United States, and 12 percent in the United Kingdom.

✔ In the United Kingdom, 41 percent of patients waited four months or longer for elective surgery, compared to 8 percent in the United States.

✔ The United Kingdom reports that 60 percent of patients wait more than four weeks to see a specialist, while in the United States only 23 percent wait that long.

✔ In Canada, self-reported wait times were four weeks for a specialist visit and for non-emergency surgery.

✔ A study by Merritt Hawkins found that wait times in the United States are increasing. The average wait time across all practices was 20.5 days, and wait times increased by 8.6 days from 2004 to 2009.

These delays in receiving care do cause premature death. In 2008, 103 British patients died waiting for a liver transplant. Twelve patients died in 2007 at one Canadian center while waiting for bariatric surgery, where wait times are more than five years.

Because wait times seem to be a particular point of contention in this debate, we must distinguish between wait times for chronic conditions and wait times for acute conditions. Countries with universal healthcare do give priority to emergency situations such as medical care for a gunshot wound, surgery for cancer, or treatment for acute heart disease.

Wait times for chronic conditions such as hip replacement are longer in countries with universal healthcare, whereas wait times for acute disease treatments are comparable with wait times in the United States. Studies have shown there is little clinical difference in outcome when patients have to wait for nonemergency surgery.

Rationing by severity of illness/likelihood of recovery

In countries with universal healthcare, care is rationed not just by time, but also based on how serious an illness is, the likelihood of recovery, and the number of years a patient can expect to live after recovery. Ethicists believe that this method of rationing care satisfies the principle of egalitarian justice. Although some might think it distasteful to put numbers on the value of life, a system such as this can help ration healthcare in an ethical way.

In countries with universal healthcare, patients who are seriously or acutely ill don't have to wait for care. There are ways to determine who needs and deserves healthcare first. Statisticians have developed tools to help apply limited healthcare resources. *Quality-Adjusted Life-Year*, or QALY, is a method used to decide how much to spend extending life by one year. This system is used in Britain, France, and Canada. The EQ-5D is another tool then used to score the ability to function. The tool uses five dimensions: mobility, pain, self-care, depression, and usual activities of life.

This type of rationing addresses another of the main inequities that occur when rationing by cost: a disproportionate amount of healthcare dollars are spent on the elderly in the last year of life. More than 40 percent of Medicare dollars are spent on end-of-life care in the last two months of life. When compared to children, the average per capita healthcare spending for seniors is more than five times greater. This injustice can be addressed by using QALY numbers to look at the quality of life and likelihood of recovery.

When using QALY, every year the patient is in perfect health is assigned the value of 1.0. If a patient has some problems walking or dressing himself, along with moderate pain or discomfort, his life may have a valuation of 0.5. Health states that confine a patient to bed or cause extreme pain or discomfort may reduce that number down to a value below 0.0.

These values are determined with studies and questionnaires. Respondents are asked to choose between risky medical treatments and the resulting benefit and to weigh different states of health with quality of life. Respondents are also asked to choose between living with various diseases for long periods of time versus a shorter lifespan lived in perfect health. As can happen when conducting a questionnaire, the responses can change depending on how the question is asked.

QALY numbers change over time because this is an ongoing practice. Doctors and researchers consider new treatments and drugs, and advocates protest some decisions. This method is subjective, which raises questions about its efficacy and fairness. And QALY numbers vary from country to country.

The identifiable victim effect and rule of rescue

The *identifiable victim effect* creates a bias in how citizens respond to QALY questionnaires. Stories about problems in rationed care in countries with universal healthcare are well known. It's easy to be concerned about a story of a patient dying of kidney cancer who is denied an experimental drug that may extend his life. We can all understand that frustration and anger and can all see ourselves in that position. The *rule of rescue* also plays a part in this effect. People will demand care when stories of patients denied care are publicized.

But when the question is rephrased, the responses are different. When people are asked if $500,000 should be spent on a dying person to extend their life by one or two months, many think that is an unreasonable cost for an uncertain benefit. Because most people aren't in that particular position, it's easier to separate from the emotion behind the decision. We don't identify as strongly with that patient, so the decision is easier to make. And general questions such as "Should we spend $200,000 on experimental treatment to save one life or on vaccinations to save 1,000 lives?" generate different responses.

Three ethics principles are relevant to these discussions:

- ✔ Do we prioritize treatments that maximize total number of quality life-years, satisfying the principles of justice and nonmaleficence?

- ✔ Do we concentrate on procedures that treat the most people with the best outcome, satisfying the principle of egalitarian justice?

- ✔ Or do we focus on procedures that significantly extend the quality and length of life, satisfying the principles of utilitarian justice and beneficence?

Cost-utility analysis, or the method of estimating the beneficence of medical care products compared to the cost of that care, is applied to each situation, and guidelines for payments of treatment are set. Ensuring medical care for the underserved must be balanced with promoting best treatment outcomes and optimizing treatment for those who can afford maximum care.

For an example, let's look at the United Kingdom. In Britain, the National Health Service (NHS) issues guidelines on which drugs should and should not be used for certain illnesses. If a person is suffering from terminal cancer, the organization may recommend that expensive drugs that extend length or quality of life by months instead of years shouldn't be offered.

Rationing by citizenship

The United States also rations healthcare by citizenship. In fact, laws have been passed that forbid illegal immigrants from receiving healthcare through Medicare and Medicaid. But the drain on emergency services and medical healthcare dollars posed by illegal immigrants has been overstated. Studies show that illegal immigrants visit the doctor far less than native-born patients, and they tend to be younger and healthier.

The Employee Benefit Research Institute estimates that the share of the health-care system for illegal immigrants is about 2 percent. Only a small portion of that is paid for by public dollars. A Rand Corporation study found that $1 billion in total government funds is spent on illegal immigrant healthcare. This amount is about 1 percent of the government spending for non-elderly adult citizens and adds about $11 to the average American's income tax bill.

The Illegal Immigration Reform and Immigrant Responsibility Act was passed in 1996. It makes all immigrants ineligible for Medicaid, which forces patients into the emergency medical system. The exception is pregnancy care, which is still covered. In 2005, the United States government began paying for emergency care to illegal immigrants in response to requests from Congress members in border states. This helped reduce the strain on public hospitals and emergency room budgets.

Illegal immigrants, because of their fear of deportation, tend to avoid doctor's visits until the situation becomes critical. We aren't going to delve into the political or ethical debate about the status of illegal immigrants. Instead, we are going to focus on how this type of rationing affects the health of immigrants, and how you as a provider can optimize beneficence and justice for these patients.

Rationing according to citizenship obviously violates the principle of nonmaleficence. Even though it is costly and risky, these patients still seek medical care when needed. Medical ethics of beneficence, autonomy, and confidentiality play a part when treating illegal immigrants.

If you find yourself treating an illegal immigrant, you should

- ✔ Treat all patients with compassion and cultural sensitivity. Use an interpreter when needed. For more information, see Chapter 7.

- ✔ Act quickly to treat and stabilize patients who present in critical condition, according to emergency care protocols.

- ✔ Consider costs for the uninsured patient when making non-emergency healthcare decisions and prescribing medication.

- ✔ Consider confidentiality when treating illegal immigrants. A provider is not forced to ask about immigration status.

- ✔ Violate confidentiality only if serious and identifiable risk to the public may occur by withholding medical information.

The obvious problems of rationing by citizenship become apparent in a pandemic. If we are going to refuse healthcare to those without citizenship, what happens if a noncitizen catches the H1N1 virus and doesn't receive any treatment? Viruses don't discriminate based on the status of citizenship or pocketbook and can be spread to all of us. If we refuse medical care to certain people on this basis, we risk harming everyone else who does get care. And is that the kind of society we want to be?

Rationing in case of emergencies

A pandemic or large-scale national disaster is a unique situation when rationing healthcare. In those situations, a *triage* system, or the process of prioritizing treatment based on needed personnel and those patients who are most critically ill, is put into place. Triage was developed to deal with injuries and death on the battlefield. In a public health emergency, you may become patient and provider.

In an emergency, the public good is more important than individual principles. Healthcare providers and emergency personnel need to be treated quickly so they can continue to help the rest of the population. The order of care demanded by the public good is:

✔ Persons who perform rescue functions, such as firefighters, policemen, and military personnel, receive treatment first so they can then return to work and protect the public. Public health practitioners and safety officials also receive priority treatment so they can continue to care for the sick and injured.

✔ The seriously injured or ill who need immediate care to survive are second in line in the triage system.

✔ The *walking wounded* receive care next. These are people who are ill or injured, but who will survive even if medical care is delayed.

✔ And finally, the hopelessly wounded or ill are assessed and given palliative care to satisfy the principles of nonmaleficence and justice.

Contagious diseases can lead to different strategies for trying to preserve the health of the public. An individual with a contagious disease may be confined to a restricted area away from the general public; this is called a *quarantine.* Quarantines pit confidentiality and civil liberty against the public good. Diseases that affect the public health must be addressed quickly and truthfully. If a public health emergency exists because of disease outbreak, confidentiality is waived. A great return on public health and safety must exist to ask patients to give up liberty in a quarantine. Public health officials make decisions about emergencies and quarantines based on several factors, including how contagious the disease is, how quickly it can be diagnosed, and how treatable it is. For example, in the 1940s, patients with tuberculosis were often confined in sanatoriums to get treatment and prevent the spread of the disease. And in the 1990s, 200 patients in New York City were detained to prevent the spread of drug-resistant tuberculosis.

The risk of quarantine and resulting stigmatization can lead patients to avoid care even when they are very sick. Quarantines must be handled fairly and equitably in order to avoid violating the principles of autonomy and nonmaleficence, and be put in place only in dire emergencies.

Vaccine rationing has been a hot topic, with the H1N1 flu outbreak. In an emergency situation, it takes at least six months to develop an effective vaccine for a new virus or bacteria. How should a limited supply of vaccine be ethically distributed? If a pandemic develops, the National Institute of Health and the Advisory Committee on Immunization Practices has recommended the *investment refinement of lifecycle principles including public order* (IRPOP). In this approach, vaccines will be provided to front-line and medical responders first, in addition to the military, then to 13- to 40-year-olds, including healthy members, and finally the very young and the elderly.

In the case of each illness, however, the ethics of vaccine distribution will be based on the specific disease and early statistics in the outbreak. For example, elderly are vaccinated first for seasonal flu because they are most likely to die from this infection. But in the case of H1N1 influenza, the disease was more lethal for children and young adults, so they were preferentially vaccinated. Fortunately, a true pandemic has not occurred recently, but one will likely occur again in the future, and we need to resolve some of the difficult ethical issues of vaccine rationing before the outbreak occurs.

Looking at Healthcare in the United States

Almost every human being will, at some point, develop an illness that requires treatment. No diet or lifestyle guarantees perfect health throughout life. A 7-year-old child can have a chronic disabling health condition, whereas a 100-year-old man can suddenly die from a heart attack with few previous health problems. These different needs underscore the fact that distributing healthcare fairly over a diverse population is difficult.

Healthcare costs are increasing five times faster than the rate of inflation in the United States. That pace is unsustainable. Most countries have decided to control healthcare costs and issue guidelines for the healthiest population at a reasonable cost. Universal healthcare is the most common form of control.

In this section, we examine the current system and the ethical issues and challenges it presents. We also look at the Patient Protection and Affordable Care Act (PPACA) that was signed into law in the United States in March 2010, and what it does and doesn't do to improve healthcare access. And we look at future options for healthcare reform and examine what universal healthcare really is.

The case of Rebecca: Using U.S. healthcare

Rebecca was a 46-year-old single mother of two teenagers. She worked as a nanny for a neighbor and had no health insurance. She had hypertension and took an inexpensive drug once a day for this. She went to a local free clinic to obtain samples of this medication when it was available. One day she discovered a lump in her breast. After being seen at the free clinic, she was sent to the local hospital for mammogram and subsequent biopsy of the lump. Unfortunately, she had breast cancer. She knew the cost of the surgery and treatment would exceed $50,000, and she had no idea how she would pay for this. Her nanny job plus a small amount of alimony made it impossible for her to qualify for Medicaid. She underwent surgery, radiation, and chemotherapy and was declared cancer-free. Unfortunately, she had to sell her home to get enough money to pay her medical bills and then move her family into a small apartment, losing her main source of financial security.

The current system and its ethical challenges

If you can afford it, the United States offers some of the best healthcare in the world. Hospital care, surgeries, medications, and medical clinics are shining examples of excellent care that set the standard for medicine around the world. But the key statement is "if you can afford it." Healthcare is currently rationed by cost in this country, and the PPACA didn't solve that problem.

At this time, more than 45 million Americans have no health insurance because they can't afford it. And as many as 45,000 Americans die every year of treatable and preventable illnesses because they can't afford basic healthcare. Many more Americans are underinsured: that is, they can afford only bare-bones coverage that will not protect them financially in case of a catastrophic illness or injury. These facts violate the ethical principles of egalitarian and utilitarian justice, beneficence, and nonmaleficence.

The United States has several forms of universal healthcare at the current time. Medicaid, SCHIP, Medicare, and the Veterans Association provide care to many Americans. The government currently covers about 50 percent of our overall healthcare costs. These plans help satisfy the egalitarian and utilitarian principles of justice along with the principles of nonmaleficence and beneficence for the poor and disadvantaged, the elderly, children, and those who have served in the military.

✔ Medicaid is a means-tested program that covers children with family incomes up to 100 percent of the federal poverty level, pregnant women with family incomes up to 133 percent of the federal poverty level, those with disabilities, and long-term care of the elderly. No matter how poor they are, adults who don't have children in their household can't be covered by Medicaid. Different states have different Medicaid requirements.

✔ SCHIP, or the State Children's Health Insurance Program, covers children in low-income families that make too much money to qualify for Medicaid. Different states have different guidelines for applying for coverage and receiving payment.

✔ Medicare covers those aged 65 and over and disabled people under 65 who have received Social Security benefits for two years, satisfying the principle of justice. It pays about 80 percent of the cost of many treatments, surgeries, drugs, and procedures.

✔ The Indian Health Service (IHS) provides medical care to American Indians and Native Alaskan patients. This program originated from numerous treaties, laws, and court decisions.

✔ Veterans are covered with a portable medical benefits package offered by the Veterans Administration in hospitals and clinics around the country.

The clients of these programs are mostly happy with the system, although there are problems such as the Medicare prescription coverage *donut hole*, which is the medication coverage gap in Medicare Part D that has decreased seniors' use of prescription drugs. A Rand Corporation study in 2007 found that many seniors stopped taking drugs for chronic conditions such as high blood pressure and diabetes because of the plan's yearly spending limits. And there are issues with the VA plans as well, most notably poor building maintenance and upkeep in veteran's hospitals and facilities that are maintained by the Department of Defense.

Major reform of these programs will be needed as the population ages and as baby boomers retire. The pace of growth in Medicare and Medicaid payouts is increasing rapidly and funding to pay for these programs is decreasing. Medicare trustees warn that the fund is going to be broke by 2018.

The reformed system and potential ethical speed bumps

In 2010, sweeping healthcare reform was passed in the United States Congress for the first time in the country's history. While the Patient Protection and Affordable Care Act of 2010 (PPACA) was being debated, arguments both for and against it raged.

The PPACA does address some of the problems patients in this country currently face:

- Insurance coverage will be provided to 32 million more Americans by 2019.

- Subsidies to help patients pay for insurance will begin in 2014, when purchasing health insurance becomes mandatory.

- Insurance companies will be forced to reduce overhead, in the form of profit and salaries, from the current amount of 30 percent of each healthcare dollar to 15 percent of each healthcare dollar. This may help control the skyrocketing costs of premiums.

- Healthcare exchanges, which help individuals buy insurance plans from a collection of private companies, will be added in 2014. This is supposed to add competition among plans and reduce prices.

- Some reforms of the healthcare insurance industry will become law, such as prohibiting rescission (dropping patients who develop expensive illnesses), banning pre-existing condition limitations, and banning yearly and lifetime caps on coverage.

But many important factors that limit poorer American's access to healthcare were not addressed in the PPACA, including the following:

✔ The market still sets policy prices, which puts many insurance policies and healthcare treatments out of reach of the average American. There is no public option or single-payer plan in the new bill, which would have provided direct competition to private insurance companies.

✔ In 2019, despite subsidies and increased coverage, 32 million American will still be without insurance, according to studies released by the Kaiser Family Foundation.

✔ Medical costs will continue to rise unchecked because the free market still sets prices. The Congressional Budget Office estimates that in 2016, the average yearly health insurance bill for a family of four will be more than $20,000, not including out-of-pocket expenses and deductibles.

✔ Healthcare exchanges won't be available until 2014, and only the uninsured and some small businesses will be able to join in the first year. Plans are now being tested that offer very controlled choices of providers.

✔ Existing insurance plans are *grandfathered* in, meaning they don't have to comply with new regulations such as not allowing insurance companies to deny benefits based on pre-existing conditions.

✔ The reform doesn't address issues such as adult vision or dental care, which many Americans forgo because of cost.

✔ There is no definition of minimal benefits. Many insurance companies put restrictions in their policies that will limit available care for patients, such as higher copays for certain treatments and drugs, and extra charges for admission to top-rated hospitals.

It seems that healthcare reform will help the situation in this country a little bit, but there are still many obstacles, mostly financial, in place that keep many Americans out of the healthcare market. One organization, Remote Area Medical, which was originally designed to bring healthcare to third world countries, is now operating in the United States. In fact, their founder Stan Brock says that 64 percent of the organization's efforts take place in America. And free healthcare clinics, funded by private donations, have appeared around the country. The National Association of Free Clinics is a nonprofit group that sponsors more than 1,200 free clinics in the United States.

The providers who work for these organizations are following the principles of justice and beneficence. But the fact that people are turned away from these free clinics because there aren't enough providers to help them highlights the fact that serious reform is still needed in the United States and that PPACA did not address many of the problems millions of Americans face in their quest for healthcare.

The case of Timothy: Using Canadian healthcare

Timothy was a 72-year-old man with severe hip arthritis. His hip was so painful that it was difficult for him to walk. He needed an elective hip replacement and was placed on a five month waiting list for this procedure. Because he was so sedentary during this time, he developed a blood clot in his leg and had to go on blood thinner medication. Fortunately, this was caught before it went to his lungs, a potentially lethal condition. However, this clot delayed his surgery for another six months. Finally after ten months and a great deal of suffering, he was able to obtain the surgery which significantly improved his hip pain and function.

Examining universal healthcare

Universal healthcare is a system where a country's government manages the healthcare network in order to make basic care available to every citizen. Out of 33 developed countries in the world, 32 have universal healthcare. Which one doesn't? You guessed it — the United States.

Even after PPACA was passed and signed into law, the United States healthcare system still doesn't qualify as universal healthcare. For example, there is no public option, which is a low-cost program run by the government that everyone can join, that is in direct competition with private insurance companies. And there is little to no control over cost, which at this time is the way healthcare is rationed in the United States.

In fact, PPACA is more a health *insurance* reform act than a health *care* reform act. The tenets of the act have focused on limiting insurance company's practices that discriminate against patients in poor health. There will be a nationwide pool for high-risk individuals that begins in 2014, but, as with the other protections in the act, politicians can get rid of it in the intervening years.

Every country's healthcare system is a little different from the others. But in general, universal healthcare means:

✔ Lower out-of-pocket expenses for care for the individual.

✔ Almost all citizens have access to basic healthcare, through public or private health insurance options.

✔ Costs are paid through funding from taxes, copays, and fees, which satisfies the principle of distributive justice.

✔ Availability of publicly funded care is set by the government, which is determined by citizens voting. Citizens have a chance to be heard and vote out politicians who aren't serving their best interests.

> ✔ All citizens have the right to reach the *decent minimum* of care, and longevity increases, as measured by the World Health Organization in 2000.
>
> ✔ Guidelines help ensure uniformity of care.
>
> ✔ Longer wait times often exist for doctor visits and elective procedures.
>
> ✔ Some limits are set on certain expensive treatments requested by patients, such as transplants, experimental treatments, and end-of-life care.

In countries with universal healthcare, governments set up committees to decide how healthcare is distributed. Difficult but practical decisions, such as deciding how much to pay for an extra year of life, are made. Payments for procedures, surgeries, and drugs are discussed and set by committees.

So what about the ethics of universal healthcare? This type of system leads to rationing based on time and scarcity of providers rather than cost. This can reduce beneficence and autonomy for those who are wealthy and currently have access to all medical treatments. But if the system lets patients pay for more healthcare if they can afford that, that frees up the public system and satisfies beneficence and autonomy.

From the standpoint of justice, however, universal healthcare provides for more equitable distribution of resources for all people. If everyone is guaranteed some level of care, life expectancy can increase. If patients have access to primary care and basic health screening tools, diseases that can be treated and cured early, such as hypertension, won't develop into more expensive, life-threatening conditions such as a stroke or a heart attack. And that can help reduce the overall cost of medical care.

But does universal healthcare affect costs? This system does control government expenditures on healthcare, but may lead to higher taxes. The United States is currently spending 16 percent of its gross domestic product (GDP) on healthcare, and that number is expected to double by 2035, according to the congressional budget office. It remains to be seen if PPACA will slow that rate of growth. Countries with universal healthcare spend much less, such as 11 percent of GDP in France and 8 percent in the United Kingdom, yet achieve health outcomes that are better than those in the United States.

But will adopting a universal healthcare system in the United States place an undue burden on taxpayers? Taxes for healthcare are much higher in countries with universal healthcare than in the United States. The French system has been in the red since 1985 despite charging about 20 percent of a worker's salary. In the UK the national insurance tax adds 5 percent of income to the tax burden. And in Germany, workers pay 8 percent of their income into a sickness fund. Americans currently pay 7 to 12 percent of their income on healthcare through private insurance, copays, and out-of-pocket expenses.

Healthcare systems in other countries

Each country's healthcare system is different. Some rely on a combination of private and public insurance, and some are strictly single-payer. This means one group, usually the government, finances the system, but care is provided by private doctors. And the principles of justice and beneficence are satisfied because most, if not all, of these country's citizens have access to healthcare.

✔ **Canada:** Lifetime health insurance is provided to all residents, in plans monitored by each province. If a particular service is covered by the public plan, patients cannot buy private insurance for that service. Long wait times to see specialists and to have elective surgery are common. In 2004, the government agreed to an overhaul of the system. They set medically acceptable wait times for five areas of care: diagnostic tests, joint replacements, cancer, heart treatments, and cataract surgery.

✔ **France:** France also has a single-payer system, paid for with taxes and fees. Everyone must participate in the system. Sécurité Sociale is funded with a payroll tax and a general income tax. Patients pay for care and are reimbursed. Patients who suffer from chronic conditions do not pay for services. More than 90 percent of the population has supplemental insurance. Co-pays in France are 30 percent of the total cost of care, which controls overuse of the system. But employers feel they are paying too much into the system. And patients think there is a lot of bureaucracy in the system.

✔ **Germany:** Germany combines universal coverage with private insurance. Everyone is required to have insurance. The state sets overall standards, but the system is operated at the regional level. "Sickness funds" are paid for by region and employers. Insurance is portable and moves with the patient from job to job. Containment of cost is an issue in Germany. The country has recently set spending caps for drugs and hospital payments.

✔ **Sweden:** The healthcare system in Sweden covers the entire population, paying 98 percent of medical costs. It is funded by the government and paid for by taxes. Whereas the government establishes principles, counties and municipalities provide the care. Patients are guaranteed care by the government, with urgent cases receiving the highest priority. But the government rations what it deems "unnecessary benefits." Waiting times are longer, and the generous system can be abused. And the taxes to pay for care are high.

✔ **United Kingdom:** This country has a complete single-payer system using taxes and fees on employers and employees. Doctors work for and are paid by the government. Private care is an option. All procedures and drugs are paid for by the government. There is no connection between employment and health insurance. But quality of care and wait times are criticized. Care, especially expensive treatments for the terminally ill, is rationed.

It remains to be seen if the United States will make healthcare reform more robust. As providers and as citizens, it is now our responsibility to engage in continued reform by using ethical principles to work toward a system that results in the fair distribution of healthcare resources, while providing a decent minimum of care and maximizing outcomes for all citizens.

Chapter 7

When Spirituality and Cultural Beliefs Affect Care

In This Chapter

▶ Limiting or banning healthcare services based on religion

▶ Understanding cultural differences that affect healthcare services

▶ Working with the patient who refuses treatment

*E*thics and religion intersect in many instances. The idea of doing good, preventing harm, and promoting justice are principles in both disciplines, but sometimes religious beliefs can be in direct conflict with medicine. What are you supposed to do when that happens?

In this chapter, we look at religions that limit or ban healthcare services, and how you can still treat your patients and respect their autonomy while accommodating those beliefs. And we look at alternatives to care that religions may sanction. We also look at how someone's faith practices can be beneficial in their medical treatment and integrated into their care plan.

Cultural differences can also play a big part in patient treatment. It's helpful for healthcare workers to understand different cultural beliefs so they can give their patients the best care possible. Any cultural or religious beliefs that differ from the standard in your community should be respected and integrated into your patient's care.

Finally, what should you do when a patient refuses treatment based on religious or cultural beliefs? How can you tell if the patient really understands the risks of forgoing treatment and the seriousness of the situation? Sometimes you need to go beyond informed consent to communicate well.

This chapter focuses on adults who may refuse treatment for themselves. In Chapter 8, we discuss dealing with parents who refuse critical treatment for their children on the basis of religious and cultural beliefs.

Accommodating Religious Beliefs

Religion is a major source of comfort to many people, and doctors and all providers should respect those beliefs as part of respecting the patient. It's important that no matter what your patients believe or don't believe, you respect those choices as a function of autonomy.

In this section, we look at how you can accommodate all religious beliefs and treat your patients with care and compassion. We also look at alternatives to care that are still ethical and may be more acceptable to the patient when their faith is in conflict with best practice medicine.

Because there is such a wide range of religious beliefs in most countries, especially the United States, providers must be careful to not let their own religious beliefs compromise or interfere with patient care.

Religions that limit or ban medical care

Some religions literally forbid their members from seeking medical attention. In faith traditions that strongly object to medical intervention, in almost all cases, people believe that prayer and, in some cases, natural remedies will save a person's life. They generally oppose both diagnosis and treatment. Some of these faiths include

- Faith Assembly
- First Church of Christ, Scientist (Christian Science)
- Christ Church
- Followers of Christ
- Church of the First Born
- The Body

If a competent adult patient refuses treatment, you must honor their wishes, even if it means the patient may die. But situations with minor children are different. In the United States, courts have established that parents cannot refuse lifesaving treatment for their children for religious and cultural reasons. For more information on this issue, see Chapter 8.

Many religions do accept modern medicine but object to certain specific treatments on spiritual grounds. Here are a few examples:

- **Jehovah's Witnesses:** This denomination objects to blood transfusions.
- **Catholic Church:** The Church opposes abortion in most cases, and most forms of birth control. It also objects to some vehicles for assistance in

conception, including IVF and fertility treatments, cloning, and euthanasia. See Chapter 10 for more information.

✔ **Protestants:** Some evangelical branches of this church are strongly pro-life and object to abortion and some forms of birth control, especially the morning-after pill and the IUD, because they believe they are forms of abortion. Some branches also object to active euthanasia. Most mainline Protestant denominations do not hold these same objections.

✔ **Scientology:** This church, which is often confused with Christian Science, believes that 70 percent of all recognized diseases are psychosomatic. They believe that Dianetic therapy or auditing can cure most ills, although they are not opposed to taking prescription drugs or seeing a medical doctor for treatment. Some in this church require that a member seek permission from the church before seeing a doctor. They are opposed to psychiatry and psychiatric drugs.

✔ **Islam:** Strict interpretation of Islam limits female patients to seeing only female doctors. If a male doctor is the only physician available, the patient's husband must be present during the visit.

✔ **Orthodox Judaism:** This faith stresses extending life, which can conflict with palliative care for terminal patients. Some also object to artificial insemination and IVF. And this faith tradition sanctions abortion only when the mother's life is threatened by the pregnancy. Other sects of Judaism don't object to these interventions.

Not all members of all faiths strictly adhere to the teachings of the faith. Some religions teach certain precepts and then leave it to their individual members to decide how to interpret the teachings in their own lives. Others are much more strict, expecting obedience from members. Don't make assumptions about your patients, even if you know that they practice a certain faith.

Discussing religion and understanding objections

In most simple clinic visits, such as for strep throat or hypertension, faith practice doesn't enter into the encounter. However, with more complex situations, such as a woman carrying a baby with a severe congenital malformation or a man facing hospice care for terminal cancer, it becomes an important part of the person's experience.

When a patient brings up religious beliefs, encourage more discussion, especially as it relates to healthcare. You, too, can start a conversation about religious beliefs with your patients. Ask an open-ended question, such as "Are you comfortable telling me about any beliefs that may affect your medical care?" If the patient answers "yes," more questions about beliefs or restrictions on treatment can follow.

Handling your own objections ethically

Religion can play a part from the provider's perspective. If a treatment is legal and your patient wants it or needs it, but you believe it is immoral or against your beliefs, referring the patient to another provider is the ethical thing to do. We talk about providers refusing to provide certain types of medical care that are against their religious beliefs in Chapter 3.

You can certainly explain your objections to the procedure, drug, or treatment, but not informing a patient of a medical option because of your beliefs doesn't respect patient autonomy. The patient's right to complete medical care as understood by current medical practices is absolute. Reasonable delays are okay, but denying treatment is not.

I will often ask the following question: "Do you have any spiritual practices that are important to you during this time?" Often, the patient will give me some background on their faith practices. I then encourage them to tap into resources available in this area, such as visits from a rabbi, priest, or pastor, or other caring ministries available through their church congregation. It helps me better understand their approach when faced with difficult decisions. It is important to integrate all aspects of a patient's being — physical, mental, and spiritual — in the healing process.

It's also important to understand when an objection to a treatment, drug, or procedure is being rejected on religious grounds or on cultural grounds. In some situations, objections on cultural grounds are more easily accommodated than objections based on religious beliefs or edicts.

Chaplains and other religious representatives can play an important part in patient care. These leaders can be partners to your patients and to you. In many cases, clergy can help your patients as they navigate their way through the healthcare system. In fact, in some cases, clergy can help explain a situation to a patient who may be resistant to treatment.

Chaplains can answer questions about religious guidance, and help unravel what may be a complicated response to an illness. Sometimes a religious patient has misunderstood a guideline against a particular treatment, and clergy can help the patient understand the real meaning of the guidelines.

Offering alternatives to care

In many cases, it is possible to negotiate some type of care that will be acceptable to you, the provider, and to your patients. Some religions may make exceptions for some treatments, so it's important to have clergy from your patient's faith involved in discussion about their care.

Some high-risk patients who object to some types of care can be accommodated with just a little more planning and communication. For example, a woman who belongs to Jehovah's Witness congregation who must have major surgery could still receive good care without a blood transfusion, with closer monitoring and special care in the operating room, or her own blood banked ahead of time. Some doctors have developed *bloodless surgery* by operating in stages or using medications instead of blood transfusions. Recycling the patient's own blood is another option. Blood substitutes can be used in emergencies and surgeries. And some adults can accommodate a lower hemoglobin level naturally, especially if fluid replacement is used.

Respecting Cultural Diversity

Different cultures respond differently to illness, healthcare, and medicine. Because so many countries embrace many different cultures, providers have a responsibility to learn about the prevalent cultures in their area. Every hospital, clinic, and doctor's office should have some type of training that guides staff in dealing with patients from other cultures.

All patients need to have their beliefs and preferences respected to fulfill the principle of autonomy. In this section, we look at some of the different attitudes and beliefs that may affect care. We also offer suggestions on how to communicate with non-English-speaking patients and look at different ways to adjust care to embrace cultural diversity.

Although respecting different cultures and beliefs is important, generalizing based on appearance can seriously compromise a patient's health. For example, if you assume a Hispanic patient cannot speak English and wait for an interpreter before seeing the patient, there may be a costly time delay in the start of treatment. Not all members of all cultures adhere to specific beliefs. Communication is key.

The case of Sameera: Balancing religious beliefs with medical needs

Sameera was a pregnant patient from Saudi Arabia who was a strict practicing Muslim. Her faith tradition stated that she would be *made haram* (commit a punishable act) if she was attended by a male physician. Her OB/GYN doctor was a female, but Sameera was concerned that when she came into the hospital in labor, she would be forced to see a male doctor if the partner on call was a man. Her husband forbade this as well. To honor her religious practice, an induction of labor was arranged ahead of time on a day when a female physician was on call. After the baby was delivered, a "No Males Allowed" sign was put on her hospital door when she removed her head covering to nurse and spend time with her baby.

Attitudes and beliefs that affect care

Different cultures have many different rules, both written and unwritten, about how their members coexist with each other and interact with each other. And many of those rules affect healthcare. Some cultures think that discussing death, even making a living will, can invite death to the person who is ill. And people from some cultures will never tell a person with a life-threatening illness that she is ill, believing that this will so demoralize the patient that she will give up.

Different ways of looking at life should always be respected. Forcing a patient into a certain treatment or regimen will usually be detrimental to their health and will compromise the doctor-patient relationship. These are some of the rules and cultural differences for some cultures:

- **Vietnamese:** The father or son is the family spokesperson. Women will defer to their husbands or fathers for medical decisions. A female family member will want to stay with the patient most of the time to offer support and comfort. Most Vietnamese are Buddhists with great respect for authority, so eye-to-eye contact can be considered impolite. One common lay treatment is *coining*, or rubbing coins on the body to draw out illness. This can result in welts and scars that those unfamiliar with the culture may think are related to the disease or the result of abuse.

- **African-Americans:** Many older African-Americans prefer to be addressed by an identifier and their surnames. Direct eye contact is important. End-of-life planning may be seen as giving up. And because many members of this group distrust the medical profession, honesty and clear communication is essential.

- **Koreans:** Many people in this culture believe that telling someone about a serious diagnosis puts too much burden on a person who is already ill. The elderly in this culture are very respected. Herbalism is practiced, especially the use of medicinal mushrooms. Acupuncture and aromatherapy are also highly regarded.

- **Hmong:** Many people of this culture use herbal remedies instead of, or in addition to, conventional Western medical treatment. Sometimes patients seek traditional medical attention when the disease has progressed to late-stage because of cultural barriers to healthcare. Many Hmongs object to being touched by non-family members.

- **Hispanics:** Religion is an important part for members of this group. Patients may want to include religious items and icons in their hospital room. Prayer is important, especially praying together as a family. In some Hispanic families, consent of the husband or father is needed before a woman will consent to treatment.

- **American Indian:** Nonverbal communication is very important to this group. Direct eye contact is considered disrespectful. Traditional healers and healing ceremonies are important. And technical jargon will probably be difficult to interpret or translate into native languages such as Navajo or Lakota (Sioux).

✔ **Japanese:** The Japanese culture is quite interdependent, based on conforming to the group and relying on others within their family and cultural groups instead of reaching out to support in the community. Many men are waited on hand and foot by female relatives, and parents may rely on their children for interpretation and outside contact. Many express pain only by clenching the jaw because complaints are seen as a sign of weakness.

✔ **Arabs:** Dress requirements and modesty can be an issue among patients, especially women. The practice of Islam governs every part of their daily life. Mandatory cleansing with running water is a daily necessity. Muslims pray five times a day and will not respond to anyone else during prayers.

✔ **Russians:** This group may use natural remedies and prefer homeopathic treatments. Bad news about diagnoses is always first shared with family members and then with the patient. And most Russians think that psychiatric illnesses are shameful and should not be acknowledged.

One of the more poorly understood facets of cultural diversity is the expression of pain and complaints. In some cultures, loud exclamations and noisy conversations are normal and to be expected. In others, stoicism is valued.

If you are treating a patient from a more stoic culture, and he is complaining and voicing discomfort, the fact that he is violating the precepts of his culture may mean that his pain is severe. Here's where the family can provide important information. They know the patient better than you do, so they can tell whether or not complaining or not complaining really means something to that particular person.

Foua's case: Concealing pain

Foua was a 23-year-old pregnant Hmong woman who presented in active labor at an inner city hospital. A new resident was on call that evening. The resident had just completed a previous rotation at a hospital that served mostly Caucasians and African-Americans. When Foua arrived at the desk she said she was about to have her baby. She didn't appear to be in significant discomfort. The staff asked her to wait in the lobby to complete the paperwork and get her room ready. The resident was called to the lobby stat to deliver the baby. Despite very little sign of discomfort from Foua, he quickly realized that the woman was ready to deliver. Hmong patients do not verbalize or show other signs of pain as much as women from other cultures. Trusting the patient's demeanor doesn't work when judging how labor is progressing among women from this culture. Instead, the patient's cervix should have been checked on admission.

Hiring culturally diverse staff may be the best way to ensure that differences are recognized, understood, and respected. Have members of your staff teach the rest a few phrases in their native language, especially forms of greeting, which demonstrates respect for the other cultures.

Communicating with non-English-speaking patients

Non-English-speaking patients are becoming a larger part of the healthcare provider's patient base. When there is a large group of non-English-speaking patients in your community, you are ethically obligated to learn about the beliefs and traditions of their culture as it relates to medical care. If you can't communicate effectively and clearly with a patient, you may risk violating all of the ethical principles: Autonomy, if the patient doesn't understand a diagnosis, nonmaleficence, if you can't understand an explanation of the patient's symptoms, beneficence, if the patient doesn't understand the treatment, and justice, because everyone deserves to be heard.

Even if a patient does understand English, there is a difference between fluency in everyday English and fluency in medical English. Patients may lose some of their fluency under stress. Also, some health care providers and patients overestimate their skill with another language. And some doctors are uncomfortable with how information can change when an interpreter is used, either through misunderstanding or differences in translation.

There are certain skills you can use when communicating with non-English-speaking patients:

- ✔ Speak slowly and clearly and don't rush.
- ✔ Don't raise the volume of your voice.
- ✔ When a patient doesn't understand a sentence, repeat it word for word. Changing words may confuse the patient.
- ✔ Don't try to explain too much or give too much information in one session. Even patients fluent in English remember only one or two points in each doctor's visit.

An interpreter may be necessary in some cases. Many hospitals and clinics do not employ interpreters. Another healthcare practitioner, another patient, or a member of the patient's family can be used. When using an interpreter:

- ✔ Be sure the interpreter is fluent in English and the patient's language.
- ✔ Make sure the interpreter will keep the information private, or get consent from the patient to reveal this information.

✔ The interpreter should be able to listen and translate all symptoms without embarrassment to himself or the patient.

✔ Explain the diagnosis and treatment in plain English, and avoid medical jargon as much as possible.

✔ Allow for much more time for a visit with an interpreter.

A trained translator from a medical translation service is best to accurately and precisely transmit information, so use them when possible. When in doubt, encourage the patient to use a trained interpreter.

There are other ways to communicate with non-English-speaking patients. AT&T has a toll-free language service that will connect you with a translator in 140 languages. Cell phone technology can link interpreters to sessions. Audiotapes for physician and patient education exist in many languages. And hospitals that receive federal funding are required to hire more trained interpreters.

Discussing cultural beliefs

Probably the best way to address cultural differences and be able to communicate effectively with your patients is to simply ask them about their cultural beliefs and practices. Let them educate you about their beliefs and rituals.

When you're treating a patient from a different culture, you can address the issue of cultural differences with the questions you ask. For instance, ask:

✔ How do you think this disease or illness started?

✔ Do you know of anyone else who has this disease or condition?

✔ What do you want to be told about your illness?

✔ How involved should family members be in your diagnosis and care?

✔ How have you handled your illness so far?

✔ How would your ancestors have dealt with this illness?

✔ What results do you want to see from conventional medicine?

✔ Is there a healer in your community who could play a part in your medical treatment?

✔ Is there anyone else I could speak to who might help me understand your beliefs?

Relevant information should be noted on the patient's chart and kept updated as new preferences, needs, and responses to situations are uncovered. A person's mindset based on culture can have a significant effect on their healing.

Juanita's story: Skipped in translation

Juanita was a 68-year-old Hispanic patient who came to an after-hours clinic for blurred vision. An interpreter wasn't available, so her son came with her to act as one. A simple test of her blood sugar revealed that she had diabetes. The doctor began instructing her on the diagnosis and danger of high blood sugar and the possible complications of diabetes. The doctor noticed Juanita's son was saying a lot fewer words than the doctor was using. When Juanita visited her regular doctor a few days later, she had the vague idea that she had high blood sugar. She was unaware of the diabetes diagnosis or complications. It became clear that Juanita's son had not given his mother all of the information at her previous visit because he didn't want to worry his mother and give her bad news.

As discussed in the section "Communicating with non-English-speaking patients," the use of interpreters is essential when the patient doesn't speak English or English is their second language. Using family members to interpret can be problematic, especially when telling a patient bad news is forbidden in certain cultures.

When the Patient Refuses Treatment

It can be heartbreaking for a healthcare provider when a patient refuses treatment, especially when statistically there's a good chance the treatment will save a life. But autonomy must be respected, as long as the patient fully understands and has the capacity to understand.

Decision-making capacity (DMC) was discussed in Chapter 3. Mental competence is one thing, but if religious and cultural differences are creating misunderstandings, it's the provider's responsibility to try to overcome those barriers. Sometimes a simple language barrier or difficult translation can be all that stands between your patient and renewed health.

In this section, we look at how you can determine competency, a critical factor in informed consent. We look at ways to figure out if a patient truly understands his diagnosis and treatment possibilities, and how you can validate his concerns and ease his fears.

Adults can choose to forgo any medical treatment; however, it's not legal for a parent to refuse lifesaving treatment for their minor child based on religious beliefs. If a child needs treatment and the parents refuse it based on religious or cultural grounds, you are ethically allowed to override the parents' wishes and treat the child as necessary. See Chapter 8 for more on parental rights and settled law on this matter.

Determining competency

Competence is a legal term that means the patient has the mental and legal ability to make decisions. Some patients have the capacity to understand their diagnosis and treatment options but don't understand the language. So how can you tell if a patient is competent but doesn't understand because of language barriers, or if they lack competency for other reasons?

To be considered competent, the patient must be able to

✔ Communicate her choices with you

✔ Understand the risks and benefits of treatment and refusing treatment

✔ Be able to make a reasonable judgment about treatment

✔ Understand the seriousness of her condition

One of the best ways to determine competency is to ask the patient to describe her condition and possible treatments and outcomes to you. She'll probably provide clues to her refusal. Stay alert to any comments that indicate a cultural or religious refusal, and be sure to follow up on those statements.

If a patient isn't competent or doesn't have the capacity to understand, a surrogate can be appointed by the court to make decisions for him. For more information on surrogates, see Chapter 13.

If you're not sure if a patient is refusing treatment or not cooperating because of cultural differences or because of mental competency, it may be wise to solicit the help of another doctor or provider. A mental health professional might be brought in to judge competence and capacity to understand.

There are quite a few questionnaires you can fill out with your patient to determine capacity. Many of these questions focus on everyday activities, such as keeping up personal hygiene, planning meals, and adhering to a schedule, and how the patient handles them. The Patient Competency Rating Scale (PCRS) is one example. Other forms can be given to relatives to help decide capacity.

Making sure the patient understands

So how will you know when the patient understands the diagnosis, treatment possibilities, and prognosis? Communicating with patients from your culture is difficult enough. What happens when language and cultural differences add more barriers to communication?

Some issues that can help clarify understanding include:

✔ **Cultural differences:** In some cultures, older people are considered more knowledgeable. If you are younger than your patient from one of these cultures, the patient may not take what you say seriously, so it may be a good idea to ask an older colleague to deliver the news

✔ **Religious differences:** Sometimes a patient may misunderstand a treatment or protocol. You could ask to speak to your patient's clergy or religious leader to try to sort out differences.

✔ **Communication styles:** Some cultures value direct communication, whereas others prefer an indirect style. Even if a patient has questions or doesn't agree with your diagnosis and proposed treatment, in some cultures it's considered rude to disagree.

✔ **Silence:** Silence doesn't always mean acceptance. It can mean that the patient has given up trying to understand, or that they just want to end the visit because they are so uncomfortable.

✔ **Body language:** In some cultures, such as those from Sri Lanka, Vietnam, and Bulgaria, nodding doesn't signal agreement; it is meant as disagreement.

Noncompliance can be a clue that something is wrong in your communications with your patient. Before assuming that the patient just doesn't want to follow a certain protocol, investigate cultural differences to see if the problem is simply one of misunderstanding.

Validating concerns and assuaging fears

Any person who walks into a doctor's office or clinic is going to have concerns and fears. And one of your jobs is to empathize with the patient and reassure them. If religious or cultural differences are a barrier, this job becomes more difficult. It's important for patients to feel that they have been understood.

Part of your role as a healthcare provider is to validate concerns patients have about their physical and emotional well-being. Feedback from you to your patient and from your patient to you is critical when communicating with any patient, but especially one from another culture. Be sure that you listen carefully, ask questions, and, as we describe in Chapter 3, use a mirroring technique to help you understand.

Many times patients have fears that can be unrealistic, especially if the norms of their culture are different from yours. Part of your job is to reassure, whether you tell someone that their symptoms are not life threatening, or that you can help them feel better.

Listening carefully and in a nonjudgmental manner, doing your best to overcome boundaries set up by religions or culture, and taking the time to get to know your patients will help you create a successful and satisfying practice for you and your community.

Accepting refusals

If a patient refuses your treatment based on cultural beliefs, and that patient is competent and an adult, there's little you can do. If the patient is open to more discussion, it may help to bring in someone else from their culture to see if traditional medical methods may be acceptable in their case.

Some hospitals and clinics ask that patients who refuse care to read and sign an *informed refusal* document, indicating that they were informed about treatment but chose to refuse it.

If you can't help the patient and you are accepting of the patient's decisions, you can continue to care for them in the ways that they will allow. If you continue to care for the patient, trust in the relationship may grow and you may be able to help the patient with a serious condition as the disease progresses. If this is troublesome to you as a provider, you may want to refer them to a colleague who is willing to work with them. On rare occasion, the trust relationship is so compromised by the differences that it is best to recommend that a patient seek care elsewhere. Remember to never abandon a patient without helping them find an alternative provider who is more acceptable to them. And remember to always be respectful of their decisions, even if you are in disagreement.

Chapter 8

Parental Guidance and Responsibilities

For parents, the joy of raising a child is accompanied with many rights and responsibilities. The parent must act as legal guardian and make decisions about medical care and treatment.

Under the laws of most countries, minor children are considered incompetent. This doesn't mean they can't understand what is happening to them; it means they simply don't have the life experience to make an informed and responsible decision about their medical care. This changes as children grow and mature. Children who demonstrate competence and a high degree of maturity can and should take part in medical decisions.

In this chapter we look at a parent's rights and responsibilities, the treatment of impaired infants, the importance of vaccination and various ethical dilemmas associated with that issue, and childhood endangerment. We also look at the rights of teenagers and adolescents regarding privacy, patient rights, and the rights of emancipated minors.

Opinions of parents and healthcare providers sometimes clash, and this may result in dramatic and tragic results. There are exceptions to a parent's control over her child's medical care. In many cases, the court has overruled a parent's opinion, which is often influenced by religion or cultural beliefs, if it endangers the child. The best interest of the child will override a parent's wishes. Laws that recognize the rights of minors, emancipated minors, and mature minors are on the books, and in a medical emergency, providers can override a parent's wishes with no fear of reprisal.

Acknowledging Parental Rights to Choose or Refuse Care

Parents have moral and legal responsibilities for their children as well as the right to care for them. This right still exists even if society doesn't consider the parent a good parent.

A parent must be competent in the eyes of the law. A parent suffering from mental illness that impairs her decision-making ability, an abusive parent, or an incompetent or neglectful parent may have her decision-making rights terminated. The important point is that the incompetence must have a direct bearing on the medical matter at hand.

Society has an interest in children's welfare. When a medical intervention can save a child's life or greatly enhance the quality of life but a parent refuses it, the courts have ruled that healthcare professionals can step in to override a parental decision. Parents can refuse treatment in non-life-threatening situations, such as not getting their children vaccinated, but they can't refuse treatment that may save a child's life.

There is a separate issue here too: *assent.* That means that approval for the procedure comes from the child, separate from the parent's approval. This is a lesser standard than informed consent. Assent becomes more relevant as the child grows and matures.

Under the age of 6, children don't have the reasoning skills or life experience to make informed decisions about their care. Between the ages of 6 and 12, they do have some ability to be involved in the decisions about their medical care. Children age 13 and older should be included in decisions about their health according to their level of maturity.

In this section, we look at parents' responsibilities toward their children, how much choice parents have when deciding preventive and lifesaving care for their child, and when a parent's preferences can be overruled. We also explain how to decide whether to treat severely impaired newborns.

Responsibilities of a parent

Parents have legal responsibilities for their children. These include

- ✔ The responsibility to provide the child with the necessities of life and make day-to-day decisions about her care
- ✔ The responsibility to provide a safe environment for the child

- ✔ The responsibility to control and supervise the child
- ✔ The responsibility to educate and train the child and instill social and moral values

The responsibilities exist even if the parents are not married to each other, and these responsibilities last until the child is 18 years old. A parent loses all rights and responsibilities for a child who is given up for adoption.

Medical care is considered a basic need or necessity of life. When a child needs medical treatment, the parent should

- ✔ Accompany the child to the doctor's office or hospital.
- ✔ Provide accurate information about symptoms, chronic conditions, previous illnesses, and medications.
- ✔ Tell healthcare providers if a diagnosis is not understood.
- ✔ Cooperate in administering care and medicines prescribed by the doctor.
- ✔ Take responsibility for consequences if treatment protocol is refused or not followed.

 In some cases, a parent may have a mental illness or a condition that limits her ability to properly care for her child. If the parent's decisions are dangerous to the child's health, or are abusive or neglectful, healthcare providers can step in and overrule the parent. In some cases, a court order can be obtained to keep the child away from the parent.

Weighing parental choice against a child's best interest

Many state statutes require parents to provide medical care for their children, but parents do have some choice in the medical care given to their children. That choice can be overruled by doctors and the courts if the treatment is considered straightforward and the child will be harmed if the treatment is refused. For instance, if a child is injured in an accident and needs a blood transfusion to save his life, and the parents refuse because that practice violates their religious beliefs, doctors can overrule the parents and perform the procedure.

Your ethical responsibility as a healthcare provider is primarily to the child. The parents' wishes can be respected up to a point, but the child's best interests outweigh the parents' wishes.

 The *best interest* standard is important when deciding parental control over a child's care. The best interest standard reflects quality of life, whether a treatment has a good chance of succeeding, and whether a reasonable person would want to live the kind of life resulting from that treatment.

States have a vested interest and duty to protect citizens, but cannot infringe on rights granted to parents by the Constitution. These two interests must be balanced and weighed when a parent doesn't want to follow doctor's orders or recommendations.

Some religions and cultures believe that medical care interferes with parental rights and the will of God. Many children have died after their parents refused medical care because of these practices, and some parents have been convicted of child abuse, child endangerment, and homicide. Courts around the world have ruled that parents don't have the right to harm their children.

If you find yourself in this situation, first try to talk to the parents about their beliefs and their child's illness. They may be willing to let you treat their child. But if the parents resist treatment, and you know that leaving the child untreated will cause harm or even death, tell the parents that you are required to treat the child. If they still resist and the situation is critical, treat the child and deal with their distress later. If there's time, you may want to go to the medical ethics board for assistance. As a last resort, you can go to the courts and let a judge handle the situation.

Some states have allowed religious exemptions for some preventive medical treatments. At this time, 48 states allow parents to avoid immunizations for their children for religious reasons and allow exemptions for standard newborn metabolic tests. In these cases, doctors and healthcare providers must weigh the child's best interest and contact an ethics board or the hospital legal department to determine if parental choice should be overruled.

The state must provide a high standard of proof to overrule a parent's decisions about a child's medical care. The outcome of the illness weighs heavily on this decision. If the treatment's success rate is good and the child will be harmed or die without it, the courts will usually overrule the parents. If the treatment's success rate is not good and the child's life is not at risk, the courts will usually side with the parents.

The case of Karen and her newborn

Karen came to her obstetrician for pregnancy care. It was her first pregnancy, and as her due date drew near, she told her doctor she was a Jehovah's Witness and would refuse a blood transfusion in case of a life-threatening hemorrhage during delivery. She brought a signed document in accordance to her faith to be attached to her chart. Her doctor agreed to abide by her wishes. But her doctor told her that if the baby had any blood loss requiring transfusion, it would be performed in accordance with the law. At the end of her pregnancy, the baby was in a breech presentation, and an elective C-section was performed. Fortunately, all went well and no transfusion was needed.

Caring for a child when parents disagree with you

Parents are becoming more aware of medical issues, and they often research information about care and treatments online, from sources with varying credibility. This can cause conflict if a parent disagrees with a doctor about diagnosis or treatment. Because doctors have less time to spend with patients, especially in managed-care situations, communication can quickly break down.

When parents disagree with a diagnosis or treatment, three ethical principles may potentially come into conflict: beneficence, autonomy, and nonmaleficence. Beneficence is shown when doctors and parents want what is best for the patient, in this case, the child. The parents want the autonomy to decide what is best for their child, and the doctor, parents, and society want no harm to come to the child (nonmaleficence). But doctors and parents can disagree about what exactly causes harm. For example, some parents believe that traditional medical treatments, such as chemotherapy, cause more harm than good. Some parents believe that alternative treatments are best for their child, despite evidence to the contrary. A recent case that showcases this ethical dilemma is Daniel Hauser, a child whose parents refused chemotherapy for a treatable cancer in favor of alternative treatments. This case is reviewed in more detail in Chapter 19.

Clear communication and full disclosure can go a long way to resolving disputes between healthcare providers and parents. The disagreement may stem from a simple misunderstanding. When no agreement can be reached, a hospital ethics committee can get involved.

If there is a clear-cut benefit with little risk in the case of critical or life-saving treatment, the treatment will be supported by law, and the provider should proceed with treatment. Conflict will most likely occur when the odds of a good outcome aren't very high and risks associated with the treatment are fairly high. To be ethical, withholding treatment must also have a significant benefit for the child.

Sometimes the opposite situation occurs. A child may be very ill and further treatment is deemed medically futile. In that case, the child won't be helped by a treatment, and the treatment may actually cause harm, pain, or distress. Some parents insist on treatment for their children no matter if it is futile or not. Again, good communication with the family is critical. Having a team meeting with the family and members of the child's care team can sometimes help the family come to terms with stopping aggressive treatments. If conflicts can't be resolved, the hospital ethics board can make recommendations as well.

Most situations in which parents and providers disagree about what treatment is in the best interest of the child can be resolved through good communication. However, when a disagreement persists, having the ethics committee review and discuss the case with involved parties can be helpful. This step can be requested by the providers involved in the child's care or the child's family. The ethics committee won't make decisions about the care, but it can make recommendations and help clarify decisions for the patient and his family.

Some hospitals have implemented mentoring programs and hired liaisons. A liaison attends doctor's appointments and treatment sessions along with parents and children. The liaison can help catch missed questions and clues and guide the parents through a stressful situation. Mentoring programs are used to help staff interact with parents and children so they communicate better.

Knowing when and how to treat impaired infants

One of the most difficult situations in medicine is to be involved with a family who is facing the birth of a severely impaired infant. More than a half million premature babies are born in the United States each year, and some of the preemies have very serious defects.. Other babies are born at term with anencephaly or severe spina bifida, profound mental retardation, or other serious defects.

These situations raise some very difficult ethical issues. How much intervention or resuscitation should be performed on very premature infants, ages 22 to 25 weeks, when 26 weeks is considered compatible with life? Is it ever ethical for parents to allow a severely impaired infant to die without aggressive therapies? Who decides what constitutes severely impaired? This issue also brings up questions of personhood and sanctity of life versus quality of life, which are addressed in Chapter 11.

An important ethics case that led to changes in how impaired infants are treated was the case of Baby Jane Doe. Baby Jane Doe was born in 1983 with severe defects — spina bifida and hydrocephalus. The doctors initially gave her a grim prognosis, and her parents decided to forego surgical treatments and give her comfort care. However, the news media became aware of the story and soon a suit was filed to force treatment. (For more about Baby Jane Doe, head to Chapter 19.)

Her case eventually led the government to enact Baby Jane Doe regulations and ultimately revise the Child Abuse Prevention and Treatment Act, which labels nontreatment of Baby Doe cases as child abuse.

There are three exceptions to this rule:

- When an impaired infant is "chronically and irreversibly comatose"
- When a child is inevitably dying
- When treatment would be "futile and inhumane"

So in the case of disabled newborns, parents have very little autonomy to make decisions about their child's care. On the other hand, some babies who may have died have gone on to have meaningful lives because intervening with lifesaving treatment was in the best interest of the child.

So what does this mean for providers caring for an impaired infant and their parents? Unless the child meets one of the three listed criteria, full medical care must be given to the infant. Parents can be involved in all treatment decisions other than choosing no treatment, and should be supported during this difficult time. If it appears that treatment becomes "futile and inhumane," then a comfort-care approach should be considered.

A different scenario, however, is the mother who presents in active labor between 22 and 26 weeks' gestation. Because the child is unlikely to survive at this young gestational age, treatment options range from full resuscitation to a brief attempt at resuscitation to no resuscitation at all — these are all considered reasonable and ethical. A provider can help the family make this decision with clear and compassionate discussion, noting that no matter the approach, the baby is unlikely to survive.

Vaccination: The Evidence and the Ethics

Vaccines have saved more lives than any other medical intervention. Before vaccinations, many people died of infectious diseases, and pandemics ravaged entire populations. In fact, there has been a 95 percent reduction in cases of preventable diseases since vaccines were introduced in the 20th century.

The ethical principles of autonomy, beneficence, and nonmaleficence play a part in vaccination. A patient (or parent) should have the right to decide if a vaccination is given. Doctors know that vaccinations prevent disease and save lives. Not vaccinating can make people sick and be a potential starting point for pandemics, endangering society as a whole.

Some parents object to vaccinating their children either because of religious or cultural beliefs, or because they fear the vaccination will cause more harm than the disease it prevents. However, because vaccinations have nearly eradicated many of the diseases they prevent, most parents have never witnessed the potentially devastating effects of these diseases.

In this section, we look at the evidence of vaccine efficacy and the ethics of choosing not to vaccinate a child. We look at vaccination as a public health issue.

We also look at the importance of full disclosure between a healthcare provider and a parent concerning a child's vaccination status and risk of disease, along with other options parents might consider.

Understanding vaccination as a public health issue

Because children are often most vulnerable to diseases such as measles, mumps, polio, and pertussis (whooping cough) and because they most likely have not been exposed to them, they benefit the most from immunization. Vaccinating large numbers of a population also creates *herd immunity*, which is the protection of the community as a whole. This is an important societal benefit.

In the United States, all states require that children must receive a series of immunizations before they can attend school. These vaccines are tied with school attendance because this requirement reaches a large number of children. Children are required to present immunization records or a form stating the reason for refusal when they start school.

At this time, the United States does not have a *mandate*, which is a legal requirement for vaccination without exception. The last time a mandate was issued was in World War I for the Spanish flu pandemic. In the United States, vaccinations are required for school-age children, but parents can seek exemptions for religious or cultural reasons.

Parents can object to these vaccinations for religious reasons or personal beliefs, but not because of cost or inconvenience. All 50 states have these vaccination requirements, but 48 states have created exemptions for religious reasons, and 20 states have granted exemptions for personal reasons. There are no legal penalties for refusing vaccinations, but if an unvaccinated child contracts a disease and then infects another child, the parents may be civilly liable.

Most Americans have been vaccinated against common diseases. As a result, smallpox has been eradicated. A child who isn't vaccinated does have a reduced chance of catching a particular disease because of herd immunity. However, unvaccinated children still can contract diseases that have not been eradicated, like measles, mumps, or varicella. Some of the consequences can be tragic. A study in the Journal of the American Medical Association found that children who weren't immunized were 35 times more likely to get measles and almost 6 times more likely to contract pertussis. Complications from these diseases can include pneumonia, encephalitis, seizures, and death.

Considering risk-benefit analysis

Risk-benefit analysis is applied to drugs, treatments, and medical procedures. Vaccinations do prevent disease, so every individual who is vaccinated will benefit, but vaccination isn't without risk. The exact benefit of a certain vaccination changes over time and with individual characteristics. Some people develop severe clinical symptoms when vaccinated.

The ethical standards of beneficence and nonmaleficence come into play in risk-benefit analysis. Vaccination does a great amount of good by preventing disease and death. But some people react adversely to vaccines, and some of these reactions cause great harm. Risk-benefit analysis states that, to be ethical, the benefit of a vaccine must outweigh the risk.

Risk-benefit analysis is conducted on all vaccines. In fact, the Federal Drug Administration has a department that regulates vaccines in the United States. The Center for Biologics Evaluation and Research (CBER) sponsors the process that vaccine manufacturers must follow before a vaccine can be approved.

For each vaccine, a risk level is set. If the risk level is considered too high, researchers can work to develop new vaccines. For example, the Urabe-strain MMR vaccine, given to children until 1992, carried a risk of developing aseptic meningitis. The risk was listed as 1 per 12,000 children. A new vaccine was developed that reduced the risk to 1 in 27,000.

Vaccines do save lives, many more lives than are lost due to vaccine complications. It currently takes about ten years to bring a vaccine through development and testing to the market. Critics say that vaccine clinical trials should be longer and include a larger and more varied population. But delaying vaccines that have been shown to have a good risk-benefit ratio costs lives and increases expense.

Understanding full disclosure

Doctors should always reveal all of the risks and benefits of any medical procedure to patients. This is known as *full disclosure*. The problem with full disclosure is that listing the risks of vaccination, which are small, may scare some parents into refusing vaccinations.

You, the doctor, must inform parents of all risks and benefits of vaccines before vaccinating children. Although the side effects of vaccines can be serious, the risk of not vaccinating has to be emphasized. Because these diseases are now rare due to vaccination, parents are no longer familiar with the serious complications and deaths these diseases cause. Full disclosure is not meant to scare parents into vaccinating; it is meant to inform them of all of the risks and benefits so they can make an informed decision.

The CDC has created Vaccine Information Sheets (VIS) that are to be given to patients or their legal guardians when a vaccine is administered. In fact, it is United States law that this information is given with each vaccine administered. A 2001 study by the American Society of Pediatrics found that doctors don't often discuss risks of vaccination or contraindications. Telling parents to read the information sheet before vaccinating their children helps doctors meet the guideline of full disclosure.

Vaccination is viewed as routine. However, some people feel that the risks involved in vaccination outweigh the benefits, despite risk-benefit studies. Opponents to vaccines sometimes quote the Declaration of Helsinki (see Chapter 2), which is used as a guideline for human medical research, to support their opposition to vaccines. This Declaration states:

> Considerations related to the well-being of human subjects should take precedence over the interests of science and society.

The problem with using that statement from the Declaration to oppose vaccines is that society's interests in preventing disease and pandemics have been judged greater than the individual risk of vaccine reactions and side effects. In fact, by protecting all of society, each individual is protected. Because the risk of the disease is so much greater than the risk of the vaccination, most people feel current vaccination policy is in accordance with the Declaration.

Healthcare providers and manufacturers are required to report adverse reactions to vaccines. The Vaccine Adverse Event Reporting System (VAERS) was set up under the 1986 National Childhood Vaccine Injury Act. (That act, by the way, was designed to protect vaccine manufacturers against financial liability, not to improve vaccine safety, as the name implies.) The system covers the entire population of the United States, including adults. Doctors, parents, and manufacturers can submit reports of patients' adverse reactions to vaccines.

The HPV vaccine and informed consent

Sometimes informed consent around vaccines is not completely straightforward. A vaccine against human papillomavirus (HPV) is given to girls, starting as young as 9 years old, before they become sexually active. Researchers estimate that HPV causes 70 percent of all cervical cancer cases, so the goal of the vaccine is to prevent cervical cancer. When doctors tell parents and their daughters about this vaccine, it can prompt discussions about how the virus is transmitted and becoming sexually active — a discussion that parents may not be comfortable undertaking. Would a 15-year-old girl be willing to discuss this in front of her mother at her sports physical?

It is important to educate both the parent and the patient about this vaccine and have the consent of both parties. A parent can be asked to leave the exam room during the physical exam, and the girl can be given the opportunity to ask further questions and disclose additional information. If the patient is over 13, she is a mature minor and should have an active role is deciding about the vaccine. It may be best to discuss the risks and benefits of the vaccine, and then give the family time to review Vaccine Information Sheet information. The patient can proceed with the vaccine or discuss it with her family and return for the vaccine at a later date. It is important that parents and their daughters be educated about this vaccine even if it leads to more difficult conversations.

Elijah's case: Vaccines and autism

Elijah is a 2-year-old who was diagnosed with autism. His parents started becoming concerned when he was 15 months old, just at the time he received the MMR vaccine. He did not make eye contact with his parents and did not interact with others. He could not say any words by 18 months. Evaluation by a developmental pediatrician revealed the diagnosis of autism. Because of the timing of his symptom development, the parents wondered if the MMR vaccine caused the autism. The parents have stated they won't get any more vaccinations for any of their children.

As with any medical procedure, there are risks associated with vaccines. In the last 30 years, a subculture decrying vaccination has risen. Some parents are convinced that vaccines cause autism. The U.S. government set up a vaccines court that heard evidence about the vaccine preservative thimerosal, the MMR vaccine, and development of autism over a course of several years. The court looked at all available studies about the preservative. In 2010, the court ruled that thimerosal does not cause autism. Vaccine manufacturers stopped using thimerosal in 1999, but autism rates have continued to increase. That points to a lack of causal effect between vaccinations and autism development.

Many of the adverse reactions reported after vaccination, such as fever, muscle aches or rash, can also occur in the unvaccinated population. It can be difficult to tell whether the vaccine caused the adverse event. If an adverse reaction is reported after vaccination, more studies are needed to determine if that reaction was caused by the vaccine or if it was a coincidence.

There is no independent vaccine safety board. A National Vaccine Safety Board, which would consist of doctors, researchers, industry experts, and statisticians, has been proposed. It would focus on improving vaccine safety, reducing adverse effects, and gathering relevant information quickly.

Addressing parent opposition to vaccines

If you are practicing pediatric care, it's not uncommon to have parents who refuse vaccines for their children or are quite anxious about possible side effects. Much of this is due to fear spread by the media and certain Web sites. The ethical dilemma as a provider is that clearly the most beneficial path for the patient and society is to proceed with immunizations. But the parents' autonomy supersedes your desire for beneficence for the patient.

For parents who are concerned about adverse vaccine reactions, there are ways to help them feel more comfortable. Parents can opt out of vaccinations. This is their right under the law and must be respected because of autonomy. The herd immunity factor decreases the risk that their children will contract one of these diseases, but you, the provider, must stress the risk of avoiding vaccinations.

There are ways to help prevent the risk of adverse vaccine reactions. These include

- ✔ Spread out vaccinations over several months.

- ✔ Don't administer many vaccines at one time. This will cost more and involve more doctor's visits, but some parents will feel more comfortable with this method.

- ✔ Limit combination shots. Some of these combination shots, such as MMR, can be given as individual doses over time.

- ✔ Delay the Hepatitis B vaccine routinely given to newborns.

- ✔ Check immunity levels in the blood before giving booster shots. Some children don't need booster shots if their immunity level is high.

Some doctors have developed alternative vaccine schedules. The American Academy of Pediatrics has told doctors to work with parents who want different schedules for vaccination. You should be open to different vaccination schedules if they are medically advisable.

There are other things you can do to make your patient more comfortable. Make sure that the child drinks plenty of water before a vaccination because fevers can occur, and hydration helps the body handle fever. A mild pain killer and fever reducer can be given after the vaccinations. Tell the parents to make sure that their insurance company will pay for a different vaccination schedule. And be prepared for more fussiness and crankiness from the child from mild vaccination reactions.

Child Endangerment: The Healthcare Provider's Role

It's a sad fact that many children are abused and killed by parents, relatives, and acquaintances. More than 3 million reports of child abuse occur every year in the United States.

As a healthcare provider, you are a *mandated reporter* — someone who is required by law to report abuse or neglect of a child. Healthcare providers must make this report even though it breaches confidentiality. The point is to catch abuse at a relatively early stage so damage is minimized. Mandated reporters are professionals, like teachers, doctors, nurses, police officers, clergy, probation officers, and firefighters. Each state sets its own standard for reporting.

If you suspect child abuse or neglect, a report must be filed with your local Child Protective Services (CPS) office. Mandated reporters can't file an anonymous report, but they are granted immunity as long as the report is done in good faith, and their names are kept confidential.

File a verbal report as quickly as possible; file the paperwork within 48 hours. CPS will investigate the claim and take further action as needed.

Child abuse doesn't have to be violent. Child abuse occurs at every social level and in every economic and cultural group, and most abused children know their abusers, either intimately or casually.

In this section, we look at how to recognize the signs of child abuse and neglect. We examine how to best work with CPS and social workers.

Discovering signs of abuse and neglect

It is very troubling to discover signs of neglect and abuse in children, but that's part of your role as a healthcare provider. When child abuse or neglect is caught early, the child has a much better chance of making a full recovery. Minimizing long-term emotional and physical damage to the child is of paramount importance. There are different kinds of abuse; all are harmful.

Physical child abuse is actual physical injury to the child. It can be a secondary result of discipline or punishment, or may be a deliberate action to harm the child. The signs of physical abuse include

- Frequent injuries and bruises, including burns, bites, black eyes, and broken bones
- The child exhibits sudden changes in behavior
- Fading bruises or healing injuries after an absence from school
- Injuries with a pattern, such as marks from a belt or stick
- The child wears clothing inappropriate to the season to cover up bruises and cuts
- The child flinches at sudden movements or pulls away from touch
- The child is cautious and watchful in the extreme

Emotional child abuse is more difficult to detect. It consists of humiliating or belittling a child, bullying and threatening, calling the child names, or exposing the child to violence. The signs of emotional abuse include

- The child isn't attached to the parent
- The child has learning problems not caused by physical problems
- The child exhibits actions inappropriate to age, such as being more mature or regressing to thumb-sucking or bed-wetting
- The child exhibits behavioral extremes, either being very docile or very aggressive
- The child has delayed development, either physical or emotional
- The child is very withdrawn, anxious, and fearful

Sexual abuse is any sexual contact with a child. The signs of sexual abuse include

- The child refuses to change clothes in front of appropriate persons
- The child tries to avoid a specific person or persons
- A pregnancy or STD under the age of 14
- Sudden change in weight or changes in appetite
- A young child has problems sitting or walking
- A young child exhibits seductive behavior or interest in sex
- The child runs away from home

Child neglect is a pattern of not caring for a child, either physically or emotionally, that threatens the child's well-being. The signs of neglect include

- Dirty clothes that don't fit or are inappropriate for the weather
- Untreated illness or lack of medical or dental care
- The child steals food or is constantly hungry
- Untreated injuries
- Poor hygiene
- Frequent school absences or tardiness
- The child is left alone at a young age

Parents can give clues to the existence of child abuse or neglect, too. You may suspect child abuse or neglect if a parent

- Is very protective of or limits contact with the child
- Is very isolated or secretive

✔ Behaves irrationally

✔ Abuses controlled substances, including drugs and alcohol

✔ Blames or denigrates the child for problems, injuries, or illnesses

✔ Offers a weak or no explanation for injuries

✔ Is depressed, apathetic, or indifferent to the child

Parents who abuse their children are adept at offering excuses or reasons for injuries or symptoms. You must be on the lookout for warning signs of abuse and neglect.

Although it seems like it would be easy to pick up abuse based on the many possible signs and symptoms, it's actually quite difficult. I've never had a parent come in and admit to abusing a child or a child report a parent's abuse. The signs can be quite subtle, and the picture may have to develop over time. But there is an urgency to intervening because the health and even the life of a child may be at stake. This is one of the biggest ethical dilemmas in medicine. Obviously, your primary concern for the pediatric patient is nonmaleficence and beneficence, so reporting your concerns if you suspect abuse seems like the right thing to do. But what if a father is spanking a child and leaving marks? Is this within his right as a father, and should his autonomy be honored? When in doubt, I sometimes anonymously call CPS and review the case, without reporting it, to get advice and recommendations.

Reporting abuse and working with Child Protective Services

Child abuse is a common problem, and it is up to you to help protect children in any way possible. Reporting suspicions of child abuse is one of your ethical duties as a healthcare provider.

The type of report you must file and the phone calls you must make vary from state to state. On these forms, authorities usually ask for your relationship with the child, what you have observed, any suspicions about abuse you may have, and how to contact the child and her parents.

Sadly, many child abuse cases go unreported. A study in the United States that looked at 15,000 child-injury doctor's visits found that 27 percent of doctors who believe injuries were caused by abuse didn't report them to authorities.

Doctors do not diagnose child abuse or report it for several reasons:

✔ Fear of breaking up a family.

✔ Lack of confidence in authorities to stop abuse.

✔ Uncertainty as to the cause of the injury.

✔ If the patients are boys, abusive fractures are often misdiagnosed. Injuries are more common for boys, so the assumption is the fracture is accidental.

✔ Fewer abuse cases are diagnosed in a primary care setting than in an emergency room.

✔ Diagnosing fractures caused by accidents is more difficult than diagnosing fractures caused by abuse.

Always check for other abuse risk factors when a child has a fracture. Any child with a skull fracture should have a skeletal survey to rule out abuse.

Many hospitals have special team of medical providers experienced in dealing with abuse cases and collecting evidence; someone on the team is always on call should a suspicious case present in the Emergency Department. Some large hospitals even have a branch of CPS in the building. The special team or agency can review cases and provide counseling when needed, especially during emergency admissions.

When investigating a family situation, if CPS finds that abuse of any kind has occurred, CPS staff can bring children to a hospital or doctor's clinic without parental permission. Children aren't always removed from a home unless there is threat of imminent harm.

If a child is removed from the home or a family member prosecuted, you may be called to testify or asked to provide more information if a case progresses. In some states, you are required to call CPS after making a written report. Your medical relationship with the child and the family may change after CPS investigates. If possible, try to maintain your professional relationship with the child even if his living situation changes. The child needs someone whom he can open up to and who will not abandon him during a difficult time.

Child abuse hotlines

There are many hotlines you can call if you suspect child abuse. State agencies provide one line of defense, but there are other places to call, either for more information or to report abuse.

✔ National Center for Missing and Exploited Children: 800-843-5678

✔ ChildHelpUSA National Crisis Hotline: 800-4-A-CHILD

✔ National Domestic Violence Hotline: 800-799- SAFE

✔ National Referral Network for Kids in Crisis: 800-KID-SAFE

Confidentiality, Care, and the Adolescent Patient

The Health Insurance Portability and Accountability Act (HIPAA; see Chapter 4 for more details) has established laws for adolescent confidentiality and privacy in the United States. Many states have granted teenagers rights to confidentiality in certain situations.

There are some situations where an adolescent may not feel comfortable discussing a medical problem with a parent. The courts have decided that adolescents do have a right to seek medical care independent of their parents' decisions. This helps ensure that adolescents get needed medical help even in difficult situations.

In this section, we look at the adolescent patient's rights and how you, as the provider, must keep information confidential. We look at the balance between the patient's rights and the parents' right to know. We see how to teach teens the concept of informed consent, and we deal with the legal situation of the emancipated minor.

Understanding adolescent patients' rights

As children grow, they are allowed more decisions and input into deciding their medical care. Even when a child is still classified as a *dependent minor* they are legally allowed some privacy and have a certain amount of autonomy.

In the United States, most states have given minors the right to be treated for sexually transmitted diseases and alcohol and drug abuse. The courts recognize that in some cases, minors will not seek treatment at all rather than tell their parents. In some states, minors can consent to five services:

✔ Minors can get contraceptive services in 25 states.

✔ All 50 states allow minors to be tested for STDs, including HIV, without parental permission.

✔ Minors can get outpatient mental health services in 20 states.

✔ Minors can get confidential counseling and care for the abuse of drugs or alcohol in 44 states.

✔ Minors in 27 states can get prenatal care and obstetrical services, including delivery, without parental consent or notification.

Abortion is a different matter. Just a few states allow a minor to obtain an abortion without parental consent or notification. Most of the other 48 states allow the minor to go to a judge for consent. This is called a *confidential alternative* and is required by the Supreme Court to protect the right to privacy. Many of these laws are being decided in court now or have been blocked by the courts. As of August 2010, Connecticut, Maine, Maryland, and the District of Columbia allow minors access to abortion without parental consent.

Some states that require parental permission for an abortion don't require permission to let a minor continue her pregnancy and deliver. Many states let a minor place a child for adoption without her parents' knowledge or permission.

It's important to understand the family dynamic when a minor child comes to you for care without her parents. Encouraging the minor to talk to her parents is a logical step, but may not be practical in some situations.

Balancing privacy and patients' rights

HIPAA privacy rules also apply to a minor patient's rights. When a minor child visits a doctor for one of the services protected by law, confidentiality about his records can be compromised.

Problems and confusion can arise in several areas. States often have different laws about privacy and confidentiality. You, the doctor, must be knowledgeable about the confidentiality laws for minors in your state. HIPAA regulations specify that state laws determine parental access to their child's medical information. HIPAA laws supersede state laws, unless the state laws are more stringent.

Doctors, clinics, and hospitals can't demand that minors let parents see confidential information as a condition for eligibility for treatment, insurance enrollments, treatment, or payment for services.

When a minor child must be informed of test results, it can be difficult to communicate with the patient without informing the parents. You can communicate with minor patients by text messages, e-mail, or notification via another phone number such as a cell phone. You, as the doctor, are required to accept these requests and abide by them as long as they are reasonable.

Finally, communication with insurance companies can be problematic. Minors are usually part of their parents' healthcare plans, but HIPAA doesn't require that insurance companies get a minor patient's written permission before disclosing information. HIPAA says that insurers must honor an alternative communication request if the minor says that this information may endanger him if his parents learn about it.

Sarah's case: Keeping a teen's request confidential

Sarah is a 16-year-old who came to her family physician requesting birth control pills. She had become sexually active and said her parents would "kill her" if they found out. She was also having painful periods. After an exam and negative pregnancy test, her doctor gave her a prescription. He encouraged her to talk to her parents. He coded the visit with the diagnosis of "dysmenorrhea" rather than "contraceptive counseling" so that when her parents received the insurance statement, the complete reason for the visit would remain confidential. The patient paid for her prescription rather than running it through her parent's insurance. Otherwise, confidentiality about the patient's reason for the visit could not have been ensured.

Minors should receive written notice of your clinic's privacy standards and practices. Minor patients have the right to file a complaint if they feel their privacy has been violated, although they don't have the right to sue that organization through HIPAA.

Talking to teens about informed consent

As children grow and become more educated and more aware, they can start participating in their medical care. Most doctors believe that children who are age 12 and older should be included in discussions about healthcare. Still, parents must give consent for many procedures, including most surgeries, for children under the age of 18. The principle of autonomy should be respected.

Informed consent is a moral and ethical responsibility and a contract between a doctor and patient. For a teenager to give informed consent, some standards must be met. These standards include:

- ✔ The document should be written at the minor's reading level.
- ✔ The teen must be competent and rational enough to make a medical decision. The child must state that she understands the healthcare choices available to her.
- ✔ There must not be any coercion forcing the teen into the treatment.
- ✔ The teen must be able to compare the outcomes of different treatments and be able to choose the best one for her situation.
- ✔ If the teen needs emergency treatment, consent for emergency procedures is presumed.
- ✔ The teen must understand the risks and benefits of treatment, and the risks and benefits of forgoing treatment.

It is the doctor's judgment whether a minor patient has the capability to make a decision about informed consent. It's important to remember that your first duty and responsibility is to your patient. In many cases, this duty exists regardless of parental wishes.

When adolescents refuse treatment, an ethical dilemma occurs. You, the doctor, must weigh the risks and benefits of the treatment. If a treatment has a low success rate, is elective, or is considered futile, there is no need to pursue parental permission. If the risks are low and benefits high or if the adolescent's life is in danger and the adolescent refuses the treatment, healthcare providers have an ethical responsibility to pursue the matter.

There aren't clear guidelines about the procedures when minors, parents, and doctors disagree about medical intervention. In some cases, mediation may be the best option. Intervention of the courts should be the last step.

Mature minors and emancipated minors

Some minor children can be treated without consent of their parents under the *mature minor* exception. This is a legal status called *judicial bypass*. If the court decides that a minor child can act in his own best interest, he can make medical decisions without parental involvement. This refers only to medical decision-making. There is not an absolute age for a child to be considered a mature minor. A court must decide the child is mature enough to give consent for his own medical care. Mature minors are usually age 14 or older.

In some cases, a child under the age of 18 is judged mature enough to live on his own, independent from the protection and control of his parents. The child is then known as an *emancipated minor*. An emancipated minor is usually between the ages of 16 and 18. He can make all medical decisions, in addition to other legal decisions, for himself without parental consent or opinion. This standard is set by the states. A minor is considered emancipated in several scenarios:

- ✔ If he is self-supporting or not living at home, or declared emancipated
- ✔ If the parent has consented to the emancipation and has surrendered rights and responsibilities
- ✔ If he is married or has a child of his own, or is in the military

Part III
Ethics at the Beginning and End of Life

The 5th Wave   By Rich Tennant

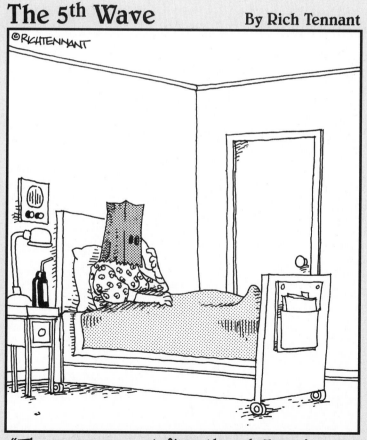

"The surgery went fine, though I can't say much for their post-operative sensitivity."

In this part . . .

When does a human being become a person? And when does personhood end? These critical questions are some of the most interesting and affecting in medical ethics at the beginning and end of life. Abortion, assisted reproduction, surrogacy, end-of-life-care, and euthanasia are the hot button issues that can be addressed with medical ethics, even if on a case-by-case basis.

The combination of science and sex has produced some amazing results, including pre-implantation genetics, surrogacy, and in vitro fertilization. So, what are the ethical issues surrounding these procedures? Who gets to decide what happens when conflicts arise?

The end of life presents some difficult scenarios, too. We look at how to ensure your patient gets the best end-of-life care through advance directives, relief of suffering, and withdrawing life-sustaining treatment.

Chapter 9

Two Lives, One Patient: Pregnancy Rights and Issues

*P*regnant women are a special subject in medical ethics. Technically, there is only one patient, but two lives are in the balance. Healthcare providers must weigh issues such as medication, treatments for disease, and autonomy of both patients.

Sometimes what is good for the mother is not good for the fetus, and vice versa. Because their rights may sometimes compete, doctors must understand the ethical and legal challenges of that balancing act. The rights of the mother may automatically be diminished if it's decided that the fetus has the same rights as a full person.

In this chapter, we look at the rights of the mother and the rights of the fetus from a legal and an ethical standpoint, which sometimes conflict. We examine fathers' rights, the ethics of birth control, and the issue of fetal abuse. Finally we look at the ethics of prenatal and genetic testing.

Medical Intervention: Rights of the Mother versus Rights of the Fetus

Most women choose to be pregnant and consent to treatments offered them. But in some circumstances, some women won't consent to medical interventions that restrict their freedom or endanger their health during a pregnancy, even if these treatments may be in the best interest of the fetus. A few women have even refused treatments that may save their fetus's life with little risk or inconvenience to themselves. In the United States, the courts decided in *Roe v. Wade* that a fetus is not a full person and doesn't have the same rights as a person until it is born.

Abortion is not a part of this particular debate. Chapter 11 is devoted to consideration of the ethical, legal, and medical aspects of abortion. Here we're talking about medical treatments that may save the life of the fetus. An example would be a mother with preterm labor who is placed on strict bed rest at 22 weeks gestation to try to get her to 36 weeks gestation so the baby can be born safely. As the fetus grows and reaches viability, it is granted more protection under the law. But a pregnant woman's autonomy is considered to be so important that providers must go to a judge and obtain a court order to force her into treatment against her will. Some judges have done just that and put the rights of the fetus ahead of the mother's autonomy.

Unless a court intervenes, until the baby is born, the mother's decisions about medical care (other than abortion) take precedence, and providers are legally bound to abide by her wishes.

Of course, as with all medical ethics issues, individual cases are far more complex than the law. What may be decided in the courts or may play out in a medical setting may not be the best decision from a purely ethical standpoint.

In this section, we look at the Fourteenth Amendment and how it influenced *Roe v. Wade*. We also try to understand self-determination, an issue in autonomy, and the role of technology in the mother's rights and the fetus's rights.

Setting forth rights with the Fourteenth Amendment

The Fourteenth Amendment to the United States Constitution defines citizenship. It was added after the Civil War as one of the Reconstruction Amendments, overruling *Dred Scott v. Sanford*, which held that slaves were not citizens and, therefore, had no rights. The amendment defines a person as "someone who has been born or naturalized in the United States." It sets forth the concept of personal liberty and places restrictions on state actions that restrict liberty.

Two important clauses in that amendment are *due process*, which outlines certain steps that much be taken before a person is deprived of their liberty, and *equal protection*, which forces states to treat people equally.

This amendment relates to pregnant women in several ways. Because a fetus has not been born, it is not considered to be a person with all of the legal rights. The right to privacy in *Roe v. Wade* came from the due process clause, and states cannot limit abortion beyond this ruling due to the equal protection clause.

As we discuss in Chapter 11, in the United States a woman can terminate a pregnancy in the first trimester with no reason. In the second and third trimesters, the interest of the state in the health of the fetus increases, so states can set limits on abortions, as long as exceptions are written to protect the life and health of the mother. *Roe v. Wade* was an important ruling with respect to abortion, but it also guides us in other situations where maternal and fetal rights conflict.

Understanding self-determination

Self-determination is primarily a political concept. In short, a person should be allowed to determine her own actions without external forces influencing her. Under the principles of autonomy, bodily integrity, and sovereignty, women as well as men have legal and ethical control over what happens to their bodies. If the concept of self-determination applies fully in a given situation, a woman can refuse treatment of any kind for herself and for her fetus, even when that treatment is in both of their best interests.

The life of a fetus carries a substantial moral value, but should that value infringe on the mother's legal rights? This is a difficult but important question when determining the rights of a fetus in certain medical situations. One of the most important ethical issues in this discussion is the concept of personhood. When is a fetus considered a full person? Ethicists argue full personhood from the point of conception to the point of birth (see Chapter 11). From a legal standpoint in *Roe v. Wade,* the Supreme Court's ruling seemed to acknowledge that the state's interest in the fetus increases as the pregnancy progresses. It's rare that a mother's rights are ever overruled by a legal decision in the fetus's best interest, but when this does occur, it is usually late in pregnancy.

The other critical ethical concern is the autonomy of the mother. Pregnancy affects a woman's health and life; if she makes a choice, for instance, to smoke during pregnancy, she has the right to do so without intervention. But is this right to autonomy absolute? As long as the fetus remains in the womb, the mother's decisions about medical care take precedence and must be respected unless a court intervenes and orders treatment.

What if a mother in preterm labor at 22 weeks refuses to go on bed rest to prevent premature delivery? The baby will not survive if born at this point. Is restricting the mother's freedom by forcing her to be on bed rest so unethical that it should mean the difference between life and death for her fetus? In certain circumstances, we may have to decide whether restrictions can be placed on the mother's autonomy in the best interest (beneficence) of the fetus, depending on the mother's competence or other extenuating circumstances.

The case of Samantha Burton: Hospitalizing a pregnant woman by court order

Samantha Burton was a pregnant unwed mother of two children who experienced premature rupture of membranes in March 2009 at 25 weeks gestation of her third pregnancy. She sought care at Tallahassee General Hospital in Florida. Her obstetrician ordered her to be hospitalized on bed rest to prevent the preterm birth and almost certain death of her fetus. She wanted to leave the hospital to care for her two children. She also had two jobs to maintain.

The case was immediately brought to the Leon County Circuit Court. Ms. Burton was forced to argue her case by telephone from her hospital bed without proper legal representation. The court ordered Ms. Burton to remain hospitalized and undergo "any and all medical treatments" that her physician deemed necessary. Three days after her court-ordered treatment, the patient underwent an emergency C-section, and the baby was born dead. In August 2009, Ms. Burton, along with the ACLU, filed an amicus brief charging that the state deprived her of her physical liberty, right to privacy, and autonomy. The case was decided in Ms. Burton's favor in August 2010 by the Florida District Court of Appeals.

Where do medical groups stand on the issue of self-determination? The American College of Obstetrics and Gynecology states that doctors should not perform procedures on pregnant women who don't want them done, and that the courts ideally should not be brought into the situation to resolve a conflict. The focus should be on doing what is medically ethical and in the best interest of the patient in a given situation. The AMA states that going to court to override a pregnant woman's medical decision, as long as it made with informed consent, is inappropriate and does not respect her autonomy.

Balancing treatments for a woman and fetus

Given these ethical considerations, you, the provider, must balance the health of the mother and fetus during a pregnancy.

Some over-the-counter (OTC) medications and prescription medications are fine for the mother and fetus; others should be taken only when necessary, and others should be avoided.

There are medical treatments for the mother that can harm the fetus. They include

- Treatments for maternal cancer
- Diagnostic tests such as x-rays or CAT scans

- ✔ Prescription medications such as accutane, tetracycline, valium, warfarin, some blood pressure meds, and sulfa antibiotics
- ✔ Live vaccines, including measles, rubella, and yellow fever

And there are medical treatments for the fetus that have the potential to harm the mother. They include

- ✔ Forced caesarian sections
- ✔ Keeping a terminally ill mother alive through medical intervention to keep the fetus alive until viability
- ✔ In-utero operations on the fetus

In the past several decades, some pregnant women have been given blood transfusions, been forced to undergo surgery, and detained in hospitals when their doctors thought they were violating medical advice. Many courts will consider the fetus's right to life, especially in the third trimester when it is in conflict with a woman's right to privacy and autonomy. An unintended consequence of these decisions is that at-risk women may avoid prenatal care for fear of being forced into treatment against their will.

Many courts have issued different rulings about fetal rights versus maternal rights. This sets contradictory precedents and can be confusing for providers who are trying to care for their patients. At this time, there isn't a consistent standard about the legal status of a mother who endangers her fetus by refusing medical treatment.

There are also problems with medical uncertainty. You often will advise a patient based on what is likely, but not guaranteed, to happen. In some cases where a pregnant woman has refused medical advice, her baby was born healthy, without the problems or issues the doctors predicted.

You, the provider, should talk to your patient and explain the situation and possible outcomes. It's important to stress the relative risks and benefits of any medical procedure, both to her and her fetus, as well as the risks and benefits of choosing to forgo the procedure. Most women want to deliver a healthy baby and will undergo significant risk to achieve that goal.

The role of technology

In the last 50 years the point of viability where the fetus can live outside the womb has been reduced from 28 to 24 weeks gestation. But, the fetus still requires extensive mechanical support to survive at that point. Technology has developed so the fetus can now be seen as it grows in the womb. A fetus can be monitored, diagnosed, and treated — even operated on — before birth. There are many prenatal diagnostic tests that literally open a window into the uterus.

The ethical principles involved here are justice and autonomy for the mother, and nonmaleficence and beneficence for the mother and fetus. If we force a pregnant woman to undergo some type of treatment because of the fetus she carries, we are imposing an obligation on her that we don't impose on men or nonpregnant women, which is unjust. Are pregnant women autonomous in the same way that men and nonpregnant women are? On the other hand, she has, in most cases, chosen to be pregnant and carry a fetus, and we want medical care to provide the greatest benefit to both of them.

Fetal surgery is the latest technological advance that poses the most risk to the mother. There are two types of fetal surgery: open and fetoscopic. Open surgery means the uterus is cut open and the fetus operated on. In fetoscopic surgery, also called *key-hole* surgery, fiber-optic instruments are inserted through small openings cut into the uterus.

In 1990, "Baby Blake" underwent major surgery while in the womb, and was born healthy seven weeks later. This was the first time a fetus was treated as a *second patient*. In the early years of in-utero surgery, most of the fetuses did not survive. It is now effective only for a small number of birth defects. This type of surgery is performed only about 600 times a year in the United States, and only some of those surgeries are successful.

Doctors do not perform in-utero surgery on fetuses that have incurable health problems. Prolonging the life of a fetus in that state is unethical. And fetal surgery is performed only when the benefits of surgery clearly outweigh the risks of the procedure to both the mother and the fetus.

Fetoscopic surgery, similar to arthroscopic surgery, is more promising. This is a minimally invasive procedure done by inserting a fiber-optic endoscope through small incisions into the uterus. Ultrasound is used to guide the surgeon's instruments. Fetoscopic surgery holds less risk for the mother and the fetus, although preterm labor can occur. Open womb surgery risks include bleeding, preterm labor, complications with anesthesia, and infection.

These technological advances have changed our view of pregnancy, making a gestation more accessible to doctors and more manageable. This also led to the idea that if the fetus can be treated apart from its mother, and has medical needs of its own, it should have legal and moral interests of its own. In fact, some doctors call the uterus after a fetal surgery "the best possible intensive care unit."

What does this mean for our ethical dilemma of maternal versus fetal rights? Usually mothers will choose these procedures because it is in the best interest of the fetus. But does this place the same ethical and moral status on the fetus and the mother? Does this give the fetus, who by law is not a full person, autonomy? Could a procedure such as fetoscopy be forced on a mother for the sake of the fetus even against the mother's wishes or her own autonomy? These are difficult questions that have yet to be resolved. Ethics just seems to get more complicated with the advancement of technology.

Considering a Father's Rights

Peg Bracken once wrote that she thought men who were expecting a baby should undergo some type of physical change as well, such as enlarged hands or feet, so they could understand the process and be easily identified to all. We all know this doesn't happen, although men can wear the Empathy Belly that simulates pregnancy.

Men do not have legal rights in a pregnancy or any decision-making power or rights over the fetus while it is in the womb.

Paternal rights relate to confidentiality. Should a woman tell a man he is a father? Can someone be forced into a paternity test? And what about genetic testing kits, sold over the Internet, that claim to establish paternity?

In the 1990s, paternity testing rates in the United States doubled. Paternity testing can be conducted on the fetus in the womb between 10 and 24 weeks gestation, using chorionic villa sampling (CVS) or amniocentesis, but it's most often done after the birth of the baby. There are risks to the mother and fetus with the prenatal procedures.

Paternity testing through DNA test can be ordered by the court system. Until paternity has been established, and if there is no legal father, anyone undergoing a paternity test is called a *putative father*. The state has an interest in the welfare of the child and wants the father to support the baby.

In 2005, British researchers wrote in the *Journal of Epidemiology and Community Health* that 4 percent of all fathers in that country were raising children who were not their biological offspring. Learning that a child you thought was your own is actually someone else's can destroy families and change lives. Counseling and support services should always be available when this information is obtained.

Sam's case: A man struggles with his girlfriend's decision

Sam was a freshman in college who visited a doctor at the college health service. Since the beginning of the year, he had struggled with depression and insomnia. Upon discussion with the doctor, he shared something. In his senior year of high school, his girlfriend of two years became pregnant. Although he wanted to keep the pregnancy and help her raise the child, she did not. She was afraid to tell her parents and wanted to go on to college. Even though he disagreed with her decision, he went with her when she had the abortion. The relationship ended, and he was feeling guilt, grief, and sadness over his loss. The doctor referred him to a counselor to let him work through his feelings.

Counselors are concerned about the well-being and even safety of the women and children involved in contested paternity cases. Paternity tests can be requested by the mother, the father, or the child, or, with a court order, by men who think they may have biological children.

What's the healthcare provider's role in all this? Confidentiality. If a woman comes to you and says her husband is not the father of her fetus, this must remain confidential. Mothers who request paternity tests do not have to share the results with the father. Standards of confidentiality apply in this case. No healthcare provider should share the results of a paternity test with anyone without the express written consent of the mother. It's important to discuss the results with the mother and encourage her to share the information with interested parties. But your role ends after counseling your patient.

When a man is involved throughout a woman's pregnancy, caring for him is also important, especially if you are caring for the whole family. Even though fathers don't have many rights in pregnancy, they may be emotionally involved in it. The primary ethical issue here is beneficence.

Birth Control

The advent of the birth control pill changed women's lives forever. In fact, the advent of accessible and reliable birth control has changed society. Birth control has given women a more reliable way to prevent both unwanted pregnancies and dependence on one particular man because of a shared biological child.

There are two kinds of birth control: one prevents fertilization, such as the pill and barrier methods, and the other prevents implantation, such as the IUD and morning-after pill. Some people feel that this second type of birth control is actually abortion because rather than preventing the egg from being fertilized, these forms of birth control prevent a fertilized egg from implanting in the uterine lining.

In this section, we look at counseling a patient on birth control, providers who are opposed to certain forms of birth control, and religious views on birth control.

Educating your patient about birth control

Parental consent isn't required to treat minors in certain situations such as sex education and prescribing contraceptives. In some states, minors can seek an abortion without parental permission. *Mature minors,* or minor children who are old enough to understand the consequences of sexual acts, can get treatment for STDs, prescriptions for birth control, and other treatment related to sexuality. (See Chapter 8 for more on adolescents and parental consent.)

Establishing policies among partners for prescribing birth control

It's important to think about how your personal religious views affect the way you practice medicine and how this will affect your partners. I have some physician friends who are opposed to prescribing birth control because of their religious faith. They feel this is wrong and can't in good conscience write these prescriptions. It is important for these doctors to follow their beliefs, but also to recognize how this affects their patients and partners. It can be difficult for patients get the medicine that is legally available to them, especially in emergency situations.

This can also place an extra burden on their partners in practice who find themselves filling a lot of birth control prescriptions for patients they have never seen. And what happens when one of these doctors is on call and gets a request for emergency contraception? The group must have a backup plan in place. This can lead to divisions within a group of providers.

In my experience, it works well for providers who share a similar view to work together in a practice. And the patient must be told about these views when they walk through the door of a clinic. For instance, a Christian clinic could be set up where prayers are offered with patients, abortions are not offered, and birth control is not prescribed. Patients who share these views are often happy to have a clinic where their religious practice can be a part of their medical experience.

The ethical issues of autonomy and informed consent come into play here. A teenage girl and adult women should receive all of the information necessary to make the best decisions about her health.

When counseling a patient about birth control, you should tell her:

- ✔ How to use the method, and if there are any special precautions
- ✔ How reliable that method is
- ✔ Any risks of the method, including risk of STDs
- ✔ Side effects or other health concerns, including the circumstances under which it should not be used
- ✔ Any health risks involved in that method
- ✔ What to do if the birth control method fails

When a patient requests a certain type of birth control, you should provide it unless there is a medical reason not to. If you object to counseling or prescribing any type of contraception, refer your patient to another doctor who can tell her about all of her options.

The age of consent in most states is 16. A person younger than the age of consent may verbally agree to sex, but that person is considered too young to understand all of the implications of sex. When a girl under 16 becomes pregnant by an older teenager or an adult, this is called *statutory rape,* and the man can be prosecuted (for example by the girl's parents), even if she consented to sex. In fact, medical providers are mandatory reporters if statutory rape is suspected.

Balancing your beliefs about birth control with a patient's rights

A difficult ethical situation arises when a medical professional, such as a doctor or a pharmacist, refuses to prescribe or fill a medication based on personal or religious beliefs. It seems unethical to force a provider to go against deeply held personal standards. But on the other hand, the ethical principles of patient autonomy, beneficence, and nonmaleficence are violated when a patient is refused a medical treatment or prescription that they need and have a right to by law.

For example, a pharmacist may refuse to fill a prescription for a birth control pill based on his religious beliefs. This dilemma may be solved by simply transferring the prescription to another pharmacy. But what if that pharmacy is the only one in town? What if the patient needs the prescription urgently for emergency contraception? What if a physician in a group refuses to prescribe birth control and his partner requires the patient to be seen again before writing the prescription? All of these scenarios place an undue burden on the patient for simply obtaining a legal medication. Is this ethical? This is currently an ongoing discussion, not only in ethics, but in law and politics as well.

The American Pharmacists Association has taken the position that pharmacists can refuse to fill a prescription if it violates their personal standards. But if they do, someone else must fill it, or the prescription must be transferred to another pharmacy without delay. Two states have laws, called *conscience clauses* or *refusal laws,* that protect pharmacists and other medical providers who will not fill birth control prescriptions based on personal beliefs.

Understanding religious ethics and birth control

Religious ethics and edicts play a large part in the lives of many people. Devout members of some religions choose to forgo medical treatment. Some religions prohibit certain types of treatment. And religious ethics can play a large part in birth control. In any case, it's important for you, the provider, to understand different religions' points of view about this issue so you can treat your patient. And you must respect your patient's decision about whether to use birth control and which type to use.

The different religions and their views on birth control include:

- ✔ **Catholic Church:** Formally, the Catholic Church opposes all forms of artificial birth control because they believe that human beings should not oppose or thwart the natural God-given end of human sexuality, which is the procreation of children. They support birth control through abstinence and natural family planning (NFP), or the rhythm method, which follows the natural pattern of fertility in the woman, to avoid pregnancy. Not all Catholics adhere to this standard.

- ✔ **Judaism:** Jews have several views on birth control, depending on their branch. Orthodox Jews approve of birth control when a couple already has some children. Conservative Jews allow birth control in more situations, and Reform Judaism lets its followers use their own judgment.

- ✔ **Protestantism:** Most liberal Protestants such as Presbyterians and Anglicans hold that birth control is entirely acceptable and a matter of personal privacy and conscience between the individual and their god. Some Evangelical Protestants disagree with this view. They condemn the type of birth control that works to prevent implantation of the blastocyst, such as the IUD. Some consider that an abortion.

- ✔ **Islam:** The Islam faith does not oppose birth control, except to state that in a marriage, birth control should be used with the full knowledge and consent of both parties. They oppose permanent sterility.

- ✔ **Hindu:** Hindu scholars do not ban birth control. They do believe that there is a duty for adults to have children at a certain stage of life.

- ✔ **Sikhism:** Sikhs do not object to birth control, considering it a private matter relevant only to the parties directly involved.

It's important to remember that religious beliefs about birth control are important to both patients and providers. But your personal beliefs should not interfere with your patient's right to the care they want and deserve. If you are a firm believer in birth control and abortion, but your patient is not, it is unethical to lecture them about this stance, and vice versa. You can talk about the medical facts, but the final decision about the type of birth control used, if any, is up to your patient.

Fetal Abuse

Fetal abuse is a relatively new area of medicine. This concept goes hand in hand with *fetal rights,* the idea that fetuses should have the same legal rights and protections as children. In other words, under certain conditions, pregnant women could be arrested and charged with fetal abuse.

Homicide is the number one cause of death of pregnant women. In 2004 in the United States, the Unborn Victims of Violence Act (UVVA) was signed into law. It made killing or injuring a fetus while attacking a pregnant women a crime against the fetus. The law does not apply to abortion, to any type of medical treatment, or any act or omission of an act by the mother. However, some are concerned that this law grants an independent legal status to the fetus and may lead to criminalization of a mother's behavior while pregnant.

These laws are based on the principle of nonmaleficence toward the fetus. But, in certain circumstances, the concept of "do no harm" to the fetus can infringe on the mother's rights or autonomy, if, for instance, the mother is hospitalized against her will or prosecuted for conduct that endangers the fetus.

Women's rights advocates do not like this trend toward charging mothers who may neglect or abuse their bodies, and therefore their fetuses. Advocates believe that this standard limits a woman's autonomy and will make many pregnant women avoid healthcare altogether, resulting in more problems for mothers and children down the road.

In this section, we look at maternal behavior that some think should be called crimes against the fetus, such as maternal drug abuse. We also explain how to detect fetal abuse and the provider's ethical and legal obligations, as well as the issue of limiting maternal freedom for the health and well-being of the fetus.

Maternal drug abuse or neglect: Crimes against the fetus

In the late 1980s, the story of *crack babies* (babies whose mothers used crack cocaine while pregnant) got a lot of media attention. More than 30 states in America started charging female crack and cocaine users with child abuse and even manslaughter. Many of these cases were thrown out of court because the precedence of *Roe v. Wade* has established that a fetus is not a person and, therefore, crimes cannot be committed against it. That is changing; 30 states now have some laws on the books protecting the fetus from harmful behavior by its mother.

As long as a woman is competent, she has autonomy and can make decisions about her own body. But are there conditions where a mother's competence is questioned? How about a severe drug addiction or mental illness? Nonpregnant patients can be committed based on these conditions if they pose a significant harm to themselves or others. How about if they pose a significant risk to the fetus? We are right back to the ongoing conflict between a mother's autonomy and the concern for the principles of nonmaleficence and beneficence for both the mother and fetus.

Crack babies and fetal alcohol syndrome

While prosecutors were charging pregnant drug users with crimes against their fetuses, the most common drug use that causes the most birth defects went unpunished: alcohol. Some early studies about crack use were alarming, leading many scientists to believe that this drug was causing a serious problem with newborns. However, the huge onslaught of crack babies never occurred. Hospitals never reported a huge increase in drug-addicted children.

So what caused the uproar? Researchers have found that pregnant women who use crack and cocaine are more likely to drink alcohol, smoke cigarettes, use other drugs, get less prenatal care, and have poorer nutrition. Those factors were causing many of the problems doctors were seeing. And the ethical issue in this problem is that although crack mothers were arrested and prosecuted, mothers who drank alcohol and smoked cigarettes were not. It's worth noting that the majority of women who are prosecuted with these crimes are poor and minorities. One study in Florida showed that black women were ten times more likely to be reported for drug use than white women. And both groups of women used drugs during pregnancy. It's also problematic that there are far more charges of fetal abuse brought against drug users than alcoholics because fetal alcohol syndrome is the number one cause of preventable birth defects in America.

Detecting fetal abuse: Ethical and legal obligations

Healthcare providers walk a fine line when they suspect fetal abuse, and detecting fetal abuse can be difficult. A mother rarely admits to a behavior that can harm the fetus.

Here are some clues to look for when seeing a pregnant patient:

- ✔ Poor fetal growth on abdomen measurements or ultrasound
- ✔ Poor weight gain of the mother
- ✔ Fetal tachycardia suggesting stimulant use
- ✔ History or signs of maternal alcohol or drug abuse
- ✔ History or signs of anorexia or bulimia
- ✔ Worsening depression or apathy toward the pregnancy
- ✔ History or signs of domestic abuse

Ellen's case: Intervening when drug abuse is suspected

Ellen was a pregnant patient suspected of relapsing into heroin addiction. When she presented to the hospital in active labor, a concerned family member made an anonymous phone call to the doctor, telling him that the patient had been using narcotics heavily, including just the past few days. A toxicology test at the time of the delivery was positive for narcotics.

According to state law, the doctor notified Child Protective Services. The baby was immediately taken from the mother, and after receiving treatment for narcotic withdrawal, was placed in foster care. The mother was sent to an in-patient drug treatment clinic for 30 days. Upon successful completion of the treatment, the baby was returned to her. Social Services continued to be involved, and she received outpatient counseling.

The AMA states that because there are not enough drug treatment centers and services for pregnant women, criminal charges against them on the grounds of child abuse are unfair. They punish a woman for not seeking treatment that is usually unavailable. These punishments are also not applied fairly across race, sex, and economic status, which violates the principle of justice.

Healthcare providers should ask all of their patients about drug and alcohol use, and educate them about the risks and harms of that use. But reporting a pregnant drug user to the authorities is indicated only if she poses a severe threat of harm to herself or others. The AMA states that: "Pregnant substance abusers should be provided with rehabilitative treatment appropriate to their specific physiological and psychological needs." However, as the fetus approaches viability, concerns about its well-being become more urgent. A baby born addicted to heroin or methamphetamine, for example, requires preparation for resuscitation and ongoing NICU treatment after delivery. A mother who has a positive toxicology screen in labor may be reported to Child Protective Services, and they will assist with alternate care for the infant while the woman undergoes treatment.

The problem with a legal punishment approach to the problem of pregnant women taking drugs and alcohol is that punitive measures such as jailing a woman do not allow for ongoing prenatal care or treatment of the addiction. Doctors worry that if they start policing pregnant women and must report them to the authorities for drug and alcohol abuse, those women will just avoid medical care altogether, which would mean more harm for both mother and fetus. These laws and statutes also interfere with the confidential relationship between a doctor and patient.

Educate your patients *before* they become pregnant about the danger of drug and alcohol consumption while pregnant. If you suspect a pregnant woman is drinking or abusing drugs, talk to her about it in a nonjudgmental way. Offer help, counseling, or referral to clinics or other providers with specific experience in this area.

Some states do have statutes that require providers to report the use of controlled, illegal substances by pregnant women. Toxicology tests are routinely given to some newborns, and those reports are given to law enforcement. Some babies have been taken away from their mothers after these tests have showed positive results.

Limiting maternal freedom for fetal well-being

In some pregnancies, mothers are advised to stay in bed to help the fetus mature until birth. Other times they must take certain medications, or undergo some type of treatment. In some cases the courts have been involved and have imposed medical care upon pregnant women.

It's important to communicate with a pregnant woman who refuses treatment that will help the fetus. If the treatment doesn't impose an undue burden on her, you should make sure she understands the situation. If necessary, a psychiatrist can be brought in to evaluate the woman's competence, and if she is found to be incompetent, the courts can be brought in to help clarify the situation.

Always document all discussions with your patient and recommendations about actions or behaviors that could cause prenatal harm. If your patient continues to persist in harmful behavior despite your advice to stop, you can

- ✔ Continue care, if you feel your relationship with the patient is good and referring her to another doctor might compromise the patient's health or continuity of care.

- ✔ Refer the patient to another doctor if you feel that the outcome may be better for the patient.

- ✔ Talk to an ethics committee and, as a very last resort, the legal system about an intervention. You may discuss getting a court order for an order of commitment or protective custody if there is a risk of serious harm to the fetus that a medical intervention will prevent.

Limiting the freedom of pregnant women for the well-being of the fetus is a last resort and should only be tried when there is significant risk of harm to the fetus. The circumstances for this type of action should be very narrowly defined. Courts are more likely to restrict maternal freedom when the fetus is at or very near the point of viability.

The issue of brain-dead pregnant women is also relevant here. If a woman's body is going to be kept alive just so her fetus can develop to the point of viability, certain conditions must be met. They are:

- ✔ The family, preferably the father of the fetus, should agree. Providers should ask about what the mother would have wanted.

- ✔ There should be a reasonable chance that the fetus will reach viability in a reasonable amount of time. Keeping a brain-dead woman on life support for months is usually inappropriate.

- ✔ The dignity of the woman must be preserved.

- ✔ Each case should be decided individually.

And finally, forced Caesarean sections do limit maternal freedom. In some cases, women have been forced into a C-section to purportedly save the life of the fetus, or if providers are concerned about a problematic lifestyle, like drug abuse. In 1987, the *New England Journal of Medicine* published a study which found that when courts have ordered Caesarean sections over the objections of the mother, 81 percent of the women were black, Asian, or Hispanic, and 100 percent of the women were poor. These statistics have serious implications for the ethical principle of justice. If forced Caesareans are going to be indicated, they must be applied equally across all factors, including race, income, and marital status.

Seeing into the Future: Prenatal and Genetic Testing

Prenatal and genetic testing has offered a wonderful window into the womb and has led to the birth of many more healthy babies. But there are ethical issues and risks associated with these tests. Patients need to be informed of the risks and benefits of each procedure. And counseling should always be part of genetic testing. Initial testing can be done with blood tests and obstetric ultrasound. Then, if needed, more invasive testing can be used to further clarify a diagnosis.

Invasive genetic testing may be recommended for several reasons:

- ✔ A problem noted in an ultrasound

- ✔ A family history of a genetic disease

- ✔ Abnormal maternal serum markers (quad scan) test or nuchal scan

- ✔ A previous child diagnosed with an abnormality

- ✔ Maternal age, because the risk of a baby with birth defects increases over the age of 35

✔ If a woman has already had two or more miscarriages

✔ If a child has been stillborn with genetic abnormalities

✔ If the mother or her partner are carriers of a dominant gene for a disease such as Huntington's Disease

✔ If the mother and her partner are carriers of a recessive gene for a disease such as cystic fibrosis

The decision about testing and any further procedures is up to the woman. Even if a woman has risk factors for some of these diseases, she can choose not to have testing done because of the ethical principle of autonomy.

In this section, we look at the ethical use of prenatal testing, the risks and benefits of these tests, and how to share results of prenatal and genetic testing with parents.

Many women who receive a diagnosis of a compromised fetus will choose to continue their pregnancy, but all women should be told that abortion is an option if they choose it, with no restrictions in the first trimester, but with restrictions after that, depending on state law.

Prenatal testing can be offered to all pregnant women, but is more strongly indicated in certain situations. Every woman who needs testing should be able to get it, whether it's because her family carries a genetic disease, she is an older patient, or a diagnostic test suggests it. But providing prenatal testing to every pregnant woman just to learn more about her fetus may not be a good use of our limited healthcare resources. Some providers are also worried that repeated ultrasounds and other tests may prove harmful to the fetus. And some ethicists feel that overuse of testing may pressure women to consider abortion if problems are found.

Understanding the ethical use of prenatal testing

Some type of noninvasive screening should take place before prenatal or genetic testing is offered. These tests include ultrasound and maternal blood tests. It's important to remember that although there are no proven risks of ultrasound, it may not be without risk to the fetus. Ultrasound should not be used for vanity purposes, or just to get a picture of the developing fetus for a scrapbook.

Before any invasive prenatal testing is done, the parent(s) should be informed of all of the risks and benefits relating to the procedure. They need to be told how the test will be conducted, when to expect results, what the test will tell them, and their options after the test.

Some women who undergo prenatal testing get this information with the idea of terminating a pregnancy if a serious defect is found. Some want to know about their child's potential condition so they can be mentally and financially prepared to take care of it. Financial and logistical planning to care for a disabled child takes time and effort.

Whatever choice parents make about their unborn children should be respected. They are the ones who must raise the child. It's also important to remember that when a high-risk pregnancy is suspected, prenatal testing can reassure the parents with negative results, or there may be an opportunity to repair the fetus in-utero.

Some of the genetic diseases we can screen for include late onset diseases, or diseases that present relatively late in life. For example, we can now screen for breast cancer genes. If a woman has these genes, her chance of developing breast cancer is greatly increased, although it is not a given. Screening for potential future diseases raises ethical issues. Should abortion be offered for a fetus that carries a breast cancer gene? Many ethicists think that making a choice for the fetus regarding something that may happen years in the future is unethical and voids the autonomy of the future person.

What about diseases such as Huntington's Disease? If the fetus has this gene, the person will develop this devastating disease, for which there is no cure. The disease usually manifests between the ages of 30 and 50. Any child of a person who has Huntington's has a 50 percent chance of receiving the gene. Because most geneticists believe that a 10 percent risk of a disease is high, a 50 percent risk is too high for many. Many ethicists think that people with Huntington's disease should undergo in vitro fertilization and choose a fetus without the Huntington's gene in preimplantation diagnosis. For more information about the ethics of these procedures, see Chapter 17.

But what if the parents want to know that the fetus does or doesn't have the gene? Do they have a right to this information? There are several issues relevant to this question.

- ✔ The autonomy of the parents need to be balanced with the autonomy of the fetus now and the potential person later.

- ✔ Can a provider refuse to give a medical test to a patient who requests it without being paternalistic?

- ✔ Should any diseases or disabilities be considered severe enough to defend selective abortion, and if so, which ones? Who gets to decide?

- ✔ Who is the patient: the woman or the fetus?

- ✔ Should parents be allowed to make decisions for their future child about diseases that present later in life?

We must also remember that most birth defects and disabilities are caused by poor prenatal care, exposure to drugs, alcohol, cigarettes, poverty, and poor nutrition — all issues that can be addressed without prenatal testing. By spending so much of our resources on prenatal testing, we may not be addressing the biggest risk factors to a fetus's health.

Understanding tests and accuracy issues

Currently, pregnant women are offered a number of different screening tests in the first trimester. Fetal abnormalities can be detected by checking certain markers in the mother's blood and by doing early ultrasounds on the spinal cord (nuchal cord translucency). The most commonly used test in many practices is the quad screen. This is a maternal blood test performed between 16 to 18 weeks gestation to determine if there is an increased risk of Down syndrome, trisomy 18, or neural tube defect. If any of the early, less invasive tests suggest problems with the embryo or fetus, further, more invasive testing may be recommended.

In amniocentesis, amniotic fluid surrounding the fetus is withdrawn using ultrasound-guided insertion of a needle through the abdominal wall. The cells are cultured, and chromosomes from those cells are studied to see if abnormalities are present. There are risks associated with this procedure, so it is usually not performed unless a woman is older than 35, or there is a history of genetic abnormalities in her or her partner's family. There is generally a 1 percent risk of miscarriage during amniocentesis. The procedure is performed between 15 and 20 weeks, well into the second trimester. Amniocentesis can check for 40 of the 4,000 known abnormalities.

Some genetic abnormalities that can be tested for using amniocentesis include

- Down syndrome, or trisomy 21
- Tay-Sachs disease
- Sickle cell anemia
- Muscular dystrophy
- Trisomy 13 and 18
- Turner and Klinefelter syndrome
- Cystic fibrosis
- Neural tube defects like anencephaly and spina bifida

There is another method for diagnosing genetic abnormalities in the fetus. Chorionic Villus Sampling, or CVS, is used to detect chromosomal disorders such as cystic fibrosis or sickle cell disease. The doctor removes some of the villi, or hair-like projections, from the placenta and tests them. The miscarriage rate for CVS is slightly higher than for amniocentesis.

CVS does not detect neural tube disorders, so it doesn't have the scope of amniocentesis. The CVS test is performed in the first trimester, so an abortion, if requested, can be performed earlier. Some women want to have this test before their pregnancy is externally visible, so if ending it is the best choice for them they can keep the decision private.

Test results from amniocentesis and Chorionic Villus Sampling are very accurate. Amniocentesis results are usually 99.4 percent accurate. And CVS results are usually 99 percent accurate. The tests are not 100 percent accurate because in rare cases the doctor can't collect enough amniotic fluid or cells to perform a test, or the cells may not grow after harvest.

In addition to the risks associated with each test, the risks of false positives and false negatives is a reality, too. More than one diagnostic test should be offered to women who are classified as high risk, especially if the results are positive in early tests. It's important to note that there is no prenatal test, or group of tests, that can detect all types of abnormalities, genetic diseases, and birth defects.

Although these tests can diagnose genetic abnormalities, they cannot predict the severity of the resulting disorder. Some children with genetic abnormalities can live a fairly normal life. And in some cases, diseases such as hemophilia only present in a male child.

Some birth defects can't be detected through any available test. A child who is born blind or deaf or with a cleft palate cannot be diagnosed with these tests. So even though these tests can offer some peace of mind, it's important that you, the provider, let the family know that having good results on these tests does not guarantee a perfectly healthy baby.

It's important to remember that these tests are very stressful and draining for the parents and family. Genetic counseling both before and after the test is highly recommended. If the results are bad and the mother wants to abort, time is of the essence. Still, giving the patient space and time to come to the correct decision for her is ethically mandated.

Genetic counseling and sharing results with parents

Counseling should always be offered, if not mandated, when prenatal testing is done. Your responsibility to your patient extends beyond taking care of her physical body. You must offer support and compassion for her emotional needs as well.

The National Society of Genetic Counselors was established in 1979. Screenings for genetic and birth defects raise ethical questions, and the counselors are trained to explain screening results and the choices that arise from those results. Most women should go through counseling with a genetic counselor before and after testing is done.

Genetic counselors have their own standards of ethics. The codes that relate to interaction with clients include

- Serve patients who need your services without bias and objectively.
- Respect your patient's beliefs, circumstances, feelings, cultural traditions, and family relationships.
- Work to help your patients make informed decisions, with no coercion.
- Provide the facts, clarify the alternatives, and list the consequences.

Counselors should not let their own beliefs and biases enter into counseling any patient. Autonomy should always be respected, and patients should be told the truth. This is called *client-centered, nondirective counseling. Directive counseling,* or counseling with suggestions or unsolicited advice, is only ethical when the person(s) involved cannot give informed consent.

Because the results of prenatal testing can be devastating, counseling should always be paired with the genetic tests. Test results should always be revealed in face-to-face meetings, never through a phone call, letter, or e-mail.

The possible results should be discussed before the actual results are available, so your patient has an idea what may happen and can prepare herself. Information about prognosis, long-term care for a child with a disability, and assessment of psychological needs is also important.

Counselors should also stress that there is no such thing as the perfect baby. And no test can guarantee that a baby will be perfectly healthy, no matter how many tests are performed or how well the mother takes care of her body during pregnancy.

Chapter 10

When Science Supersedes Sex: Reproductive Technology and Surrogacy

*I*t's not nice to fool Mother Nature! Remember that margarine commercial? Well, doctors and scientists fool Mother Nature on a regular basis these days, especially when it comes to reproductive technology. When Louise Brown was conceived in a test tube (actually it was a petri dish) in 1977, some people believed that she would have serious physical, emotional, or psychological problems because of the way her life began. As it turned out, Louise is now 32 years old, healthy, and has a son of her own. And Louise is not alone. Since then, the number of children born by assisted reproductive technology is estimated at 3 million babies.

Assisted reproductive technology (ART) has come a long way since that time. Now infertile couples or single women can have a biological child in several different ways. In vitro fertilization, artificial insemination, and surrogacy can improve the chances of having a child for anyone who can pay for it.

If science helps a woman produce a biological child she would not otherwise have, is assisted reproduction ethical? One answer lies in autonomy or individual choice. If science can help an infertile couple have a child, they can afford it, and that is what they want, some people feel no one else should have the right to interfere in a personal decision or deny a legal medical treatment. If we look at ART more closely, however, the ethical arguments against it center on harm. As we will see, there is increased risk of potential harm to a child born through ART. Is it ethical to endanger a child before that child has been brought into existence? Is there harm that can come to the mother as well? The potential harm to mother and fetus must be weighed against the mother or couple's autonomy.

In addition, some of these procedures create embryos that may never be implanted or will be discarded. What is the moral status of these embryos? We spend a great deal of time in Chapter 11 looking at the ethical arguments around personhood and how this relates to termination of embryos, so this won't be discussed here, but this issue is essential to the ethical critique of reproductive technologies.

In this chapter, we look at the ethics surrounding these techniques. We look at in vitro fertilization (IVF) and some of the objections to this procedure. What about *pre-implantation genetic diagnosis* (PIGD), which is evaluating embryos for genetic defects before implantation? Is it ethical to discard embryos with genetic defects to prevent children with these defects from being born? We also look at the type of risks that are both acceptable and unacceptable to the woman involved in these procedures. And what happens when IVF works too well, and suddenly a woman is carrying six or more embryos? Is selective reduction, or removal of some of the embryos so that others can live, an ethical practice? We also examine the ethics of artificial insemination, which is a much more widely accepted practice. Surrogacy, however, has been a contentious subject. And sterilization, whether voluntary or not, is examined.

In Vitro Fertilization

In vitro fertilization is one of those topics of medicine that seems to provoke all kinds of opinions. Before Louise Brown, most laypeople thought that we would never be able to make babies by artificial means. (For more on Ms. Brown, see Chapter 19.) Yet today IVF is an accepted and almost routine form of conception.

In vitro fertilization works like this: A woman is given fertility drugs and then eggs are harvested via a surgical procedure. The eggs are combined with sperm from the father under just the right conditions in a petri dish in a lab. If the father's sperm have motility problems, the sperm can be injected directly into the egg, in a process called *intracytoplasmic sperm injection* (ICSI). The resulting *blastocysts* (what the fertilized egg becomes before it grows into an embryo) are then examined for genetic defects, and healthy ones implanted in the woman's uterus. And hopefully, a baby is born in about nine months. Each IVF session has about a 25 percent chance of success and costs between $5,000 and $10,000. Insurance doesn't pay for this technology.

In this section, we look at the ethical questions of IVF and genetic diagnosis of blastocysts. We try to understand acceptable versus unacceptable harm to the women involved in this procedure, what to do when IVF results in a multiple pregnancy, and the ethics behind embryo storage and destruction. And what about cost? IVF is extremely expensive, and the chances of success are low. This violates the principle of justice regarding equal access to healthcare. But then again, as we state in Chapter 6, not all people can receive all the healthcare they want. Even in a universal healthcare system, some treatments are rationed by cost. And choosing to have a child seems ethically different than being treated for an illness such as cancer.

IVF is a much more precise procedure than it used to be. Multiple pregnancies from this type of conception have decreased, although there are still more multiple births than with natural, or spontaneous, conception. Most clinics now will not implant more than three embryos at once for women under the age of 35. If the woman is older, more embryos are usually implanted. Other ways of inducing ovulation are much more likely to result in multiple pregnancies.

Understanding acceptable versus unacceptable harm

In IVF, the mother, fetus, and any egg donors all face some degree of risk. In this section, we cover some of what's at stake. Harm is really at the core of some of the ethical arguments around IVF. A mother has the autonomy to choose IVF, but does she really understand the potential harms that can come to her and her baby?

Helping couples cope with infertility

In my experience, one of the most difficult medical situations for a couple is infertility, both from an emotional and physical standpoint. I make sure counseling is part of my patients' treatment when discussing reproductive technology. I also keep in close contact with my patients so they have another ally during a very difficult journey. Infertility can be all-consuming. The emotional highs and lows are very difficult. A woman tries to conceive and then waits with hope, excitement, and fear for the first pregnancy test. If it's negative, there's a huge sense of grief and loss. There's also plenty of self-blame. Questions I have heard are "Is it my fault?" "Am I too thin or fat?" "Is it because of bad habits in my past?" "Did I wait too long to try to get pregnant?" "Is God punishing me?"

Infertility is also very hard on a couple's relationship and intimacy. And then there are the invasive medical procedures, such as artificial insemination and egg harvesting for in vitro fertilizations. The hormones that women must take contribute to mood swings and other physical symptoms. Most good infertility clinics include regular counseling as part of the treatment.

Harm to the woman

In IVF, harm to women can occur in many ways. Emotional and psychological suffering can occur throughout the rigorous treatment. The hormone shots can cause mood swings. The surgery to harvest the eggs is invasive. And the stress of trying to conceive, after months or years of infertility, can be enormous. The financial burden can also be significant.

Most women think that those risks are worth it, if they can become pregnant. But women must be completely informed about other risks. Even with pre-screened, apparently healthy embryos, there isn't a guarantee that a healthy and normal baby will be born. That's a risk all pregnant women take, but it must be stressed with IVF.

Other risks and harm can be serious. Before any woman goes through an IVF procedure, these risks must be clearly explained for informed consent.

✔ Drugs used to create more eggs in the ovaries can cause Ovarian Hyperstimulation Syndrome, which can cause abdominal pain, fluid retention, and more severe symptoms such as difficulty breathing and clotting problems. A few deaths have been reported. These drugs may increase the risk of future problems. For example, the use of Clomid (clomiphene), a drug that induces ovulation, increases the risk of ovarian cancer.

✔ If a multiple pregnancy is created with IVF, the mother's health and very life can be at risk. Complications from high blood pressure, gestational diabetes, and the stress on the body from carrying multiple fetuses are significantly increased. The risk of miscarriage, stillbirth, or complications from Caesarean sections is fairly high.

✔ And the financial, physical, and emotional burdens of caring for many babies at the same time can be overwhelming.

And what about older women? In 2010, a 54-year-old postmenopausal woman gave birth to a child through IVF. Is this ethically acceptable? When this child graduates from high school, the mother will be in her late 70s. This is, of course, a private decision to be made by the mother. But society does have an interest in this issue. The older a pregnant mother is, the greater her risks of preeclampsia, gestational diabetes, and other pregnancy-related health problems, which is a cost to society and a harm to the mother. And the odds of a child losing a parent increase as the parent ages, simply because the risk of disease and death increase as we get older. Will a woman in her 70s be physically or emotionally able to care for a teenager? Many clinics have an upper age limit on IVF patients because of concerns about elderly parents and health issues.

Also, women who donate eggs and even embryos for use in IVF must be considered. Eggs and embryos should always be freely donated, in an uncoerced manner, and with reasonable financial reimbursement. Because human eggs are very difficult to freeze (unlike sperm), donors must go through surgery to retrieve eggs just before fertilization. Creating a market for reproductive tissue is problematic. Selling and buying human beings, even embryos and fetuses, is unethical and illegal because it's attaching a dollar value to life. Producing and harvesting human eggs takes a physical toll on a woman. And there may be psychological attachment to embryos that couples may donate or sell.

Risk to the fetus

We also have to consider the risks and harm to the embryo, which directly affect the woman. Babies conceived through IVF can have more problems than babies conceived naturally. In general, babies conceived through IVF have twice the normal rate of birth defects.

- ✔ About 5 to 10 percent of these babies can have abnormal DNA methylation, which affects the expression of genes and can lead to birth defects.

- ✔ These babies usually have a lower birth weight, which is associated with an increased risk for diabetes, cancer, and hypertension.

- ✔ They also are more likely to be born with neurological problems, such as cerebral palsy and developmental delays.

This doesn't mean that people conceived through IVF *will* have these medical problems; there's just an increased risk. The oldest person born through IVF is only 32 at this time. No one knows what, if anything, will happen as these people age. This is where the concept of harm enters into the argument. Is it just to expose a child to harm before he is even born? Proponents for IVF use the ethical concept of *baseline harm* to defend IVF, which states that a being must exist before it can be made worse off. Therefore, IVF is ethical because a person created by IVF cannot be harmed by the procedure that brings them into existence. Without IVF, this person would never have existed.

Opponents of IVF use the ethical concept of *abnormal harm* to argue against IVF. This concept states that someone can be harmed by being brought into existence if the person bringing them into existence causes harm by an act or an omission. In this case, IVF, chosen by the parents, can harm a baby if it causes some defect or medical problem that the baby otherwise wouldn't have had. And whether or not harm to the child exists, it still must be weighed against the autonomy and the beneficence of the mother or the couple having the child as we discuss the ethics of IVF.

Other ethical concerns about IVF have to do with treatment of the embryos created. Some people feel that embryos have the same rights as a full person. Others feel embryos have some value as potential person. Others feel embryos have no rights. The status of embryos is important as we look at pre-implantation genetics, selective reduction, and embryo storage and destruction.

Pre-implantation genetic diagnosis: Choosing which embryos to implant

Pre-implantation genetic diagnosis (PIGD) is literally negative selection, where we screen for negative genes or traits so they don't enter the population. Blastocysts or embryos specifically created in the lab with genetic defects or those that are not healthy are discarded. Before doctors were able to diagnose a blastocyst, they took what looked like the healthiest blastocysts or embryos and implanted a bunch of them. Now, doctors can remove one cell from a blastocyst without harming it, culture that cell in the lab and then examine the chromosomes for genetic defects. Only healthy blastocysts free of genetic damage are implanted, and doctors use fewer of them today.

This procedure helps raise the odds of a healthy baby, which is good, right? Well, yes. But, as always, there's a catch. What genetic defects are serious enough to prevent implantation? What happens to the embryos that aren't implanted? They often are destroyed. Pro-life advocates are opposed to discarding embryos because they believe this is morally wrong (see arguments on personhood in Chapter 11), and, therefore, are usually opposed to IVF and PIGD. They also think the practice of disposing the embryos with genetic defects smacks of eugenics (addressed at the end of the chapter), and destroys a human life. But, as we discuss in Chapter 11, these procedures also focus on the individual choices and the individual lives of private people, not society as a whole. We don't prevent people with disabilities from reproducing, and we don't force women who are carrying fetuses with birth defects to abort. The ethical principle of autonomy plays an important part in the right of a patient to shape her life and her family.

There are some ethical concerns about pre-implantation genetic diagnosis:

- ✔ Most people agree with screening embryos for genetic diseases such as Tay-Sachs, which is crippling and leads to an early death. But should we screen embryos for late-onset diseases such as cancer or heart disease? Having the BRC1 gene for breast cancer, for instance, means that a woman is more likely to develop the disease. It doesn't mean she will get cancer, and if she does, she may survive it. Is it right to destroy an embryo based on something that *might* happen 30 or 40 years from now?

- ✔ Others feel that if a woman, or a couple, is going through the risk and expense of IVF, they should use every means possible to ensure that the baby or babies born from that procedure are as healthy as possible. In this view, the couple's autonomy is the primary concern.

- ✔ What about screening embryos so the child's blood or an organ can be used to save a person who has already been born? Some couples have conceived children to become donors for children they already have. Isn't that placing a huge burden on the child even before he is born? Is it ethical to create another life primarily to save another? A child created to save another has automatically lost autonomy.

✔ Sex selection is another issue. Most clinics that offer PIGD don't have a policy against sex selection. Sometimes sex selection is done to eliminate embryos with sex-related diseases, such as fragile X syndrome or hemophilia. But implanting only female embryos if the couple wants a girl and destroying male embryos seems to be in conflict with the ethical principle of justice due to discrimination based on gender. Doesn't each one of these embryos have a right to life, no matter their sex?

✔ As this technology advances, we are going to face more ethical dilemmas. If we can create and screen ten embryos for implantation, what is going to happen when we can create hundreds? One can picture a literal audition for your next child with dozens of embryos competing for a chance to be born. Which are you going to pick, and which will be discarded?

And we're not sure if pre-implantation genetic diagnosis works 100 percent of the time. PIGD hasn't increased the number of IVF live births. The single cell extracted from the blastocyst may not be representative of the remaining cells, leading to missed diseases. Some of these embryos don't implant, even if they seem healthy, because there are hidden genetic and physical problems or for unknown reasons.

Multiple pregnancy reduction: When IVF works too well

Women can only carry one, or perhaps two, fetuses at once for the best possible outcome. We've all heard stories of five, six, even eight babies born from the same pregnancy. It can happen, but there are almost always serious medical consequences for the babies and for the woman. For instance, carrying triplets instead of twins can be very risky. Three fetuses more than double the risk of preeclampsia and other maternal diseases, and the babies are usually born two months premature, which can sometimes lead to severe physical and mental disabilities.

Fertility drugs have also resulted in multiple fetuses. Before these drugs are administered, the potential parents should be told that there is a chance that multiple embryos will result from these drugs, and that selective reduction may be recommended. Of course, the principle of autonomy still takes precedence: if a woman wants to carry six or eight fetuses, she can. And her doctor should support that decision, although referring her to a specialist would be a prudent move.

When fertility treatments create a multiple pregnancy, sometimes doctors recommend *selective reduction*. We touch on this issue in Chapter 11. This is a very difficult issue, ethically and emotionally. The procedure, usually done at the end of the first trimester, terminates one or more fetuses so the others have the best chance to thrive, or sometimes just survive. This could be seen as a kind of *lifeboat ethics*: throwing some over the side so others have a chance at life.

Can we ethically kill an embryo or embryos so others can live? This is really an abortion of one or more embryos. As we state in Chapter 11, from a legal standpoint (*Roe v. Wade*), this is always legal in the first trimester based on a mother's right to privacy and autonomy. As the pregnancy proceeds, there must be compelling physical or emotional reasons for aborting a fetus.

Many people oppose termination of embryos as potential human life. An embryo ethically seems to have more moral value than, say, a rock because of its potential to become a human being. They argue that it should not be disposed of for trivial reasons such as position in the uterus or gender. On the other hand, some people take a utilitarian approach to selective reduction, "the greatest good for the greatest number of people." In this case, if selective reduction loses one life to save four lives, for example, instead of having the entire pregnancy fail, it is ethically the right decision.

Selective reduction is a unique situation in ethics. All ethical principles are applicable here. Where is the mother's autonomy if she isn't allowed to make decisions about her pregnancy? Where is the nonmaleficence and justice for the fetuses who are *selectively reduced*? How can we maximize beneficence for all? In some situations, that just isn't possible. The woman and her medical team must consider how to proceed to obtain the best outcome for the mother and the most fetuses and make decisions based on ethics, the patient's feelings and autonomy, and medical facts.

Fetuses that are eliminated are specifically chosen for this procedure for specific reasons. There are lots of rules for selective reduction and many tests that are run before it is performed. They include:

- ✔ Chorionic villi sampling is done to see if any of the fetuses have a genetic disease. That would be the fetus to eliminate.

- ✔ Ultrasound is performed to check on nuchal fold transparency, which can indicate Down syndrome. The doctor also needs to see if any of the fetuses are smaller than others or not developing normally.

- ✔ Fetal position is also a factor. The fetuses that are easiest to access, as cold as that sounds, are the best candidates for the procedure.

- ✔ Sex selection can be a factor. If all of the fetuses are normal, reduction for sex selection is practiced by many fertility clinics.

Using ultrasound, potassium chloride is injected into the fetuses selected for reduction. The fetus or fetuses are not removed from the womb. They just stop developing, and gradually are absorbed into the placenta. There is a 5 percent risk of miscarriage — losing all the fetuses — during the procedure.

Any women who goes through IVF has already been through an emotional wringer. She has tried to get pregnant for a long time and then has endured the invasive IVF procedure. To make matters worse, experts in the field believe that selective abortion should not take place until the 11th or 12th week of gestation, just in case one or more of the fetuses is spontaneously aborted. Miscarriages are most common before the 12th week of pregnancy (the end of the first trimester). The woman may have seen the embryos on ultrasound and heard their heartbeats at this point, so she may be emotionally attached to all of them.

Women and couples who have gone through selective reduction as a result of IVF need counseling before and after the procedure. Women quickly become attached to fetuses, and having to abort one of more of them is emotionally painful. This decision is not reached lightly. A significant number of these women do suffer from depression, which can adversely affect their attachment to the surviving infants.

One solution to this problem is that IVF doctors no longer implant large numbers of embryos in each round. More clinics are choosing to transplant only one or two embryos at a time, instead of the five or more that were transplanted when the procedure was first used. The higher number is used for older women because the chance of a successful pregnancy decreases as the mother ages.

Selective reduction is a difficult ethical issue. Some people feel fertility treatments such as IVF are unethical because they have the potential to lead to selective reduction. Others feel that the reason for the selective reduction is what is important: that it is acceptable only if used to improve the chances of a healthy pregnancy for the mother and a chance for life for the remaining fetuses. And others, based purely on the autonomy of the mother feel that selective reduction is the private choice of the mother, the one most affected by the pregnancy, even if it is for more trivial reasons such as sex selection.

Decoding embryo storage and destruction

Not all embryos created through IVF are implanted. Most fertility treatments yield at least a dozen eggs, and most of those are fertilized. What happens to them? Most are frozen, using a cryopreservation process called *vitrification*. This means freezing without the formation of intracellular ice crystals, which can disrupt cell structure when the embryo is thawed. The embryos are frozen at the one cell stage up to the blastocyst stage, about a week after fertilization.

This is the ethical issue of freezing. Embryos that are not implanted are called *leftover*, a designation that doesn't sit well with pro-life advocates. Most times, these embryos are not used because they are not deemed as healthy as embryos that are implanted: that's another issue parents and doctors must face. Leftover embryos can be frozen indefinitely, used for research, or discarded. People opposed to any type of abortion oppose IVF because it does create blastocysts and embryos that will not become human beings.

Doctors who run IVF clinics have an ethical responsibility to tell women that there will be leftover embryos and that not all embryos created will become babies. But the decision to use IVF and dispose or donate embryos is entirely up to the parents based on the principle of autonomy.

Religious objections and the Roman Catholic Church

Some faith traditions object to assisted reproduction. The Roman Catholic Church (RCC) is probably the best known for its objection to reproductive technologies. The RCC forbids artificial insemination, surrogacy, and IVF based on natural law, their interpretation of the Bible, and historical teachings of the church.

The basis for the Church's opposition to assisted reproduction dates back many years, but was formally outlined in an Encyclical by Pope Paul VI in 1968 entitled "Humanae Vitae." This document asserts that the sexual act between a husband and wife must "retain its intrinsic relationship to the procreation of human life." The marriage relationship is a union between man and wife, but also with God, and therefore must be open to God's purposes. The marriage act must be both unitive (sharing love in intimacy) and procreative (open to the possibility of creation of a new life). The church considers sex without both of these purposes improper. The Roman Catholic Church also believes that life begins at conception and that that life is of a full human person, so any destruction of a fertilized egg, blastocyst, embryo, or fetus is considered destruction of a human life. Not all Catholics support these stances.

The Catholic Church has the following objections to certain types of reproductive procedures:

✔ Objection to artificial insemination because it separates the sexual act from the procreative act and includes another person (the doctor) in the reproductive act.

✔ Objection to artificial contraception except for the rhythm method and natural family planning on the grounds that it dissociates the sexual act from the possibility of procreation. The RCC is also concerned that some contraceptives are forms of abortion.

✔ Morally forbids cloning because it is in "opposition of the dignity of procreation and the conjugal union." They also object to the cloned embryo because it is a product of "technology, not as a gift of God."

✔ Opposed to IVF because it interferes with the unitive nature of the marriage act, and because many of the embryos created in the process are destroyed.

✔ Morally opposed to surrogacy because it adds another person into the act of reproduction, which is considered immoral, and it separates procreation from the sexual act.

✔ Morally opposed to abortion because they believe life begins at conception and, therefore, abortion is murder. The Church's position is that the embryo and fetus are both full human persons with all the rights of a person existing outside the womb.

Unused embryos are frozen. Because they are the property of the couple that conceived them, albeit with moral status, the couple chooses what to do with them. They can be used in several ways:

✔ The embryos can be frozen indefinitely. This means they will not be destroyed, but they will also most likely never develop into human beings. And freezing an embryo will eventually compromise its health, so it may not be implantable.

✔ They can be donated to other infertile couples and implanted. But many people don't like the thought of their biological children being raised by other people. And leftover embryos are usually not implanted because there are some problems with their DNA or general health.

✔ They can be implanted during a nonfertile time of the mother's cycle, when they can't attach to the uterine lining and are miscarried. For some, this satisfies the ethical issue of embryo disposal because the loss of the embryo is considered a natural miscarriage.

✔ They can be donated to science for research. Many people object to using embryos in medical experiments, such as stem cell research, although many medical advances have been discovered through this research, including treatments for fetuses in utero.

✔ They can be buried by the couple.

✔ They can be destroyed, which does destroy a life. Whether that life is fully human remains up for debate.

In a couple of legal cases, women have won wrongful death lawsuits against clinics that accidentally destroyed their frozen embryos. Some states do have wrongful embryo death statutes, but in Arizona in 2006, a three-judge panel ruled that a couple couldn't sue for accidentally destroyed embryos. The issue is whether an eight-cell blastocyst can be considered a person that deserves a wrongful death lawsuit. Lawyers and judges against these lawsuits state that because these embryos do not have full legal rights or person-hood under *Roe v. Wade* and because we don't issue a death certificate for embryos, there is no human death.

There's another issue with long-term embryo storage. In some cases, the parents of those embryos have been lost, whether through frequent moves or problems with administrative paperwork. So who do they belong to?

And there's also the issue of custody of embryos created during IVF. Some couples have created embryos, stored them, and then separated or divorced. Court cases have established that if one partner wants the embryos to implant and the other doesn't, the negative right of not being forced to be a parent usually overrides the positive right of reproducing. We discuss this issue of negative and positive rights in reproduction in Chapter 11.

Clinics should have specific procedures and rules about embryo storage. The informed consent form should include written instructions from the parents about the treatment of stored embryos. This form should state:

✔ What should happen to the embryos in case the couple divorces or dies.

✔ What should happen if storage fees aren't paid.

✔ What should happen if the couple disagrees about embryo disposition.

✔ What should happen if the clinic loses track of the parents.

If embryos have been abandoned, the ethics committees of most clinics have ruled that the embryos should be destroyed. Donating them to another couple or to a research clinic would be unethical because the clinics must have permission from the parents before the embryos are used for any reason.

Artificial Insemination

Artificial insemination (AI) has been a reproduction method for decades. In this process, sperm from a male partner or sperm donor is inserted into the woman's uterus. It's usually performed when a male partner has sperm motility problems or low sperm count. In other cases, a single woman or lesbian couple use a sperm donor to have a child. Artificial insemination isn't as controversial as IVF. However, some people oppose interferring with the natural way of conceiving, and others oppose children being born to nontraditional families.

In this section, we look at the ethics of artificial insemination, particularly safe, anonymous, and consensual sperm donation. We also look at the issue of sex selection, and the ethics of nontraditional families that are formed with artificial insemination.

Understanding safe, anonymous, and consensual sperm donation

Men are paid to donate sperm. When they donate, they legally sign away all rights and claims to the children that may result from that donation. Informed consent is a very important part of this contract.

In a contract for a sperm donor, doctors must consider these issues:

✔ Anonymity of the donor is crucial. The donor has no legal or moral claim to any children born as a result of his donation, and the woman and child involved don't have a right to learn his identity. If the donor is known to the woman because he's a friend or acquaintance and she chooses him, he still has no rights to or responsibility for any children resulting from AI.

✔ The client should be informed about the limitations of the procedure and any complications that might arise. No sperm can be guaranteed free of disease or genetic defect. And the client is 100 percent responsible for any child born from this procedure.

✔ The number of offspring from a single donor must be limited. In most clinics, only 10 children can be conceived from one donor to minimize risk of incest. If one man is the father of hundreds of children, those children may someday meet and fall in love.

Clients can look through biographies of donors and choose characteristics, such as height, eye color, or even professions or hobbies. Because couples want their offspring to look like themselves, this selection is reasonable and ethical.

Sperm donors should be chosen with ethical criteria. Some sperm banks have more elite clients: those with advanced degrees or special abilities, even though those traits aren't 100 percent genetically determined. The women should be told that none of the criteria listed for each potential donor are guaranteed in her offspring. Selection of a sperm donor is a personal decision, and the patient's autonomy is the foremost ethical criteria. If a woman wants the father of her potential children to have blonde hair, brown eyes, a flair for music, and athletic ability, that is her choice. But is it ethical? With these choices, we start to lean toward genetically engineering children, which if taken too far can lead to eugenics. And sperm donation is expensive and only an option for people who can afford it, also an issue of justice.

Sex selection: Is it ever ethical?

Artificial insemination and IVF have increased the ability to choose the sex of a child even before conception. Sperm can be separated out so there are more sperm with X or Y chromosomes used in AI, and embryos of either sex can be selected and implanted with IVF. In AI, there is no guarantee of a particular sex. The odds of a boy or girl are simply increased.

Couples who want to select the sex of their children should be carefully counseled before the procedure. In the contract, the couple must be told:

- ✔ The procedure may not produce a child of the desired sex.
- ✔ They will accept any child that results from the procedure, even if it isn't the sex they wanted.
- ✔ They shouldn't have unreasonable or unrealistic expectations about the behavior or personalities of boys or girls.

Most ethicists are uncomfortable with sex selection in reproduction. The American Society for Reproductive Medicine says that couples undergoing reproductive assistance can choose the sex of their offspring simply because they are going through such an extensive process to conceive, but sex selection for nonmedical reasons is discouraged. The right of reproduction isn't an absolute right, and no one can receive every medical consideration in every medical procedure. And the use of medicine to select the sex of a child for non-medical reasons is a poor use of limited medical resources and many people consider destroying embryos because they aren't the preferred sex to be immoral.

When a sex-linked genetic disease is the issue, sex selection is morally permissible. Preventing the birth of a child with a serious and potentially fatal disease is ethical. Gender bias doesn't enter into this decision. The decision is made for the good of the child and the parents.

From an ethical standpoint, we also must look at the effect of gender selection on society as a whole. Traditionally, many cultures prefer males, so the issue of sex selection raises the specter of females being devalued. There is the risk of social harm if the balance of males and females is disturbed by artificial sex selection. For example, in China where females are regularly aborted, this has led to a highly imbalanced ratio of males to females of childbearing age by two to one. By 2020, there will be 1 million excess males in China. Subsequently, women are often kidnapped and sold into marriage. Gender discrimination should always be discouraged as clearly unjust and detrimental to society. The ethical position at this time is that sex selection is ill-advised unless medically necessary for a genetic condition.

Surrogacy: Carrying Someone Else's Child

A *surrogate* is a woman who carries a fetus for another woman who is infertile or unable to carry a child. The embryo is conceived through artificial insemination or IVF. There are two types of surrogacy:

- **Traditional surrogacy:** The surrogate mother is the biological mother of the baby because semen from the father is inserted into her womb.

- **Gestational surrogacy:** The potential mother donates an egg and the potential father donates sperm, which are used to make an embryo and then implanted in the surrogate's womb. The surrogate has no biological ties to the baby.

In this section, we look at the ethics of gestational surrogacy. What rights does the surrogate mother have? What about the rights of the parents who are using the surrogate? What are your responsibilities in this issue? And where does the emotional and physical health of the surrogate fit into this equation?

There have been many reported cases of surrogacy gone wrong in the past 20 years. Baby Manji, who was born through artificial insemination, was immediately placed in a tug of war between the surrogate and her legal parents. For more information on this issue, see Chapter 19. That case set precedent in the law. The laws about surrogacy vary by state. Some states prohibit surrogacy agreements, and others have mixed laws or rulings. It's important to understand the laws in your state before you become involved in this type of situation.

Paying for pregnancy: The ethics of commercial surrogacy

Some women become surrogates out of the goodness of their hearts. This is called *altruistic surrogacy*. The surrogate doesn't accept any money and gives up all rights to the baby. This type of surrogacy is fairly rare. It often occurs within a family, where a woman, for example, may carry her sister's child. But many women who become surrogates do so for money, in *commercial surrogacy*. To be blunt about it, a woman's womb is being rented.

Embryos, blastocysts, and fetuses can't be bought or sold, but eggs and sperm can be exchanged for money. So what about using another woman's womb to create your child? Is it ethical to pay someone for the use of their womb?

The Center for Surrogate Parenting estimates the cost for bringing one baby to term is about $30,000 to $60,000. Of course, this automatically eliminates those who can't afford that sum of money, and can divide prospective parents and surrogates into employer and employee. Middle- and upper-class couples tend hire the surrogates, and poor and lower class women tend to become the surrogates. This violates the ethical principle of justice, since the risks and burdens of pregnancy falls on the woman with less money. But, women aren't forced into becoming surrogates, although exploitation is still a concern because lower-class women are used to provide a service that puts their health at risk, a service that they themselves could never afford.

People who support surrogacy have the infertile couple's rights in mind. They feel that if science has progressed to the point where these people can have a biological child, at least related to one parent, they should.

So what about paying for a surrogate? Is it ethical to "rent" a womb so you can have a child? Opponents to surrogacy think that commercial surrogacy is simply baby selling that turns an infant into a commodity, which could be considered human trafficking. After all, if a woman is willing to undergo the risks and potential complications of pregnancy, only to give up the child at the end, is she freely entering into this contract if money is the incentive? Isn't money coercion to those without it? The issue really boils down to autonomy again. A woman can choose to be a surrogate if she wants to and if another person or couple wants to rent her womb.

Opponents to surrogacy believe that infertile couples should adopt. But adoption has its limitations. There are long waiting lists to adopt healthy white (and most in demand) infants. Is this discrimination against those of other races or is it a personal choice? Shouldn't people have the right to have the kind of family they want? Also, if infertile couples have been through fertility treatments for years, they risk being too old to adopt before they finally decide to give up on a biological child of their own. And in adoption, biological mothers and fathers have legal rights, so they can change their mind after the baby is born.

Some ethicists are concerned about abuses in this system. There isn't uniform federal law in the United States about surrogacy at this time. The law varies by state, so couples in one state where it's legal may advertise for a surrogate in another state, or vice versa. And because surrogacy is legal in other countries, surrogacy is becoming a tourist industry. Many wealthy people are traveling to other countries, especially India, to rent a womb for their embryos. The principle of justice can be violated in these cases, and poor women can be exploited. There may have to be new laws enacted to make sure that ethical principles are satisfied and the whole transaction is as fair as possible.

Surrogacy isn't as regulated as adoption, so it's easier to become a parent with this method. In fact, a couple and a woman can enter into a surrogacy agreement without medical intervention, using home artificial insemination.

Considering the emotional and physical health of the surrogate

The emotional state and physical health of the surrogate are central in this situation. Most agencies who manage surrogacy require that the surrogate already have one biological child. The woman should be physically and emotionally healthy and be of a certain age, usually between the ages of 21 and 39. The principles of justice, nonmaleficence, and beneficence all demand that the surrogate be thoroughly screened and up to the task of bringing a baby to term and then giving it up.

Complete family history must be taken and provided to the potential parents if the surrogate is going to be the biological mother of the baby. If the surrogate will be only a gestational surrogate who does not provide the egg, but only the womb, family history isn't as important to the parents, but is still important for her medical evaluation.

People who are opposed to surrogacy believe that there is too much stress placed on the surrogate and her family. Opponents believe that someone is usually hurt in this process, and that person is usually the surrogate. Because pregnancy can take a physical and emotional toll on women, her health should be considered at all times. Postpartum depression is common after birth, and giving the baby to another couple can exacerbate that condition.

The surrogate should have a good support system in place to help her mentally and physically, before, during, and after the pregnancy. If a surrogate isn't biologically related to the potential parents, some compensation is expected. Some of the ethical issue of paying for a baby can be mitigated when the time and effort of the woman involved is considered.

The case of Angela Robinson

In New Jersey in 2006, Angela Robinson agreed to carry twin babies for her brother Donald and his male partner. An egg was obtained from an ovum donor, and fertilized with sperm from Donald's partner. Angela gave birth to twin girls in 2007.

In 2007, Angela sued her brother, saying she had been coerced into the contract. The court ruled that she was the babies' legal mother, even though she isn't the babies' biological mother. The siblings now share visitation rights, although Ms. Robinson's status as legal parent gave her the right to seek full custody, which she did. The trial is ongoing.

How much information about the surrogate's health should be shared with the potential parents? While she is pregnant, the surrogate still has control over her body. Although she may have agreed to eat certain foods and undergo certain physical tests, she still has some autonomy. But there are restrictions on that autonomy that the surrogate has agreed to by entering into this contracted arrangement. That's why it's important for the potential parents and the surrogate that psychological screening before surrogacy is thorough and that informed consent is clearly met.

Looking at the contract and surrogate responsibilities

A surrogacy contract is usually involved, complicated, and has many stipulations. A contract can require the surrogate to

- ✔ Undergo psychological testing before the pregnancy begins. It's important to make sure that the surrogate is mentally stable and emotionally prepared to surrender the baby at birth.

- ✔ Undergo physical medical testing and testing for STDs, drug use, and even genetic testing.

- ✔ Refrain from drinking, smoking, and using drugs during the pregnancy. Most contracts have a clause about a healthy diet, and some can mandate an organic diet or other special diet.

- ✔ Obtain good prenatal care with regular checkups. The parents usually pay for medical expenses, especially if there's a problem with the surrogate's insurance company.

✔ Require prenatal genetic testing and stipulate an abortion if there is a serious genetic problem. This is a difficult issue because no court will force a woman into an abortion.

✔ Decide who is going to be in the delivery room when the surrogate gives birth, and when the baby will be given to the potential parents.

What if the surrogate isn't meeting the terms of her contract? What should you do if she skips prenatal checkups, or admits to drinking wine or smoking during the pregnancy? What about confidentiality?

Surrogate agencies state that the surrogate is allowed to choose her doctor and exercise care over her medical care. And she can share as much or as little about the pregnancy as she wants to. If the contract states certain information must be passed on and the surrogate signed it, you can provide that information to the potential parents.

And here's a really tricky issue: The surrogate can terminate the pregnancy in the first trimester, even if there isn't a medical reason for an abortion, as is her right through autonomy. This risk must be acknowledged by all involved in surrogacy. Although the surrogate has a moral obligation to continue the pregnancy, she doesn't have a legal obligation to do so. And the couple who will adopt the baby needs to be told about this fact to satisfy informed consent.

Some ethicists think that surrogacy should be managed similar to adoption. An adoption agency should be involved from the very beginning, screening potential parents and surrogates, managing the financial transactions through escrow accounts, and visiting the potential parents and surrogate throughout the pregnancy.

Understanding rights of the child

Of course, if there are problems between the couple who have contracted with the surrogate, all bets are off. There are cases where a couple has divorced while a surrogate is carrying their child, and when surrogates have changed their minds and want to keep the baby. Not all surrogacy contracts cover all situations.

If the baby is the biological child of the couple contracting with the surrogate, the parental rights are pretty clear. If the surrogate is the biological mother, things can get tricky.

In states where surrogacy is legal, such as California, parents can go through a parental rights confirmation process. This takes place in the second trimester of the pregnancy. Papers are filed with the court and a judge reviews them. The surrogate's presumed parental rights are terminated. This process is not the same as adoption.

The parties involved in this situation should have independent attorneys who have their client's best interests at heart. Some surrogacy clinics recommend that the doctor who examines the surrogate before pregnancy be different from her primary physician, and that the doctor who performs the psychological testing on all parties be independent as well to avoid any conflicts of interest.

The law is very unsettled in this issue, and just about anything can happen. Usually, the parents get legal custody of the baby and the surrogate surrenders custody and all parental rights. But some situations are different. The surrogate might want visitation rights, or arrange a situation such as an open adoption. These issues should ideally be settled before the pregnancy begins.

The doctor's responsibilities

If your patient expresses an interest in hiring a surrogate, advise her on the following:

✔ **Careful screening of the surrogate:** Almost 95 percent of all potential surrogates are rejected for several reasons, including emotional instability or complicated family situation.

✔ **A clear contract, explained to all and signed and properly witnessed:** The contract should try to cover all situations and eventualities. Make sure the state will recognize the surrogacy contract. Many of them will not uphold these contracts, so special care must be taken.

What are your responsibilities in this situation? If one of your patients wants to use a surrogate to have a baby, there are many things to consider. First of all, you do not have any obligation to be a part of surrogacy if you have religious or ethical objections to it. As noted in the previous sidebar, Roman Catholics who adhere to church teachings on surrogacy would be an example. But, as a provider, you do have to refer your patient to another doctor who can participate in this legal medical arrangement.

When helping a couple who is considering surrogacy — or when talking to a potential surrogate — there are several points to consider:

✔ Informed consent is crucial in this situation. All relevant medical information should be shared with the doctor managing the surrogacy before the pregnancy begins. The potential parents have primary responsibility for the baby after it is born. And the surrogate has primary responsibility for the fetus before it is born. You must tell all parties about all of the issues of this situation, and all parties should agree to details, such as activities the couple would like the surrogate to abstain from, before the pregnancy begins.

✔ Most ethicists believe that a couple who wants to use a surrogate shouldn't use the surrogate's eggs for the pregnancy. If the surrogate is the biological mother of the baby, she has a strengthened claim to parental rights.

✔ Potential parents should use a surrogate only if they really need it. If a woman faces a higher-risk pregnancy, surrogacy may be the ethically permissible answer. But surrogacy for convenience reasons, such as avoidance of pain or maintenance of body image, is ethically problematic because the situation involves another person's body and physical health. If a woman wants to use a surrogate simply to maintain her figure or for other trivial reasons, she is violating the principle of nonmaleficence for the surrogate.

✔ All parties must be clear on what prenatal testing is to be done, and what should be done if a genetic defect is discovered.

✔ The surrogate must not be coerced into the situation. Whether or not money is coercion remains in debate. And her partner must be informed about the ethical and legal responsibilities.

✔ The surrogacy has to be in all parties' best interests.

✔ A waiting period should be put in place before the final contracts are signed so all of the involved parties can think about this situation and make an informed decision.

✔ Counseling for all parties, before, during, and after the pregnancy is essential. In fact, if the surrogate has a family of her own, they may be included in counseling.

If you choose to be involved, contact an attorney. The law has not kept up with reproductive technology so the legal status of the surrogate and potential parents can be unclear. Even if you live in a state where courts don't recognize a surrogacy contract, going through a legal document can help all parties realize their true feelings about this issue and help those involved reach decisions that have to be made. There are so many potential minefields in these situations, and as many of them as possible should be covered before surrogacy begins.

Sterilization: Preventing Reproduction

Sterilization is a medical procedure that surgically removes the ability to procreate. Because medicine can improve a person's life and not just save or preserve it, patients can request medical procedures for reasons other than life or death. In the case of reproduction, a patient may request sterilization to avoid the health risks and inconveniences of other contraceptives, to prevent higher risk pregnancies that occur with advanced maternal age, and to have maximum control over the size of their family. The most common examples of sterilization are vasectomy and tubal ligation.

So what's your role in this issue? Usually, sterilization is a mutual decision made by a couple when they have completed their family, but sometimes the situation is more complicated. If you feel that a patient may be harming him- or herself or a spouse in choosing sterilization, what should you do? The conflicting ethical principles are between patient autonomy and nonmaleficence. A patient has the right to control his or her body, but if he or she is denying another person the choice to be a parent, that can be harmful to the partner or to the relationship.

In this section, we look at voluntary sterilization of young, healthy people and what it may mean to others in their lives. We look at the ethics of involuntary sterilization, and what conditions must be met before it is considered. And we look at eugenics and some objections to selective sterilization.

Voluntary sterilization as birth control

Do you have to provide sterilization for any patient who requests it? How do you balance autonomy with nonmaleficence in this situation? Sterilization for nonmedical reasons should be carefully considered. The risk of serious regret in this case can be monumental. To avoid being paternalistic, list the pros and cons of sterilization, make sure your patient understands the scope of the situation, and give them time to think about it.

Counseling should be offered before sterilization, especially if the patient is very young. But just because a patient is young doesn't mean they can't make this type of decision. Doctors can certainly perform some medical procedures even when they are not necessarily medically indicated, for instance, in plastic surgery for a change in appearance. And no doctor can be forced to perform a medical procedure to which he or she is morally opposed.

What if one person in a couple wants to be sterilized and not tell their partner? Patient autonomy rules in this case. Although the patient should be encouraged to tell their partner about this decision, you, the provider, must keep the decision confidential.

A patient can be sterilized after several conditions are met. The patient must be informed of all the risks and benefits of sterilization, including the possibility of regret. And the provider must be honest about the patient's best interest. Sterilization can be ethical as a voluntary medical procedure.

The ethics of involuntary birth control

Involuntary birth control is not a subject that is raised much these days. In the past, people who were judged "unfit" were sterilized without their consent. This practice, also called *eugenic sterilization*, violates a person's autonomy and concept of personal freedom. The Nazi sterilization program certainly comes to mind in this discussion. The Germans sterilized anyone who was mentally ill, handicapped, blind, deaf, epileptic, alcoholic, or potentially carried a dominant gene such as Huntington's Disease. The 1933 German Law for the Prevention of Hereditarily Diseased Offspring was another example, sterilizing more than 3 million people against their will, based on race, mental health, and capacity. These acts have been recognized as crimes against humanity.

In the United States, many states had laws in the early 1900s for compulsory sterilization of mentally ill patients. More than 60,000 Americans were sterilized against their will under these laws. These are extreme violations of justice because forced sterilization is negative eugenics. Eugenics is really discrimination against people who do not fit a society's concept of what a person should be. Nonmaleficence is violated because forced sterilization can cause psychological problems and medical harm, and autonomy is violated because no one else should decide for you whether or not you can become a parent. This should be a free choice.

Some charities have recently been offering payment to alcoholics and drug abusers to be sterilized or use long-term birth control, such as the IUD. Because the IUD cannot be removed without a doctor, it is considered involuntary birth control unless the woman has consented to its use. Many ethicists think that this is coercion and that people who submit to sterilization under these circumstances are not even capable of giving informed consent because of the forced nature of the consent.

In the past, involuntary sterilization has been an issue for adults with disabilities. Before science unraveled some of the mysteries of DNA and heredity, many felt that most disabilities were inherited. People believed that preventing the disabled from conceiving would reduce the number of people with disabilities.

The case of Jim and Joan: Encouraging conversation

Joan came to her family physician for her annual physical. She was quite distraught because her husband Jim wanted only one child, which they had, and wanted a vasectomy. He was under a great deal of financial strain trying to support the family, and didn't think they could afford another child. He had been an only child and was happy with his situation.

Joan, on the other hand, had brothers and sisters, and felt this was important for her child. She thought that after Jim had a child he would

naturally want more. Jim was planning on a vasectomy in spite of Joan's objections.

Jim called this same family doctor and asked for a referral to a urologist for the vasectomy. He acknowledged the conflict in his marriage. Their physician convinced the couple to come into the office together to talk about this decision. After this conversation, Jim and Joan agreed to using an IUD as a form of birth control, which would allow them a few years to decide what was best for their family.

Unfortunately, that issue is not very far in the past. In 2008, an Illinois woman had to go to court to avoid being sterilized. The judge in that case said that involuntary birth control restricts the fundamental personal rights of reproductive freedom and personal inviolability. Counsel for the plaintiff found that Illinois was one of 16 states that had no laws preventing involuntary sterilization of the handicapped. A new law was signed in August that banned sterilization of adults with disabilities without a court order.

There are certain legal conditions that must be met before a person can be involuntary sterilized or subjected to involuntary birth control. They are:

- ✔ The patient must be proven to have no capacity for competence, assent, or consent.
- ✔ The patient must be fertile and have some access to sexual contact.
- ✔ For women, any pregnancy must be high risk and impose an unacceptable burden.
- ✔ The patient must not be able to use any other type of contraception.

Most ethicists think that involuntary birth control and sterilization are never ethical, even when the court system has been involved and the conditions stated above have been met beyond a reasonable doubt. Involuntary sterilization may be legal in some states or countries, but that doesn't mean it's ethical because of the clear violations of the principles of justice, autonomy, and nonmaleficence.

Understanding eugenics: Social engineering

Eugenics is the engineering of human life through reproduction, or more precisely, selective breeding. Its aim is to improve the human species through genetics. It is strongly associated with Nazi Germany; millions were sterilized under that regime because they were deemed inferior or unfit. This type of negative eugenics violated autonomy, privacy, freedom, and other human rights. The most reprehensible part of eugenics was government involvement. Those types of eugenics are called *collectivist* or *totalitarian eugenics*.

There is now a movement called *liberal eugenics*. This stresses individual autonomy when deciding about prenatal testing. This line of thought favors *positive eugenics* in the form of *reprogenetics*, which includes techniques such as PIGD to choose the characteristics of embryos before implantation with IVF.

There are several problems with this stance. First, PIGD and IVF are quite expensive, so only wealthy people can afford to reproduce with the assistance of this technology. By promoting this type of eugenics for those who can afford it, we could create a two-tiered society of genetically enhanced people, pitting "designer" human beings against those who were born the natural way and could then be considered inferior. Those who might be considered lower class may face severe discrimination and even be considered expendable. We may lose our sense of compassion for those who are not "perfect." Thus, eugenics can lead to a society that is profoundly unjust. But we also must remember that these are individual reproductive decisions made by individual people, exercising their right to autonomy. This freedom must be balanced with future effects of these decisions on society.

Now, of course, we know that genetics isn't the only determining factor in what a person becomes. Environment plays a large role in human development. Although choosing superior characteristics in embryos may improve human beings, genes aren't the only force shaping people.

And there's another problem with social engineering through genetics: inbreeding. This is extreme and will probably not occur without isolation, but we know that the strongest and most healthy gene pool is varied. By having people mate with others who share similar characteristics and backgrounds, genetic mutations and abnormalities are actually much more likely to occur. Inbreeding doesn't create more mutations, but rather distributes mutations among a smaller population. Recessive genetic diseases will become more common because the chances of both parents having the same recessive gene increase when they are related.

Chapter 11

Walking a Fine Line: Examining the Ethics of Abortion

*T*here is possibly no more divisive subject in the United States than abortion. Both sides claim the moral high ground. Both sides can cite cases and examples that show they are right. There seems to be no common ground. So what do healthcare providers need to know about this issue? Although abortion is one of the most ethically difficult issues, the role of the healthcare provider is relatively simple. As in all other cases, your responsibility is to the patient.

The divisiveness about abortion extends to the names used to describe each side. For the purposes of discussion, the side that opposes abortion on demand will be referred to as *pro-life*. The side that thinks abortion should be legal will be called *pro-choice*. Although an entire book could be written arguing about these terms, we will not impose moral or ethical statements on either side; they are simply labels.

The ethical positions about abortion vary widely. Providers need to know the ethical stances of each side to provide the best care for their patients. Autonomy, informed consent, beneficence, nonmaleficence, and justice all play a part in this debate. How should doctors communicate with women who are wondering about abortion?

In this chapter, we look at the question of when personhood begins and then we examine both sides of this issue. We also look at the three types of abortion (therapeutic, selective, and voluntary) and the ethical issues of each, including what you can tell your patients in these situations. Because a patient faces different ethical issues based on the reason and type of abortion, this is probably the most meaningful way to look at abortion from an ethical viewpoint. We also look at the legal status of abortion in the United States and how the law has changed. And we sift through the religious arguments on the topic.

When Does Personhood Begin?

The question of when personhood begins is crucial to the abortion debate. An abortion stops the development of an embryo into a fetus, and a fetus into a baby. At what point does a person, with all its inherent rights and privileges, begin? Can we even decide on a point?

The establishment of personhood is important for ethical reasons and because of legal status. A person is legally protected against harm and killing because of their status as a human being. In its ruling on *Roe v. Wade*, the United States Supreme Court said that it could not set a point where personhood begins, and that, in fact, medical science, philosophy, and religion can't fix that point. The Court chose the end of the first trimester as the point where abortion could be regulated.

In this section, we examine the legal and moral status of the beginning of personhood and apply the four ethical principles to personhood. Remember, we aren't trying to change anyone's mind here. We're setting forth the parameters of each position so you understand them.

What, and who, is a person?

There are several definitions of *person*. Most include some type of interaction with the world. Definitions of *personhood* include:

- A human being who has a conscious awareness of self
- A human being, regardless of age or mental capacity
- A being who can set personal values and goals
- A human being who has been born and will die

These definitions are as problematic at the beginning of life as they are at the end of life (for more on personhood and end-of-life issues, see Chapter 12). After all, a newborn doesn't have personal values and can't set goals. We're not even sure a newborn has a conscious awareness of self, other than the basic biological drives of hunger, thirst, fear of falling, and reaction to pain. But of course, a newborn is considered a person.

Many people use the term *potential person* to describe the embryo and fetus. They state that because all of the DNA and material needed to produce a human being exist at the moment of conception, it is ethically wrong to stop this process. After all, an embryo will likely become a person who can set values and goals. Some people believe that the embryo, a potential person, should have all the rights and moral status of a person who has been born. However, at this time in the United States, a potential person doesn't have the same legal rights as a full person. As soon as you qualify the term person, should the legal standing change? The question is: What rights and status, if any, should be offered to a potential person?

It should be noted that not all human beings have full moral status or legal rights. People attain rights in degrees. Those under the age of 18 don't have the right to vote or give informed consent to most medical care. Prisoners don't have the right to vote or the right to freedom. Competent adults have more rights than those who have been found to lack the capacity to think and reason.

Gestational development

To clarify the legal and moral status of abortion, it helps to know the stages of gestation. Medical science divides a pregnancy into three trimesters of gestation, each lasting 13 weeks.

✔ **First Trimester:** When the sperm fertilizes the egg, a zygote is formed. After 5 days, it develops a hollow core with inner and outer cells and is called a blastocyst or pre-embryo. By definition, the developing baby is called an embryo from conception to the end of the 8th week of life (or 10th week of gestation as measured by doctors from the last menstrual period). After implantation, around 15 days, the primitive streak appears; this becomes the brain and spinal cord. By 5 weeks, the embryo has a tail and looks just like any other embryo, including elephants and rabbits. At 6 weeks, a heartbeat can be seen on ultrasound. At 7 weeks, pain sensors begin to appear, although it's unclear whether the fetus can feel pain. At the end of the 10th week of gestation, the embryo is called a *fetus* until the time of delivery. At 13 weeks, the fetus weighs about 1 ounce, is 3 inches long, and all major organ systems have started to develop. More than

90 percent of all abortions are performed before this date, or in the first trimester.

✔ **Second trimester:** During the second trimester, the fetus continues to grow. At 22 weeks' gestation, the fetus cannot survive outside the womb. Medical science hasn't been able to move the viability date earlier than 23 to 24 weeks because of lack of lung development. By 26 weeks, most doctors think the fetus can most likely feel pain, and its lungs are fairly well developed. Many fetuses can survive outside the womb at this point, but only with a considerable amount of medical assistance.

✔ **Third trimester:** At 26 weeks, the third trimester begins and continues to 39 or 40 weeks, when the fetus is considered full term. The fat layer forms and organs continue to develop. At 34 weeks' gestation, lung development is complete. Labor is usually allowed to progress naturally if a mother is 35 weeks or beyond. At birth, the status changes from fetus to neonate. The neonate status is continued until 28 days after birth, when the baby is called an infant.

Many ethicists think that life is a continuum: That there is no one single moment when multiplying cells become a person, just as there is often no one defined moment when a person dies. This continuum is used to decide when a person has died, so can we use it to determine when personhood begins?

Applying ethical principles to personhood

All of the ethical principles of medicine are relevant to the fetus's status of personhood. Under the principle of autonomy, a woman has the right to determine what medical procedures she chooses and refuses. But does the embryo or fetus also have the right to autonomy? Doctors must do what is best for the patient under the principle of beneficence. But who is the patient: the pregnant woman, the fetus, or both?

The principle of nonmaleficence is important, too. When an abortion would save the life or health of the mother, refusing to perform it causes harm. But performing an abortion ends fetal development and growth, harming the fetus. And justice, of course, is central to this issue. Whose rights are more important: the woman's or the fetus's?

Many ethicists have debated the abortion issue on both sides. Some of these arguments are well documented and have been discussed countless times over the years. Here we look at two famous arguments, one on each side of the issue, using the context of personhood.

- ✔ **Mary Anne Warren:** This ethicist proposes five criteria for personhood: consciousness, ability to feel pain, ability to reason, self-motivated activity, and the capacity to communicate. A being lacking all of these capacities fails to meet these *cognitive criteria* and cannot be a person. Warren argues that because a fetus does not meet these criteria for personhood, it does not have an absolute right to life. Opponents of this perspective argue it denies personhood to the severely disabled, infants, and people in PVS (persistent vegetative state) or a coma.

- ✔ **Don Marquis:** This argument supposes that a person is someone with the potential for future cognitive experiences. Therefore, what is wrong about killing an adult human is the same thing that is wrong with killing a fetus. This argument claims that it is always wrong to take a human life, no matter how young or undeveloped. He says that we are cutting off a possible future by ending a pregnancy. Because a fetus is human, and we have no way of showing that it is not human, it has a right to life. Opponents of this theory ask this question: How can you harm something that doesn't yet exist?

Looking at Each Side's Point of View

There is no way that we are going to settle the argument between the two sides of the abortion issue. What you need to know is the ethical stance of each side so you can better help your patients who are struggling with this issue. In this section, we look at the pro-life and pro-choice ethical arguments about abortion.

Even if you have a strong preference for one side of the abortion debate, try to fully understand and respect the other side so that you can give the best care to your patients. Don't hesitate to refer your patient to a qualified therapist who can help her reach a decision she can live with.

Understanding the pro-life stance

A person is classified as pro-life if they don't believe abortion should be available on demand. This side focuses on the rights and moral status of the embryo and fetus. Pro-life individuals believe that human life should be valued from conception to natural death. In most pro-life arguments, person-hood begins at conception, and this side believes that any deliberate destruction of human life is ethically wrong. Those on the pro-life side do not think that the destruction of life is ever mitigated by benefits to others. From the pro-life view, any action which destroys an embryo or fetus kills a person and that is always wrong.

This side focuses on the rights and moral status of the fetus. To this group, the rights of the fetus are paramount and outweigh the woman's rights because many believe that abortion is wrong on deontological grounds: it's always wrong because it ends a life. Many religious people define a *person* as a human being with a soul, although medical science has not been able to measure a soul or define a soul in any way.

Many on the pro-life side think that life begins at the moment of conception. Other views on when life begins include

- ✔ When the cells begin to divide
- ✔ When the primitive streak, or the beginning of the spinal cord and brain, appears
- ✔ When the heart begins beating
- ✔ When brain waves appear

- ✔ When the fetus begins to move (quickening)
- ✔ When the fetus can feel pain
- ✔ When the fetus is viable separate from its mother
- ✔ When the fetus is born and draws breath

Because all of these points are arbitrary, it's difficult, if not impossible, to pick just one. If you pick one week when you think a person exists, why didn't you pick the day before that or the week before that point? The pro-life position is that it makes sense to define life at the moment of conception because all other points are arbitrary.

An ethical concept called *the slippery slope* is used to defend the pro-life position. This argument states that a relatively morally insignificant first step can lead to a chain of related events culminating in an event with very significant moral effects. The pro-life side argues that without a clear definition of personhood, we step on to a slippery slope that ends in the disposal of inconvenient people.

If we are willing to terminate an embryo that does not fit the full definition of personhood, what about a mentally handicapped adult? If we terminate pregnancy for any reason, will it lead to termination of pregnancy for trivial reasons, such as the gender of the baby?

Many groups that support the rights of the disabled are opposed to abortion, especially abortion due to fetal defect. Some even call abortion on demand *eugenics*, which is the elimination of people who don't fit the mold of the perfect person in order to create a better society. Are we on a slippery slope toward eugenics by allowing abortion? And if we don't respect life at conception, will we eventually find those at the end of their lives disposable as well? This is also called the argument from marginal cases and is widely used in ethics. Those at the margins of personhood, such as the embryo or the disabled, must have the same moral and legal standing as people at the center of personhood.

Deontology is an ethical theory embraced by the pro-life position. This theory states that certain acts are simply right or wrong, no matter what good or bad outcomes they lead to. In the case of abortion, some pro-life proponents say that abortion is killing a person and is simply wrong, no matter what the consequences for or the opinion of the pregnant woman.

One well-known ethical position that supports the pro-life view is proposed by federal judge John Noonan. Noonan says that a genetic criteria is all that is needed to assign rights to an embryo. In other words, when sperm and egg meet and merge genes, a genetically unique person is created. The embryo has all the potential in its DNA to become a full person; therefore, it has a right to life that is absolute. This argument rests on the presumption that if you are conceived by two human beings, you are a human being and have personhood, no matter your stage of development. In this scenario, abortion is argued to be wrong because it takes the life of a genetically unique person begun at conception.

This is only a brief review of the pro-life argument. For updates or more information, visit www.nrlc.org/.

Understanding the pro-choice stance

The pro-choice stance is based on autonomy, privacy, and self-determination. This side focuses on the rights and moral status of the mother. The pro-choice side believes that because she bears the burdens of pregnancy, birth, and raising a child, a woman should be able to decide if she wants to let her pregnancy proceed. The pro-choice side argues that this decision belongs to the mother alone, and that government has no jurisdiction on this issue.

This side believes that an embryo or fetus gradually attains moral standing and legal rights as it develops, but doesn't have them from the moment of conception or during the first few months of gestational development.

As it stands now, this issue comes down to one point: Two people can't have equal rights within one body. U.S. attorney Janet Gallagher calls this issue the struggle over the *geography of pregnancy*. Because a fetus is inside a woman's body, we can't assign it separate legal rights without depriving women of their rights to bodily integrity, due process, and autonomy. Depriving women of these rights would be unprecedented under the law.

A famous ethical argument on the pro-choice side is made by Judith Jarvis Thomson. She compares pregnancy to one person being attached to another person for the purpose of survival. The existence of the first person depends on the second person giving up rights to keep the first person alive. Ms. Thomson argues that no one has the right to impose himself on another person for survival. She uses the following scenario to defend her position that abortion is a situation in which killing is morally permissible: Imagine that suddenly, without your consent, a another person who is dying of kidney failure is attached to your body to obtain kidney dialysis. That person goes everywhere with you and is dependent on you for survival. Are you required to continue this arrangement against your will? Thompson argues that you would have the right to choose to unplug yourself from this person and recover your freedom, even if it means the death of the other person. She likens abortion to this scenario.

In ethics, there are two kinds of rights: positive and negative. *Positive rights* are the right to some kind of benefit, such as the right to life. A *negative right* is the right to be left alone or to not be forced to do something, such as the right to refuse medical treatment.

The pro-choice side argues that a woman's right to be left alone to make her own decisions about her own life (a negative right) outweighs the pro-life side's right to force their opinion on her life (a positive right). And the woman's right to not be burdened with pregnancy (a negative right) outweighs the embryo's or fetus' right to life (a positive right).

The pro-choice side argues that pregnancy imposes a burden on women and carries risk. Women must give up many rights to carry a fetus to term, and some women lose their life or health in the process. Worldwide, complications in pregnancy and childbirth are the leading cause of women's deaths. Pro-choice advocates believe that picking a point when personhood begins should be an individual decision. They argue that unless a woman has control over her body, she is not really free.

And what about those who support the rights of disabled and feel that abortion is eugenics? The pro-choice side argues that that those in the movement are free to believe what they want to about themselves or about disability. But their opinions can't be more important than the decision of a woman who is carrying a child with a disability. Because no one is forced to end a pregnancy when an abnormality is detected, pro-choice advocates think that eugenics is not a logical part of the abortion debate. A woman who chooses to abort a fetus with a birth defect isn't making a statement about the purity of society. She is making a choice for herself and her child.

For pro-choice advocates, the issue comes down to privacy and autonomy. The mother must live with her decision and care for her disabled child. They reject the slippery-slope argument and say instead that it is a staircase with many steps where society can easily stop. When there are many intermediate steps in an issue, the strength of the slippery slope argument decreases. There are many steps between abortion for fetal defect and eliminating the handicapped, and the connections between those steps are weak.

Pro-choice advocates also think that because abortion is such a private issue, it's impossible to prevent. They believe that we need to individually decide our moral positions about private matters. Many women have ended their pregnancies without anyone else knowing about it because it's such an intimate issue. Pro-choice advocates think that unless we want to let law enforcement become very intrusive in intimate issues, abortion must be legal.

The pro-choice movement also uses legal and medical considerations to defend their position. They argue that if abortion were illegal, it would be impossible to enforce. Such a law would lead to increased incidence of unsafe abortions and more maternal deaths, which violates the principle of nonmaleficence. When abortion is legal, we can then work to decrease the demand for it using tools such as education and contraception. In other words, we should try to make it legal and rare rather than illegal and deadly.

This is only a brief review of the pro-choice argument. For updates or more information, visit www.naral.org/.

Therapeutic Abortion: To Protect Maternal Health and Life

A *therapeutic abortion* is defined as removal of a fetus or embryo to protect the life or health of the *gravida*, or pregnant woman. A therapeutic abortion is intentional and performed because of *compelling reasons,* or a reason that most competent people agree on.

There are two types of abortion: medical and surgical. A medical abortion is performed in the first trimester of pregnancy using drugs. It is noninvasive. The drugs are given by injection or taken orally or as a suppository. This type of abortion simulates a natural miscarriage. A surgical abortion is invasive, performed with vacuum aspiration, or dilation and evacuation.

When the Reagan administration revitalized the pro-life movement, they said that most therapeutic abortions would still be permitted. This is no longer always the pro-life position, but does suggest that some therapeutic abortions may be less controversial.

In this section, we look at the ethical issues healthcare providers face when a therapeutic abortion is recommended. Sometimes an abortion can result in the best outcome for your patient. How do you inform the patient that this procedure might be necessary? What kind of counseling should the woman and her family receive? What is the provider's role if the woman chooses abortion or chooses to continue with the pregnancy?

Reasons for therapeutic abortion

The health of the mother has several meanings in a therapeutic abortion: in addition to a woman's physical health, her mental health must be considered. Reasons for a therapeutic abortion include:

- ✔ If the woman's life is in danger because of heart disease, cancer, or other disorders. In these cases, carrying a fetus to term and giving birth carries a high risk of killing the woman.

- ✔ If the woman's mental health status is compromised. If the pregnancy is the result of a rape or incest, pregnancy and delivery may be so traumatizing that it threatens the women's mental health, which can have a profound impact on her physical health.

- ✔ To prevent the birth of a child with significant birth defects such as hydrocephalus (abnormally large head). If the fetus is carried to term, the defect could compromise the life of the mother or cause the fetus's death soon after birth.

> ✔ To end a pregnancy that cannot proceed because of a maternal medical condition. This includes ectopic pregnancy (where the blastocyst embeds in the Fallopian tube and will burst as it grows, causing bleeding) or other diseases that cause complications, such as eclampsia, HELLP syndrome (hemolysis, elevated liver enzyme levels and low platelet count), or acute fatty liver of pregnancy.

Informing the patient

Telling a woman that her pregnancy is a threat to her health is one of the most difficult tasks a doctor must perform. It's important to be as compassionate and supportive as possible. It's also important to tell the patient the truth. Even if you are personally opposed to abortion, you must tell the patient that abortion is legal and available within certain parameters. If you have moral objections to abortion, even in this situation, refer the patient to another doctor who can objectively tell the patient about all of her options.

The patient should be told of all of the risks and complications of continuing the pregnancy and ending it. When the provider is certain that the patient understands her situation, he can recommend alternatives. In this case, the doctor should be the person to deliver the news and detail medical alternatives.

After the patient has been told about the problems with her pregnancy and all of the options open to her, the decision about what to do next rests entirely with her. An autonomous patient has the right to choose or refuse medical care when she fully understands the situation. A doctor can advise, but cannot decide what happens next.

In many states, the law regarding therapeutic abortion requires that the patient state in writing that she understands her medical situation and has told her doctor her entire medical history, including pre-existing conditions. This information is important for the best outcome, no matter if the pregnancy continues or is ended.

Ava's story: A case of therapeutic abortion

Ava, a 34-year-old woman, presented to her obstetrician at nine weeks gestation for her first obstetrical visit. Her Pap smear revealed cervical cancer, and further testing revealed the cancer had metastasized into the pelvis. Her doctor recommended that she undergo a hysterectomy, even thought she was pregnant, and then intensive chemotherapy and radiation for the best chance of survival. She had a husband and three other children. Based on religious beliefs, she was strongly against abortion. However, after consultation with her doctor, her priest, and her family, she learned that the Catholic Church allows therapeutic abortion in some cases to protect the mother's life and health. She agreed to proceed with the abortion.

Maria's case: When therapeutic abortion is illegal

Maria was a 27-year-old woman who lived in Nicaragua. In 2006, Nicaragua banned all abortions, with no exceptions. Maria began experiencing lower abdominal pain and went to her doctor. She was pregnant, but the pregnancy was ectopic: located in the Fallopian tube. She could not receive an abortion because her doctor would have been jailed for two to three years. She went to traditional healers who performed surgery on her without anesthetic or sterilized instruments. She hemorrhaged and died, leaving behind three children. The government position is that it can't supply protocols or guidelines on therapeutic abortions because it can't give guidelines for criminal activities.

If a patient is having trouble deciding whether or not to proceed with a therapeutic abortion and asks your opinion, be careful. Your opinion on this issue has great weight because of your position of authority and knowledge about the topic. It is wise to tell her to seek counseling so she can make up her own mind based on her worldview, lifestyle, opinions, and beliefs rather than share your personal opinion about abortion.

Therapeutic abortion is considered a human right by international organizations. However, three dozen countries around the world ban all abortions, even when the mother's life is threatened. The United Nations Human Rights Committee and the U.N. Committee on the Elimination of Discrimination Against Women urge countries to remove legal, emotional, and physical barriers to therapeutic abortion. Amnesty International and Human Rights Watch also oppose laws prohibiting therapeutic abortion.

Counseling for the family

A pregnancy is usually a welcome event and is greeted with joy and happiness. When something goes wrong and that pregnancy must end, trauma results. Some women and families who are affected when a therapeutic abortion is necessary develop post-traumatic stress syndrome (PTSD).

Counseling both before and after therapeutic abortion is important. A woman needs to work through all of her feelings about this issue in a safe, nonjudgmental, and supportive environment. It's also important to reassure the woman and her family that studies show abortion does not lead to infertility, cancer, or increased risk of suicide.

Many women go through abortions without significant emotional or mental strain. Psychological studies have found that women who have the most emotional problems following abortion are the very young, those with past psychiatric problems, women who are isolated or who have little social or emotional support, and those who belong to a group that is firmly pro-life. Anxiety and depression are common after a therapeutic abortion, but can be addressed and alleviated with good support from you, the provider, and referral to a counselor if necessary.

The political controversy about abortion can add to the family's stress. Even when an abortion is necessary to save the mother's life, she can feel guilt over the procedure. Second thoughts, grief, and anger are also common. Post-abortion counseling is a relatively new field, but a necessary step in the recovery process. Counseling should be nonjudgmental and should allow the patient to express emotions without shame or fear.

When a patient refuses medical advice

Sometimes a patient refuses a therapeutic abortion even when it is the best choice to preserve her health or even her life. It's important that you, the provider, are absolutely sure that the woman understands all of the risks and benefits of refusing the procedure.

Autonomy is an important principle in medical ethics, even when a patient chooses to forgo a procedure that may save her life. Counseling is usually recommended in case the woman is having a difficult time making the decision, or has said that others around her are pressuring her one way or the other. Because her life or health is at stake, it's especially important to make sure she understands the situation.

If a patient refuses a therapeutic abortion, you may want to refer her to an perinatologist, who handles high-risk pregnancies. In any case, both the mother and fetus should be treated with as much help and compassion as possible. You may continue to treat her throughout her pregnancy, or refer her to another physician, depending on her choice and decisions.

Exhale

Exhale is a nonprofit group located in California that offers a national telephone hotline (1-866-4-EXHALE) to counsel women who have had abortions. They also counsel the fathers, partners, and families. The organization believes that there are no right or wrong feelings after an abortion, but that women need an outlet to discuss their emotions in a safe and nonjudgmental environment. The organization respects the religious, cultural, and social beliefs of everyone who participates. Translators are available for non-English speakers upon request.

The case of Pam Tebow: Against medical advice

During the 2010 Super Bowl in the United States, an ad from Focus on the Family told the story of Pam Tebow, mother of Heisman trophy-winning son Tim Tebow, who refused a recommended therapeutic abortion in 1987. When living in the Philippines, Ms. Tebow was said to have amoebic dysentery, an often fatal disease when pregnant. She went into a coma and was treated with high doses of anti-parasitic drugs. She was then diagnosed with placental abruption, or separation of the placenta from the uterine wall.

Due to concerns about fetal defects from the drugs and the placental abruption, a therapeutic abortion was recommended. Maternal death due to placental abruption in underdeveloped countries is as high as 38 percent. However, Ms. Tebow chose to continue her pregnancy, and fortunately her son was born healthy. But is it ethical to encourage other women to refuse medical advice on the basis of one positive and relatively rare outcome?

This discussion does bring up one important point. If a women, when finding out that her fetus has a severe abnormality, decides to continue with the pregnancy, healthcare providers should support that decision, too. As long as the woman and her family understand what the abnormality will mean for them and for the child, she is fully within her rights, and it is ethical, to bring the pregnancy to term. No judgments or statements about this decision should be expressed to the woman or her family.

Abortion Due to Fetal Defect

There are many instances where an abortion is considered because of a problem with the fetus. A *selective abortion* is performed to reduce the number of fetuses in a multiple pregnancy, to end a pregnancy when a genetic defect, birth defect, or physical impairment is detected, or because the child's sex is not desired.

All of these reasons pose ethical questions. Some women have given birth to multiples with no problem. Others believe that the need to abort fetuses in multiple pregnancies caused by in vitro fertilization (IVF) makes that procedure inherently unethical. (See Chapter 10 for more on IVF.)

Some people think that a child with a birth defect can live a perfectly happy life, and that the push to abort is a form of eugenics. However, in the case of a severe defect or likely death upon birth, selecting abortion is permissible to this group. And many people think that ending a pregnancy for nonmedical reasons, for example because of the sex of the fetus, is not ethical because it is discriminatory. In this section, we look at the reasons for abortion for fetal defect and what you as a provider need to know about the issue.

Reasons for abortion because of fetal defect

There are many known birth defects and genetic defects. Some are major and some are minor. The tests for detecting these defects include amniocentesis, chorionic villa sampling, ultrasound, and maternal blood tests. The problem with many of these tests is that some aren't available or accurate until a pregnancy is in the second trimester. This makes the decision to end the pregnancy more difficult, both emotionally and legally. (For more information and details about these issues, see Chapter 9.)

Some of the fetal defects that can be reason for terminating a pregnancy include

- Down syndrome
- Neural tube defects, such as spina bifida and anencephaly
- Trisomy 13 and 18
- Turner syndrome
- Missing limbs or organs
- Klinefelter syndrome
- Sickle cell anemia

Although tests for these defects are an important part of the prenatal process, it's equally important that you, as the provider, respect the woman's choice to continue her pregnancy, no matter how serious the fetal diagnosis. Informing her about the problems and risks and supporting her decisions are your primary roles. Often, the percentages play a strong role in a patient's decision. Any time providers can quantify the risk with reasonable accuracy, they should do so.

As we discuss in Chapter 10, amniocentesis and chorionic villa sampling are not 100 percent accurate, although they approach that point. We've all heard stories about a fetus being diagnosed with Down syndrome, but being born healthy. Those situations do occur, but they are rare.

Informed consent is at the center of medical care. To exercise their rights, patients must be told of the risks and benefits of medical procedures in an accurate, truthful, and complete manner. This is especially important when a therapeutic abortion is medically indicated. If accurate information about fetal disease or defects is not provided and a severely handicapped child is born, providers can be sued. Several lawsuits in the 1960s about babies born to mothers who had been exposed to rubella (German measles) set the standard. Doctors must always inform pregnant patients of the risks to themselves and the fetus when any disease or condition is diagnosed.

Some people accept a disabled child as a part of life and can be happy with the decision to keep the pregnancy. Others aren't emotionally or financially equipped to deal with the problems these issues present. In most states, the law provides recourse for women who choose to end their pregnancy in the second and even third trimester. Be sure that you know the updated laws in your state.

Weighing the ethics of selective abortion

So what are the ethical issues unique to selective abortion? In this case, the mother's physical life is not endangered, so we are not weighing risk to the mother versus harm to the fetus. Instead, we are looking at the fetal defect and trying to determine how this will affect the future quality of the life of the fetus and the life of the mother and the rest of her family.

This again goes back to the definition of personhood. Some fetal defects, such as anencephaly, mean that the infant will never achieve the cognitive criterion put forth by Mary Anne Warren in her definition of personhood. However, the fetus has all of the DNA of a human being and meets the definition of personhood put forth by John Noonan.

A mother will be greatly affected by the birth of an impaired infant and her autonomy and life must be considered against the rights of the fetus and its potential for personhood. Each situation must be considered individually, as each situation is unique.

Tasha's case: Abortion for serious fetal defect

A 37-year-old woman named Tasha came to her family physician for pregnancy care. She had been undergoing treatment for infertility, and this was a much desired pregnancy. Because she was over the age of 35 (advanced maternal age), she was offered a level II ultrasound with a perinatologist along with an amniocentesis.

Unfortunately, the amniocentesis revealed that the fetus had trisomy 18, a severe birth defect that causes mental retardation. The baby usually dies in utero or soon after delivery. The mother was very distraught about these results. After discussion with a genetic counselor, she decided to undergo a selective abortion.

Voluntary Abortion

Voluntary abortion, or abortion on demand that isn't medically indicated and is outside the concerns for physical health and well-being, is fraught with dissent and division. This type of abortion is usually a last resort after an unintended pregnancy has occurred. Pro-life groups vehemently oppose voluntary abortion, whereas pro-choice groups believe that a woman's body is hers to control.

We have already had an in-depth look at the ethical arguments on both sides of the abortion issue at the beginning of this chapter. In this section, we look at the restrictions on voluntary abortion in the different trimesters of pregnancy and the issue of partial-birth abortion. And we take a look at RU-486, the so-called abortion pill, and its medical and ethical considerations.

Legal definition and limitations

In the United States and many developed countries around the world, abortion is legal in the first trimester with no limitations. The decision to end a pregnancy is left up to a woman and her doctor.

More than 80 percent of all countries around the world have made the decision that the state does not have the right to force a woman to remain pregnant. However, this stance does have limitations. In the United States, the Supreme Court has ruled that a fetus does not have the same legal rights as a person, so a woman can end a pregnancy without limitation within the first trimester. But there are strict limitations on abortion in the second and third trimesters, especially as the fetus approaches viability.

In the second trimester, abortion is available when there is a risk to the life and health of the mother or there is fetal abnormality. The standard used to decide if an abortion is performed is *appropriate medical judgment.* Because most medical tests that can detect abnormality can only be performed in the second trimester, or after the 16th week of pregnancy, states allow abortions for this reason.

The state has a compelling interest in the health of the mother, and because abortions after the first trimester are generally more risky, they are limited. The state also has more of an interest in the fetus as the pregnancy progresses. Because the laws about second trimester abortion are usually determined by individual states, a woman may have to travel to another state to have a late-term abortion.

And in the third trimester, when it is likely the fetus will be viable outside the womb, abortions are strictly regulated and can only be performed if there is a direct threat to the mother's life or health, or if the fetus is so compromised it will suffer and die soon after birth. Many states require second and third medical opinions on the threat to the mother's health for an abortion at this point. Abortions on demand are just not available at this stage of pregnancy.

Janice's case: Voluntary abortion

Janice was a 27-year-old single mother of two children. She presented to her doctor after missing her menstrual cycle for about two months, although she couldn't remember exactly when her last period had been. She had been taking birth control pills up until a few months ago, but lost her job and couldn't afford the prescription. She had an on-again, off-again relationship with a man and suspected she was pregnant.

A pregnancy test in the office confirmed it. She was distraught about the pregnancy. With no job, no partner, and two children depending on her, she didn't feel that she could emotionally or financially support another child. After a long discussion with her doctor and many tears, she requested a referral for an elective abortion at a local clinic.

The term *partial-birth abortion* was coined in 1995 by the National Right to Life Committee. No such term is recognized in medicine. The procedure is called *dilation and extraction*, or D & X. It is performed about 2,000 times each year in the United States (0.17.percent of all abortions) in response to threats to the mother's health, including heart failure, renal disease, uncontrollable high blood pressure, or if the fetus is severely deformed.

The Partial-Birth Abortion Ban Act was passed by Congress in 1995 and vetoed by President Clinton. In 2003, Congress passed and President George W. Bush signed this act into law. The act does have an exception to preserve a woman's life, but doesn't have an exception for non-life-threatening health factors, such as the mother's loss of fertility. The Supreme Court upheld the act in 2007.

Some doctors point out that this ban ignores the medically indicated reasons for the procedure. Caesarean sections, which could be performed at this stage, carry more risk to the mother's life and health and are impossible in some medical situations. The American College of Obstetricians and Gynecologists has stated that in certain circumstances, the dilation and extraction procedure is the best one for the woman's health. On the other hand, this procedure is very harmful to the fetus late in pregnancy. How does nonmaleficence to the fetus factor in? This situation raises some very difficult ethical issues. Be sure to include your hospital's legal department in these cases.

A less invasive option: RU-486

RU-486, or mifepristone, is a synthetic steroid used as an oral abortifacent. It blocks the hormone progesterone and induces a medical abortion up to 63 days after a woman's last period in 60 to 85 percent of cases. After 48 hours, a second drug that causes uterine contractions can be administered to raise the effectiveness to between 92 and 97 percent. Because the drugs cause serious birth defects, if a woman does not abort within a few days, a surgical abortion must be performed.

This drug became available in the United States in 2000. Before this, surgical abortions were performed, either by vacuum aspiration or dilation and curettage. Women choose RU-486 because it is less invasive than a surgical abortion, is much more private, and is less expensive. Only certain registered medical providers can obtain this medication.

As with any new issue in the area of abortion, a great deal of controversy erupted when the FDA approved RU-486. New medical and ethical concerns were raised. Would this make abortions more common? Would patients not follow up after the initial treatment and have severely deformed babies? Would this pill replace birth control as a means of avoiding unintended pregnancy? So far these fears have not been realized, but we'll see what the future holds.

Because it is easier to perform abortions with RU-486, it has led to some difficult discussions within physicians groups about whether to offer this service to patients. And some pharmacists are refusing to fill legitimate prescriptions for RU-486. If you are opposed to the use of RU-486, refer the patient to another doctor who will prescribe it.

Roe v. Wade: Legal Status of Abortion and Ethical Implications

The current legal status of abortion according to the United States Supreme Court is: Because the fetus is part of the woman's body, it does not have the same legal rights as a person who has been born. Therefore, the pregnant woman has the right of self-determination and autonomy. She can decide whether to accept or reject the burden of pregnancy. The Supreme Court ruling about abortion in *Roe v. Wade* uses the right of privacy established by the Fourteenth Amendment as the foundation for the decision to legalize abortion.

In the 1973 Supreme Court decision *Roe v. Wade*, the justices wrote, "The Constitution does not define "person" in so many words . . . In nearly all these instances, the use of the word is such that it has application only postnatally. None indicates, with any assurance, that it has any possible prenatal application." Justice Blackmun wrote, "We need not resolve the difficult question of when life begins. When those trained in the respective disciplines of medicine, philosophy, and theology are unable to arrive at any consensus, the judiciary, at this point in the development of man's knowledge, is not in a position to speculate as to the answer."

The Court stated that as the pregnancy proceeds, the state has an interest in the pregnant woman's life and health and the fetus's life and health. This interest in the mother's health becomes compelling at the end of the first trimester. Because of this ruling, all abortions are legal in the United States in the first trimester. The Court placed this date because "until the end of the first trimester mortality in abortion may be less than mortality in normal childbirth." Beyond the first trimester, *Roe v. Wade* allows states to place restrictions on abortions in the second and third trimester. Under the Partial Birth Abortion Ban Act, the state's interest in the potential life becomes compelling as the fetus approaches viability.

In this section, we look at how states have modified the law through the years and examine the controversy over abortion counseling.

Looking at changes on the state level

In the years since *Roe v. Wade* became law, states have been passing laws that restrict abortion. In a 1992 Supreme Court ruling *Planned Parenthood v. Casey*, the justices changed the standard for judging abortion laws. The law also let states place regulations on abortion procedures as long as the regulations didn't place an undue burden on women. The question is: Who decides what constitutes an undue burden? At this time, it is politicians and lawyers who are making these decisions, not doctors or the patients themselves.

States have added laws to limit abortion rights. As a medical provider, it's important that you are familiar with the laws in your state so you can be the best guide for your patient. Some examples of these limitations include:

- **Waiting periods for abortions.** In many states, women who go to a clinic for an abortion are given information and counseling and then must leave and return later for the procedure, so they will have to think about their decision. Many women do not return because they can't afford the transportation costs or the time off work. And waiting periods may force a women to delay her abortion until later in the pregnancy, when it may be illegal in her state and will certainly be more medically risky.

- **Restrictions on funding.** Direct federal funding for abortion procedures is banned in the United States. Abortion rights are defined at the state level, and federal funding for therapeutic abortion is only available in states that are willing to make it accessible. This matter is very complicated and varies by state. It's best if you learn the statutes in your state so you are prepared to answer patient's questions.

- **State and local laws and ordinances.** Some states have enacted *fetal abuse laws*. These laws, in effect, treat the death of a fetus as a murder case. Doctors aren't sure if they would face murder charges in these states if they perform an abortion, but they may face criminal charges. In Oklahoma, legislators overrode the governor's veto of a bill that requires doctors to give pregnant women requesting an abortion an ultrasound using a vaginal probe.

- **Forced counseling.** Many states require specific counseling between a doctor and pregnant woman before an abortion is performed. In some cases, doctors are forced to tell women false information about the effects of abortion (see the following section).

✔ **Parental and spousal notification and consent laws.** In most states, minors must get permission from their parents or a judge before they can have an abortion. And in some states, women must tell their spouses about the abortion before it can be performed. Of course, this becomes a problem in cases of child abuse, incest, spousal abuse, and rape.

The problem with many of these restrictions is that they violate the principle of justice because they place most of the burden on poor women. Women with means have always been able to get safe abortions: They just travel to states or countries where it is allowed.

Accurate medical counseling

Accurate medical counseling both before and after an abortion is an important ethical issue. Unfortunately, some states are enacting laws mandating that providers tell women about abortion complications and after-effects that are not true. Some legislators want doctors and providers to tell women that the fetus can feel pain during an abortion, that abortion can cause breast cancer or can render a woman infertile, or that abortion leads to a severe mental illness. All of those statements are untrue.

These statements are called *biased counseling*, and some or all are the law in 20 states in America. You, as a provider, need to decide if you are going to put the welfare of your patient ahead of what the law demands. If you are a provider in a state where pre-abortion counseling is required and it is not medically accurate, you are put in a very difficult position. Truth telling is a critical ethical principle and an important part of the doctor-patient relationship, as we outlined in Chapter 3. You may choose to give the required information and then advise the patient on what is actually medically accurate. Remember — your first responsibility is to your patient.

Talking to a patient about abortion

I have never had a patient come into my office and flippantly request a referral for an abortion. In my family practice, a discussion about abortion is rare and serious. I try to discover the woman's feelings about each of her options: abortion, adoption, or having and keeping the baby. It is also critical to find out what type of support system is available to her. Is the father of the baby involved? Are there parents, other family members, or friends who can support her in her decision? Are there any religious or cultural views that factor into her decision? Whatever she decides, I support her with compassion, continuing care, and follow-up for the path she chooses. I want her to know she is not alone during this difficult time.

One way to think about the counseling many women seeking abortions are forced to undergo is this: Are patients generally made to consider such information before undergoing other medical procedures? How many people would have face lifts or tummy tucks if they were forced to look at pictures taken during surgery, or made to undergo invasive procedures or told about untrue risks before the surgery is performed?

There are two standards for informed consent. One is the *traditional* or *community* standard, which some consider doctor-centered, set by common and customary practices in the medical community. The other is supposedly patient-centered and favors telling the patient more about any medical procedure because some advocates believe that doctors understate risks. Informed consent is already required before an abortion is performed, according to medical standards. The American Medical Association is opposed to procedure-specific informed consent on the grounds that it is unethical and violates the doctor-patient relationship.

The Religious Divide

There will always be a divide between some religions and medicine, no matter what the topic. Abortion, however, is a special case. Because many religions state that life begins at conception, many practitioners of those religions believe that abortion is murder. The major religions have official stances on this topic. Patients who belong to a specific religion are free to agree with that stance or disagree with it.

Although most religions have positions and guidelines about the subjects of birth control and abortion, few religious texts actually mention the procedure. And those who are not religious may also have concerns about abortion. The beliefs and positions of different religions include:

✔ **Jewish faith:** Jews believe that human life begins at the moment of birth, when the baby is more than halfway out of the birth canal. There is no specific prohibition against abortion in the Torah, and in Leviticus, babies aren't valued as human beings until they are one month old. Reform and Conservative Judaism support abortion rights, especially in cases where the mother's life or health is threatened. They believe that abortion is wrong, but it is not murder. Abortion should only be considered after careful consideration and consultation with a rabbi. Orthodox Judaism, on the other hand, holds that abortion is permissible only to save the mother's life.

- **Catholic faith:** Roman Catholics believe that all abortion is murder. In fact, they oppose birth control because it is felt that interfering with the act of procreation violates God's will. In some cases, Catholics believe that abortion should not be permitted even to save the life of the mother. But the church does sometimes permit acts that indirectly result in the death of the fetus to save the mother's life, also called the *double effect rule*, such as removing the pregnant uterus in a cancer operation. For more about the church's position on reproductive issues, see Chapter 10.

- **Protestant faith:** All faiths recognize the power of God in a person's formation and take abortion very seriously. However, Protestant views on abortion vary considerably. Some faiths are strictly pro-life, such as evangelical traditions, Pentecostals, and Southern Baptists. Some of the mainline Protestant denominations, like Presbyterians, Episcopalians, the United Methodist Church, and the United Church of Christ, consider themselves pro-choice and belong to a group called the Religious Coalition for Reproductive Choice.

- **Islamic faith:** In the Islamic faith, positions about abortion vary. Some sects prohibit all abortion, others allow it up to 40 days gestation, and some forbid it after three months. That last date is the point when believers think the soul enters the body. In some branches, abortion is permitted only in cases of rape or when the mother's life is in danger.

- **Buddhist faith:** Buddhists believe that because life is a continuum with no starting point, abortion should not be permitted. Therapeutic abortion is an exception.

- **Hindu faith:** According to this faith, one should always choose the way of least harm, including the mother, the fetus, the father, and society. Abortion is practiced in India, usually to prevent the birth of females. Some Hindus think personhood begins at three months, when they believe the soul enters the body.

Whatever your patient's religion, or your own, it's important to respect another person's beliefs. Tell your patient the truth about her condition, offer to find her counseling if she is having trouble making a decision, then support that decision. Sometimes conversations with pastors, priests, imams, or rabbis can help a woman decide what to do in her individual situation.

Toward Common Ground

Given the strong feelings people have about abortion in this country, can we ever find some middle ground? There are actually many things we agree on. We all agree on the difficult decision a mother with an unplanned pregnancy faces and have compassion for her.

We all agree that babies are valued and should be wanted, and we want to support actions that encourage healthy pregnancies. The taking of potential life is something we all regret. To that end, we can learn to support all women in their legally appropriate decisions. We can learn to have respectful conversations with each other and truly listen to other views. We can learn to improve the climate that favors adoption, and make contraception education and materials more available. And we can help improve the social situations of people so they are less likely to face unwanted pregnancies.

The issue is almost unbearably complicated, but most providers won't encounter it often. The majority of patients have already formed strong opinions on this issue. When you are confronted with a question about abortion, keep these considerations in mind:

- Determine what is acceptable to you. As a provider, you may be comfortable with some abortion procedures, but not others. Decide what you are comfortable with; then refer all other cases to other providers, with as much diplomacy and as little judgment as possible.

- Make sure you know the laws in your state and that your knowledge is up-to-date. When in doubt, call in a lawyer or clinic/hospital administrator.

- Support your patient the best you can. If the patient asks for advice, focus your comments on medical issues, but be willing to discuss other aspects of her life that may enter into her decision.

- Based on the patient's religious beliefs, cultural values, and as many other variables as possible, you may want to arrange for the patient to meet with a therapist, counselor, or spiritual advisor. This is no different than calling in a specialist from any other discipline. The specialist can help the patient make the decision that is best for her.

Chapter 12

Determining Death: Not an Event, but a Process

*A*s medicine continues to advance and push the frontiers of what we know to be true, it becomes more difficult to define the end of life. The standard of death has changed over the years. Doctors have more sophisticated tools for assessing life and death at their disposal today than ever before, making it much more complicated to decide when a person has died.

Decades ago, defining death was simple. A person was dead when they were no longer breathing and no longer had a heartbeat. Now high-tech machines can keep a person "alive" when they are no longer able to breathe on their own and their heart will not work without assistance.

In this chapter, we look at the legal and medical definitions of death, including the Harvard Ad Hoc Committee Report on Brain Death of 1968. We examine the Uniform Determination of Death Act from 1981. We look at why pinpointing the moment of death is very difficult; in fact, it may be different for each person. The idea of death is easy to grasp, but the criteria for death, or the physiological conditions that occur when we die, are more difficult to understand. Clinical testing can offer guidelines for judging when death has occurred.

We look at two landmark ethical cases that have helped us define death and issues around withdrawing life support: Karen Ann Quinlan and Nancy Cruzan. We look at the physician's role in the dying process, including the controversial topics of euthanasia and physician-assisted suicide.

All of the ethical principles are important in this chapter. Beneficence, autonomy, and nonmaleficence can be violated if someone's death is painful, premature, or artificially extended past what the patient would have desired. Justice is in question when a large amount of our healthcare resources are spent on end-of-life situations that may be lengthy and futile.

Defining Death

The moment of death can be difficult to define because so many biological and mental processes come into play. Add in the concept of personhood along with individual biological differences, and it can be hard to tell when someone has died. Does death come when all biological functions cease? When you permanently lose awareness of self? When all the traits and characteristics that define you are gone?

The definition of personhood is also critical to defining death. Defining personhood at the end of life is as difficult as defining it when life begins. In Chapter 11, we list several different definitions of personhood. And, as at the beginning of life, these definitions for the end of life are problematic.

According to some standards such as the *cognitive criteria,* personhood can end before the human body actually dies, such as in the case of a person with advanced dementia. According to other standards, such as defining a person as a human being with a full set of unique DNA, a person with no brain function who is kept alive on a ventilator is not considered dead. It is difficult, if not impossible, to draw a bright line between life and death, but some type of standard is needed.

In reality, cessation of cardiopulmonary function decides most cases of death. However, failure of the heart and lungs is not proof that the brain has died, especially if the patient is on life-support systems. Combining brain death with cessation of cardiopulmonary activity is the medical and legal definition of death.

When a human being dies, the person's rights, including rights to principles of medical ethics, end with it, and the rights of the deceased begin. In this section, we look at the history of defining death and how we have come to our current understanding of death.

Using heart and lung function to define death

Until the 1960s, the accepted medical definition of death was cessation of heart-lung function. However, three advances in medicine made this simple definition untenable:

✔ The creation of intensive care units, which were started by Dr. Bjorn Ibsen in 1953 in Denmark. These units help keep patients alive by assisting with breathing, kidney function, heart function, blood pressure stability, and nutrition and hydration.

✔ The development of mechanical ventilators, or artificial respiration. These machines keep the brain and body oxygenated when breathing is impossible or difficult.

✔ Organ transplantation. If the heart of a dead person can be in the body of another and keep that person alive, the cessation of heart function is not adequate as a measure of death. Medical intervention lets doctors keep the body of a dead person functioning so organs like the liver and kidneys can be harvested.

In 1967, surgeon Christiaan Barnard transplanted Denise Darvall's heart into dying patient Louis Washkansky. The question was asked: "Was Denise Darvall really dead before her heart was removed?" Clearly, her heart was still beating when it was harvested, so a new definition of death was needed, specifically that of brain death.

Adding brain function to the definition of death

In 1968, the Harvard Medical School Ad Hoc Committee wrote a definition of death that is neurologically based. This definition, or the Harvard Criteria, is called *brain death*. It states that death has occurred when

✔ The patient is unreceptive and unresponsive.

✔ There is no movements or breathing except for spinal reflexes.

✔ No brainstem reflexes can be observed, including pupillary signs, such as fixed, midsize pupils and no movement of the eyes when the head is turned. No facial expression response to pain is observed, and the gag and cough reflexes are not observed.

✔ Apnea, or the suspension of breath, is observed and tested, by disconnecting the ventilator, delivering oxygen, observation, then measuring levels of blood pH and Paco2 levels.

✔ Conditions such as drug intoxication and hypothermia must be excluded as a cause of physical exam findings.

If there is any uncertainty, the tests can be repeated 6 to 24 hours later. If the results are the same, the patient can be declared dead. When brain function has ended, doctors must determine that this condition is irreversible. An electroencephalogram (EEG) may be given to test for the existence of brain waves, but this is not necessary if all other criteria are present.

In 1981, a presidential commission issued a report that created and endorsed a model statute called the Uniform Determination of Death Act (UDDA). All 50 states and the District of Columbia have adopted this act as the legal definition of death. The act states:

> An individual who has sustained either (1) irreversible cessation of circulatory and respiratory functions, or (2) irreversible cessation of all functions of the entire brain, including the brain stem, is dead. A determination of death must be made in accordance with accepted medical standards.

The words *either* and *or* are key here. This wording takes some of the focus off the dying patient and accommodates the needs of patients waiting for organ donation. The commission stressed that these two definitions are complementary to each other and help expand our understanding of death. They also stated that as medical technology advances, ethics demand that the definition of death may need to be revised.

Examining Brain Death

The functioning brain is more critical to life than any other organ because it regulates the other systems in the body and integrates them into a whole person with thoughts and feelings. The brain plays a crucial role in the definition of personhood. Most other organs can be transplanted and function well in another body; the brain and most of the nervous system can't.

In this section, we explain how doctors know when a patient is brain dead. We also examine the differences between the types of brain death and try to explain the reasons each camp gives for their standard of death.

A quick look at how the brain works

The human brain has three regions with three different functions:

- The cerebrum is called the *higher brain* because it controls consciousness, reasoning, memory, feelings, and thought. This is known as higher brain function.
- The cerebellum controls movement and balance.
- The brain stem is called the *lower brain* because it controls essential functions such as breathing, swallowing, and sleep. Human beings with functioning brainstems can seem quite alive. They can breathe, digest food, yawn, and react to stimulation.

Knowing these regions and their functions can help you understand the different types of brain death.

Mary's story: Acknowledging brain death

Mary was a 53-year-old who had a previously undiagnosed brain aneurysm. The aneurysm ruptured, causing extensive bleeding in the brain. She collapsed and her brain did not receive oxygen for an undetermined period of time. After surgery, Mary emerged from anesthesia in a persistent vegetative state. She was breathing and would occasionally open her eyes and move her arms and legs, but she was unable to communicate with family, get out of bed, or feed herself. The family elected to have a feeding tube inserted to provide water and nutrients. She was eventually transferred to a nursing home. After a year of no significant improvement in brain function, the family elected to stop the feeding tube. They knew Mary would not want to live this way. After two weeks, Mary died.

Looking at the types of brain death

Brain death is divided into two categories:

- **Whole brain death:** When the whole brain is dead, all three regions of the brain (cerebrum, cerebellum, and brain stem) have stopped functioning. In other words, the brain is no longer organically functioning so the body no longer works in an integrated manner. A person must be kept alive on a ventilator because the brain stem, which controls breathing, is no longer functioning. Whole brain death is the criteria used in the UDDA.

- **Higher brain death:** When a person's cerebrum, or higher brain, is dead, that person is no longer conscious, cannot anticipate pain or pleasure, and cannot think or reason, but may still breathe, have some limited movement, and go through sleep and wake cycles. This definition of brain death regards the brain not just as the control room of the body, but as the organ that defines personhood. Not all ethicists agree with this definition, also called the *cognitive criterion standard of brain death*.

When the brain stem is still functioning but the cerebrum is not, the person is in what's called a *persistent vegetative state*, or PVS. This is different from a coma, where the patient has a profoundly debilitating lack of consciousness. In PVS, patients can have low levels of consciousness and can breathe, yawn, open their eyes, and react to painful stimulation. If a patient does not emerge from a PVS within one year, the likelihood of recovery is slim.

According to the standard of higher brain death, people in PVS are dead. But it's important to remember that according to the current standard, which is whole brain death, PVS is not death and is not recognized as death in any legal system. A few people who have been in PVS have recovered.

There are different ethical opinions on which category of brain death we should use. If the standard of whole brain death is used, then patients in a coma, patients in PVS, and anencephalic infants are still alive because their brain stems are still functioning. If the standard of higher brain death is used, these same patients are considered dead because their cerebrum is no longer functioning.

Current standards of brain death

So how does a doctor help a family member make a decision about treatment in the case of a patient who is likely brain dead? A patient's death may be more of a process than an event. There are three main medical/ethical standards which are currently considered when these decisions are made: The Harvard Criteria, the cognitive criterion, and the irreversibility standard.

The Harvard Criteria (as reviewed above) are very conservative. No one declared dead by these criteria has ever regained consciousness. It is said, "If you're Harvard dead, you're really dead." Because of the conservative nature of this criteria, it has applied to relatively few patients. And those awaiting organ transplants object to this standard.

A second standard is the cognitive criterion, a definition of personhood discussed in Chapter 11. This criteria states a person must have five capacities — reasoning, self-awareness, communication, agency, and consciousness of the external world — to be alive. The problem with using this criteria is that a person with an advanced neurologic disorder, such as end stage Alzheimer's disease, could be classified as dead. However, whether they realize it or not, families often use these criteria when making decisions about continuing treatments for their loved one as a patient nears death and loses their capacities.

The third standard of brain death is the irreversibility standard. This criteria states that death occurs simply when unconsciousness is irreversible. This places a burden on the treating physician to make this judgment (which is not always clear) and then guide the family. This is also used by families making decisions about care. A common question might be, "Doc, is there any chance she will pull out of this?" The irreversibility standard is also is helpful because it falls in between the Harvard Criteria and the cognitive criterion.

Declaring a patient brain dead

The ethical implications of declaring someone brain dead are significant. Declaring a person dead cannot be done on subjective or arbitrary grounds. A declaration of death means that artificial life support will be removed and the patient has no chance of recovery. Observing clinical criteria and supplementing those observations with diagnostic testing can ethically establish when death has occurred. A doctor can legally and ethically declare someone dead without the family's consent.

When family members see that their loved one is still breathing, they may not understand that the patient is brain dead. They may think the patient is still alive and can be helped by medical intervention. If you have determined that their loved one is brain dead, you must explain to them that brain death is not reversible and no medical intervention will restore the patient to a fully functioning human being. It's important to be as informative and compassionate as possible. Answer all questions honestly, use plain language instead of medical jargon, and take the time to talk to the family until they are comfortable with reality.

Understanding Cases That Defined Brain Death

There may never be a right time to die, and each case has to be evaluated and handled differently. Just as death can come too early, it can also come too late. As discussed in Chapter 6, quality-adjusted life years (QALY) numbers for quality of life can be less than zero; in other words, sometimes living can be worse than death. What if a patient isn't necessarily terminal, but is suffering with no hope for improvement? And who gets to decide if a life is worth living? These questions are being answered every day, one at a time, as patients, their family, and providers struggle to make difficult and compassionate end-of-life decisions.

The Right to Die movement claims the concept of dying with dignity. This movement is grounded in the principle of autonomy. If someone is in terrible pain from a terminal illness or irreversible state of consciousness, should he have to wait until the disease takes its course to die? And if a patient can't communicate his wishes for the end of life, who gets to decide if and when life support is withdrawn, or if a patient should be assisted in the dying process? Family members play an important role in this process, as we discuss in this section.

There are a number of important medical ethics cases about death and the right to die that have helped define death, establish laws, and set parameters for when a patient can be ethically removed from life support. The most recent newsworthy case was Terri Schiavo in 2005. That case is reviewed in Chapter 19. But two cases in particular laid the foundation for the definition of brain death and ethically withdrawing life support — Karen Ann Quinlan and Nancy Cruzan. We look at these cases as a way of understanding how ethical thought on the right to die has evolved.

Karen Ann Quinlan

In 1975, Karen Ann Quinlan was a healthy 21-year-old who fell into a coma after excessive alcohol and drug use. After 16 months on life support with no improvement, Karen's parents went to court to have her taken off the respirator. Her doctors and the administrator of the Catholic hospital disagreed with this plan.

The court ruled that her father, as her guardian, and based on the right to privacy, could let an incompetent patient die by removing life support. The Quinlans were able to recall two times when Karen said she would not want to be kept alive on machines, and that met the standard for respecting the patient's autonomy. Karen was weaned from the ventilator, but because nutritional support, at that time not considered artificial life support, wasn't removed, she lived for 10 more years.

The Quinlan decision mainly addressed the issue of substituted judgment for an incompetent patient. In the case of a patient who is unable to express her wishes, relatives or friends could substitute their judgment for the patient. But there are ethical problems with this approach. What if the family doesn't have the patient's best interest in mind or has ulterior motives? And if competent people aren't allowed to hasten their own death (through assisted suicide, for example), should they be allowed to hasten someone else's death? It wasn't until the Cruzan case in 1990 that these questions were addressed.

Nancy Cruzan

In 1983, Nancy Cruzan was a 24-year-old with anoxic brain injury after a car accident. She remained in PVS for seven years. At that point, her parents wanted her feeding tube removed. Nancy had no living will and the family couldn't present evidence of what her wishes would be, so the state court turned down the request, ruling that the state has an interest in preserving life regardless of the quality of life. The case was appealed to the Supreme Court.

Three important declarations came out of this case:

- First, a *competent* patient has the right to decline medical treatment even if it leads to death.

- Second, withdrawing a feeding tube isn't different from withdrawing other types of life support.

- And third, for *incompetent* patients, states may pass a law requiring that clear and convincing evidence of what a patient *would have wanted* be presented before life support is withdrawn.

Missouri had this law and Ms. Cruzan's wishes were unclear, so the tube remained. Later evidence presented by Nancy's friends met the standard of clear and convincing evidence, and the feeding tube was removed in December, 1990. Ms. Cruzan died 12 days later.

Another important ethical aspect of the Cruzan case is that, in the case of an incompetent patient, it moved us away from substituted judgment by a patient's family to really focusing on the patient's stated wishes and what was in the best interest of the patient. Both the Quinlan and the Cruzan case convinced the public of the importance of living wills (discussed in Chapter 13) as a way to let a patient's wishes become known in the event that she may be unable to express them at some point.

One ethical criteria doctors use to decide if life support should be continued if to ask if the burden of providing mechanical life support outweighs the benefit to the patient. There comes a point when continuing medical intervention can actually harm a patient by keeping them alive. This is called the *principle of proportionality*. To ethically end life support, these conditions must be met:

✔ Certainty beyond a reasonable doubt that no medical goals other than simply keeping the patient alive can be met.

✔ The patient cannot express wishes or preferences.

✔ Quality of life falls consistently below the minimum standard.

✔ The family agrees that life support can be withdrawn.

Of course, there are cases when the last condition is not met. It seems like most high-profile cases are about family members who want to let their loved ones die rather than others who want to use technology to keep them alive. But that situation does arise.

Withdrawing Life-Sustaining Treatment

In the end, many people choose either to not accept or to withdraw life-sustaining treatment. This time is difficult and emotional for the patient, the healthcare providers, and the family. Sometimes the decision to withdraw treatment is clear; other times, a lot of tests and thought must go into the decision. Because the provider's primary role is to sustain life, it can be difficult to end treatment.

Life-sustaining treatment is any drug, procedure, or surgery that extends life without curing the disease or condition. It can include

✔ Artificial nutrition, such as tube feeding

✔ Artificial hydration, such as IV fluids

✔ Mechanical ventilation

✔ Blood transfusions

✔ Renal dialysis

✔ Antibiotics

✔ Chemotherapy

The question of withdrawing treatment at the end of life is controversial. In this section, we look at deciding when further treatment for a terminally ill person is futile and how to help friends and family cope with the decision.

Weighing the benefits of further treatment

Medical futility is a judgment that further medical treatment would have no useful result. Many ethicists don't think doctors should use the term *futility* when talking to a patient or a family because it has overtones of giving up or not trying to help the patient.

It's important to understand that it's usually easier to not begin using a treatment or drug than to stop using it. But at the end of life, there is no ethical distinction between the two choices.

If a treatment is not going to help a patient improve, but only sustains life, there is no ethical difference between refusing to start it and ending it. But patients and families often think that ending a treatment has more ethical significance. A patient doesn't have to be terminal to request treatment be withheld or withdrawn. As long as the patient has capacity, he can decide the course of his treatment.

There are some important questions to ask before life-sustaining treatment is withdrawn. If the patient doesn't have the capacity to make this decision, and if there is no advance directive, relatives, or substitute decision-makers need to have a meeting with the doctors and ask these questions:

✔ Will this treatment make a difference in the patient's condition?

✔ Do the benefits of treatment outweigh the burdens?

✔ Is the treatment distressful or burdensome for the patient or family?

✔ Is there any hope for recovery?

✔ If the patient can improve, what will his life be like?

If the family wants a futile treatment to continue, you will have to have some conversations with them. They need to understand that if the patient is not going to improve, continuing to provide treatment becomes a burden. Ethics committees and the courts may need to be brought in to a case for it to be resolved.

Remember to tell the family that the withdrawal of treatment doesn't cause death. The underlying illness or disease causes the death that the treatment was postponing. That's the ethical line between withdrawing treatment and euthanasia: the difference between allowing to die and actively killing.

If the life-sustaining treatment has just begun, it may be wise to let it continue for a while to see how the patient responds. Evaluating the treatment's efficacy and the patient's condition over a few days might make the situation more clear and the decisions easier. But you must be careful that the patient doesn't suffer unnecessarily while changing drugs and treatments to see how they react to different scenarios.

Counseling the family

The end of a patient's life is a major event for the family. Making decisions about withdrawing treatment, beginning terminal sedation, and issuing DNR orders are the most difficult anyone can make. It's important that you, the provider, are compassionate and offer counseling for any family member who wants or needs it.

When the family disagrees with a patient's end-of-life decisions, and those decisions are outlined in an advance directive, healthcare providers are obligated to follow the patient's wishes, in accordance with the principle of autonomy. If there is no advance directive, the family members who object to withdrawing life-sustaining treatment have often prevailed. As a provider, your responsibility is to keep the lines of communication open and try to decide with the patient if possible, and family members if necessary, what the patient would want and what is best for him.

Examining Euthanasia and Physician-Assisted Suicide

Euthanasia, or mercy-killing, is the practice of ending a life deliberately to relieve intractable suffering. As you can imagine, there are plenty of ethical issues to discuss regarding this issue. Proponents of euthanasia consider that a death filled with suffering is a wrongful or bad death and that euthanasia should be legal. Opponents of euthanasia would say that any deliberate effort to cause death is wrong.

Physician-assisted suicide (PAS) is a form of euthanasia where a doctor physically helps someone kill themselves. In this section, we look at both types of death and examine the ethical issues about each of them.

The American Medical Association (AMA) opposes euthanasia and physician-assisted suicide. The AMA states that if a medical practitioner acts in accordance with good medical practice, the following forms of management at the end of life don't constitute euthanasia or physician-assisted suicide:

- ✔ Not initiating life-prolonging measures
- ✔ Not continuing life-prolonging measures
- ✔ The administration of treatment or other action intended to relieve symptoms which may have a secondary consequence of hastening death

Relieving suffering with mercy-killing

Euthanasia, which means "good death" in the original Greek, is further divided into voluntary (with consent of the patient), involuntary (without consent of the patient), and non-voluntary (patient unable to give consent). Many ethicists think that only voluntary euthanasia has the possibility of being an ethical act.

The AMA has taken the position that euthanasia, or killing a human being, is never ethical or moral. The AMA Code of Medical Ethics states, "Euthanasia is fundamentally incompatible with the physician's role as healer, would be difficult or impossible to control, and would pose serious societal risks."

There is an ethical difference between suicide and refusing medical care. The difference is this: When refusing care, the patient is not ending her life. She is simply not allowing someone to help her live and is letting the disease progress naturally, leading to death. Suicide is a self-inflicted action. When life-saving care is refused, the disease is the cause of death.

Understanding the history of physician-assisted suicide

In 1990, the U.S. Supreme Court, in *Cruzan v. Missouri Department of Health*, established a patient's right to request removal of life support. Most nationwide polls show a majority of Americans think doctors should be allowed to help their terminally ill patients die. And in the 1990s, Dr. Jack Kevorkian took this a step further and began assisting patients in their deaths.

The first case was that of Janet Adkins, a 54-year-old woman with early onset Alzheimer's disease, whose case became public in 1990. As Adkins's memory loss progressed, she was convinced that she wanted to die with dignity before she became debilitated.

Adkins, who was from Oregon, traveled to Michigan to meet with Dr. Kevorkian, a retired pathologist. After a long meeting with Kevorkian and her family, and after signing many forms, Adkins decided to proceed with the assisted suicide.

The next day, in the back of Kevorkian's Volkswagen van in a public park, Adkins self-administered thiopental (a sedative) and then intravenous potassium chloride, which killed her. Dr. Kevorkian eventually built a machine that let patients self-administer the lethal drugs. A landslide of publicity ensued.

There was no law against physician-assisted suicide in Michigan at the time, so Kevorkian was able to continue this practice. (Kevorkian's initial interest in physician-assisted suicide was to increase the number of organs for transplantation, and he only later came to see it as compassionate assistance to the dying.) He eventually lost his medical license, which made it impossible to obtain the IV medications he needed to continue with his work. He reverted to the use of carbon monoxide gas. By 1998, the Michigan legislature passed a law making physician-assisted suicide illegal, but not before Kevorkian had assisted in over 100 deaths. He continued his practice, was arrested in 1998, and sentenced to a 10-to-25-year sentence at age 70.

Many people were surprised that a physician would be so directly involved in facilitating a patient's death. But even more surprising was the support for Dr. Kevorkian among terminal patients and the patients seeking his care. There was so much public support for this side that the states of Oregon and Washington eventually passed laws permitting physician-assisted suicide.

When a doctor aids in death

In 1994, the state of Oregon passed the Death with Dignity law, which took effect in 1997. Doctors in that state can prescribe drugs to help their terminally ill patients commit suicide. The patients themselves administer the drugs. Prescribing lethal drugs is tightly controlled. These controls include:

- The patient must be 18 years or older and a resident of Oregon.
- The patient must have capacity to make healthcare decisions and have expressed his or her wish to die.
- The decision must be made with informed consent. The patient must be told of her diagnosis, prognosis, risks of the drugs, the probable result of using the drugs, and alternatives.
- The patient's diagnosis and prognosis must be confirmed by a consulting doctor. The primary care physician might also request a psychiatric evaluation.

The patient's request is submitted in written form and is witnessed by at least two people. At least one of the people witnessing this request must not be a relative, anyone who would inherit an estate from the patient, or anyone employed by a healthcare facility. The patient should be told that they need to have another person with them when they take the drugs, and to be in a private place when they do so. The patient can withdraw the request at any time. There is a 15-day waiting period before the patient gets the drugs.

The doctor, pharmacist, nurses, and other healthcare providers in a state where physician-assisted suicide is legal are immune from civil or criminal charges when they participate. They also cannot be suspended or censured by any organization. And no doctor, pharmacist, or healthcare provider can be forced to participate in this procedure.

In 1997, the U.S. Supreme Court ruled that the states can decide if doctor-assisted suicide should be legal or not. The ethical question is if a patient has capacity, is suffering, and has a terminal condition, can the state force them to continue living? This ruling allowed the people of Oregon and Washington to keep the laws making physician-assisted suicide legal.

Physician-assisted suicide raises difficult ethical questions. Is killing ever justified? Is there a difference between killing and letting die? Should physicians, whose primary role is healing, be involved in ending a life? Does simply prescribing the medication, but not administering it, lift the ethical burden of nonmaleficence from a doctor? How far does patient autonomy go? And will this lead to a slippery slope where people will kill or allow suicide for lesser reasons than terminal illness? These questions are being asked and answered every day as we struggle to maintain ethical standards at the end of life. Currently, the AMA and other physician organizations don't support physician-assisted suicide because of some of these ethical concerns.

Oregon Request for Medication to End Life

This form states: "I, _____, am an adult of sound mind. I am suffering from _____, which my attending physician has determined is a terminal disease and which has been medically confirmed by a consulting physician. I have been fully informed of my diagnosis, prognosis, the nature of medication to be prescribed and potential associated risks, the expected result, and the feasible alternatives, including comfort care, hospice care, and pain control. I request that my attending physician prescribe medication that will end my life in a humane and dignified manner. I understand that I have the right to rescind this request at any time. I understand the full import of this request and I expect to die when I take the medication to be prescribed. I further understand that although most deaths occur within three hours, my death may take longer and my physician has counseled me about this possibility. I make this request voluntarily and without reservation, and I accept full moral responsibility for my actions." From ORS 127.800 to 127.897.

Chapter 13

Death with Dignity: The Right to Appropriate End-of-Life Care

*E*veryone has to die. That's a fact of life. But when we die and how we choose to die raise ethical questions. If a patient is autonomous, can she choose to end her life? How can she communicate her wishes for care at the end of life if she can no longer communicate? What is the provider's role in a patient's death? And what resources are available to help us die with dignity?

How and when we die has direct connections with autonomy, nonmaleficence, beneficence, and justice. A person has the right to refuse medical treatment even when he can't physically express that right. Keeping a person alive through extraordinary measures when he doesn't want them violates nonmaleficence and justice. And relieving pain, even if the methods hasten death, is ethical according to the principle of beneficence and the rule of double effect.

Since modern medicine became the standard in the developed world, people live much longer than their ancestors. Because most of us no longer die from preventable infectious diseases, untreated illnesses like diabetes, or being attacked by wild animals, it's the diseases that come with age that lead to death. And because of technological advances in modern medicine, it can take us a long time to die. Death with dignity is a difficult proposition, but one all of us want. And it is mandated by all ethical principles.

In this chapter, we examine how making a roadmap for care at the end of life is an integral part of autonomy. We also look at advance directives and DNR/DNI orders.

Relief of pain and suffering is an important issue at the end of life, too. When should drugs that could shorten a life, but also relieve severe pain, be given?

And when should life-sustaining treatment end? Who makes that decision? We also look at determining if a patient is competent to make these difficult end-of-life decisions themselves, based on their own competency or capacity, or if a surrogate decision-maker is needed.

The moment of death sometimes provides the opportunity to give a lasting gift — an organ donation. The final section in this chapter explores the ethical issues associated with organ transplantation: just allocation of organs, costs of transplantation, and finally a possible new frontier in transplantation — xenotransplantation.

Roadmaps for the End of Life

There are many activities you can do on the Internet: become an ordained minister, order 100 pounds of pistachios, and download documents that instruct your doctor about your care at the end of life. An Advance Health Care Directive, or advance directive (AD), is a document that expresses the type of care you want if you become incapacitated.

The goal is to prevent futile or invasive treatments, such as CPR or aggressive resuscitation, or other medical care at the end of life, as well as to request extraordinary measures to maintain life. Doctors and providers are required to follow the wishes set forth in this document. All advance directives are recognized in all 50 states in the United States. These documents are so important because they relate directly to the principle of autonomy.

In this section, we examine the types of advance directives and how they satisfy the principle of autonomy. Who needs them? What should be in these documents? We examine how advance directives work and why it's important that they are followed at the end of life. And we look at the physician's order for life-sustaining treatment (POLST) and when it is ethically mandated.

Understanding advance directives

Advance directives are legal documents filed in advance by the patient, detailing their wishes in case they are incapacitated. Incapacitated doesn't mean the patient has lost his mind. It just means that he can no longer communicate and express his wishes and can't understand the risks and benefits of healthcare choices. A lawyer is not required to fill out an advance directive.

Types of advance directives include

✔ Living wills, which state the type of care a patient wants or doesn't want at the end of life. A surrogate cannot be named in a living will.

> ✔ Durable power of attorney for healthcare, in which the patient can choose a surrogate to make decisions for him if he is incapacitated.
>
> ✔ DNR orders, which demand that a patient not receive extraordinary efforts to revive them, such as CPR, if they die.

The courts have long recognized that when deciding end-of-life treatment, the patient's wishes should be respected first and foremost. Then the wishes and opinions of a proxy or closest family member should be considered next, in line with the principle of autonomy.

Advance directives don't force a doctor to pull the plug on Grandma, as some politicians have stated. They give directions for that specific person's wishes for care at the end of her life, which can ease a family's stress when that time approaches and respects that patient's wishes. Dealing with the loss of a loved one is difficult enough. Deciding when to perform medical procedures, or deciding when the loved one's suffering should end, can just be too painful.

Everyone really should have an advance directive or go through advance care planning. But those people with terminal illnesses, those at risk for sudden death (strokes or accidents) and those who have a history of severe mental illness should especially be encouraged to plan ahead.

As your patient's provider, ethics demand that you should ask your patients if they have a living will or opinions about their end-of-life care. In fact, you are required by the 1991 Patient Self-Determination Act (PDSA) to tell patients about their right to autonomy and decision making in their care. This information should be entered on the patient's chart so there is an official record of it. This is especially important at a preoperative evaluation visit, when a patient enters the hospital for any reason, or when a patient is diagnosed with a terminal illness.

The case of Miriam: Importance of a living will

Miriam was a 93-year-old woman living in a nursing home in a small southern town. She had a series of small strokes, and was having trouble with dementia and swallowing. She would aspirate food into her lungs instead of swallowing it and would then develop pneumonia, which landed her in the hospital. The last time this happened, her son, a local farmer, wondered if she should continue to be hospitalized and treated with antibiotics for a situation that would only get worse. The patient's daughter from the East Coast arrived and felt differently. The daughter wanted a feeding tube placed and wanted her mother treated for every problem. Fortunately, the patient had a living will that stated she did not want a feeding tube, or even antibiotics, in a terminal situation where her quality of life was poor. Because the patient's wishes were so clearly stated, she was made comfortable and died peacefully in the nursing home, of pneumonia, one week later.

Talking with patients about their living wills

I am more than happy to spend time with a patient discussing his or her living will. This subject often comes up when patients have a terminal or chronic illness. Sometimes a patient just brings a document to file on their chart. I take extra time in that visit, or set up another visit and encourage the patient to bring a family member or friend along. We go over the document together and discuss possible scenarios. It helps me understand the patient, get to know them, and also understand their loved one's feelings. These discussions also help the patient know that their deepest desires are understood and that they have been heard. They know their wishes will be honored when the time comes. No living will can anticipate every scenario, but what that patient wants can often be inferred from the document and our intimate discussions.

If a patient is still able to give informed consent, it is unethical to use a proxy, surrogate, or advance directive to treat that patient. Advance directives of all kinds become effective only when the patient is unable to communicate his wishes or participate in medical decisions. And these documents are revocable. If a patient changes his mind, the advance directive can be destroyed and any mention of it wiped off his chart. This request does not have to be made in writing, does not need the services of an attorney, and will stand up in court. The patient must make sure that her providers, family members, and proxies know the document has been revoked. A court can invalidate an advance directive if someone challenges its validity and can prove the patient wasn't of sound mind when the document was created.

Looking at living wills

Living wills are the most common form of advance directive, in which the patient lists direct preferences for end-of-life care. These documents extend patient autonomy beyond a point where they can no longer give informed consent. The living will lets a patient outline their wishes while they are still able to make those decisions.

In an ideal world, everyone would have a living will. A living will not only states what treatments the patient would like to forgo at the end of life, it also states the treatments he wants. If the patient wants everything done to keep him alive until the last possible moment, that can be stated in a living will.

In a living will, a patient can

✔ State the amount of time (days, weeks, or months) they wish to remain in a coma or a persistent vegetative state (PVS) before life support is removed.

✔ Choose the type of treatments the patient wants and doesn't want. For instance, he can state he doesn't want to be intubated or fed through a tube.

✔ Distinguish between treatments for a terminal illness and a permanent disability, such as dementia from Alzheimer's.

✔ Distinguish among treatments for comfort, also known as palliative care and treatments that prolong life.

If a living will states that the patient wants some treatment that the doctor determines will be harmful, that directive can be ignored on the grounds of non-maleficence. The AMA states further: "Denial of treatment should be justified by reliance on openly stated ethical principles and acceptable standards of care."

But even the best written living wills don't cover all possibilities of what can happen at the end of life. Anyone writing a living will should be told that there is medical uncertainty throughout life and in any medical situation. From the AMA: "Physicians are not ethically obligated to deliver care that, in their best professional judgment, will not have a reasonable chance of benefiting their patients. Patients should not be given treatments simply because they demand them."

One of the problems with the living will is that they are usually written using ambiguous language, such as "do not unnaturally prolong my life." And patients can't foresee every problem or condition that can arise or the type of treatment that may be available at that time.

A living will is best if there are specific instructions, and many advance directive forms have been changed to reflect that. These instructions can be very detailed, as in "do not give blood transfusions" or "do not perform CPR." If they are not detailed, it's up to you, the provider, to interpret what "unnaturally prolonging life" may mean. Always keep nonmaleficence and beneficence in mind when dealing with end-of-life issues and vague advance directives.

For a living will to take effect, the doctor must declare that a patient can no longer make decisions and can't communicate wishes. Living wills are used only at the end of life, when the chance of recovery is slim to none.

Looking at Durable Power of Attorney for Health Care

The second kind of advance directive is a proxy document called a Durable Power of Attorney for Health Care (DPAHC). In this document, a patient chooses a surrogate, or proxy, to make medical decisions on their behalf. This document can be more useful for patients who don't have close family members or who are in nontraditional relationships that don't have the power of the law behind them.

Drafting your own living will

A living will is a simple form that can be completed by just about anyone. Each state has its own form. They can be downloaded for free from the Internet at sites such as www.gavel2gavel.com. And you don't need a lawyer. Most states require that a living will be signed and witnessed by at least two people. Some states also require a notary stamp.

It's important to tell your doctor and relatives that you have a living will. Having this noted on your chart is critical. And talking to your family about your living will is important, too. If you have designated a proxy, make sure he understands your wishes. These conversations aren't easy, but they are essential.

Laws about living wills vary by state. It's important to make sure that your living will is correctly written and witnessed according to local laws. There are living will registries available that will hold the document or documents until they are needed. Notification of the registration is added to insurance cards and driver's licenses. Most states have enacted laws that state a death that follows an advance directive cannot be ruled a suicide.

The word *durable* is crucial here. That word means the document stays in effect after a patient has lost decision-making capacity due to illness or injury. And decisions made by the proxy outweigh family choices.

Most patients should have both living wills and DPAHC so as many situations as possible are covered. If a living will is vague, or an issue comes up that isn't addressed in that document, the doctor should ask the DPAHC-appointed proxy to step in. This follows the principle of autonomy: first the patient's wishes are followed and then a proxy makes decisions if the wishes are unclear.

Sometimes a patient made their wishes regarding end-of-life care known to someone else before they became incapacitated, either verbally or in a written form. In that case, a proxy or relative can judge what the patient would have wanted in extreme medical situations.

The key here is *what the patient would have wanted*. Autonomy is the overriding principle in this situation. Because a patient's relationships with every person are all different, who can say what that particular patient's true wishes would be? The news is full of stories about patients in persistent vegetative states who didn't have an advance directive. Relatives fight for years over what the patient would have wanted. This is where a hospital's Ethics Committee or the courts can become involved, as in the cases of Karen Ann Quinlan, Nancy Cruzan, and Terri Schiavo.

Do Not Resuscitate and Do Not Intubate orders

A Do Not Resuscitate (DNR) order tells healthcare providers that a patient doesn't want cardiopulmonary resuscitation, or CPR, at the end of life. This order also refers to defibrillation, or shocking the heart when it stops beating. This is the only type of medical treatment this order affects. In some cases, CPR can save a person's life, but result in a life lived with brain damage, in a coma, or in a PVS. If CPR is performed on a patient who doesn't want it, the principle of nonmaleficence is violated.

A Do Not Intubate (DNI) order tells providers that a patient doesn't want a breathing tube inserted in the throat in case of respiratory arrest. This order can be given separately from a DNR order or combined with it. As with a DNR order, a DNI order can be revoked or rescinded at any time. Usually, these orders are obtained together, and if the patient rejects both forms of intervention their code status is documented as DNR/DNI.

Any patient can add a DNR/DNI order to a living will. But in an emergency situation, CPR is always performed unless a patient has a portable DNR or their documented code status with them, or if a family member has one. It's a good idea to recommend a portable DNR/DNI to patients with a terminal illness or who might die within a specific timeframe. There is jewelry, similar to ID bracelets, that patients can wear to prove they have a portable DNR. Some patients joke about having "DNR" tattooed on their chest! And similar to a living will, a DNR order can be rescinded if the patient recovers or changes his mind.

Weighing likely outcomes of CPR

At our local hospital, the admitting physician is expected to obtain a patient's code status upon admission. In a young, healthy, 18-year-old admitted for appendicitis, for instance, this is easy. They will be rated as *full code* or *full resuscitation* status because they are otherwise perfectly healthy and would likely recover completely if, for some unusual reason, resuscitation was needed.

But what about the 82-year-old man admitted with advanced congestive heart failure and emphysema? In a case like this, I explain exactly what resuscitation is — chest compression and shocking the heart, as well as putting a tube down the patient's throat to breathe for them along with attachment to a ventilator. I try to explain that although he may recover to his current level of functioning, given his already compromised health it is unlikely that CPR will be successful. Even if it is, the procedure may leave him neurologically impaired. No matter what a patient decides, if they want full code or DNR/DNI, I respect his wishes and document them on the chart.

It is vitally important that you, the doctor or healthcare provider, honor DNR/DNI requests. If you don't think this is best for your patient, arrange for another doctor who agrees with the order to take over the care of that patient.

But what if there's a conflict between a living will or DPAHC and a DNR/DNI order? It's been established that the living will has the highest authority, next the DPAHC has precedence, and the DNR/DNI order is last.

Physician's Order for Life-Sustaining Treatment (POLST)

Since 1995, in the United States, a new type of voluntary advance directive has been gaining popularity. A Physician's Order for Life-Sustaining Treatment (POLST) is a set of medical orders developed by a doctor and patient that set forth the patient's wishes about end-of-life treatment. This document is similar to a DNR order but broader in scope because it also addresses the type of treatment the patient does want. This document is also called a Medical Order for Life-Sustaining Treatment or Physician Order for Scope of Treatment.

POLST programs are patient-centered and satisfy the principle of autonomy. Because they are a doctor's orders, they have more weight than advance directives. The Order turns wishes about end-of-life care into actual medical orders. No one is talked into any type of treatment, and no one is encouraged to use less or more technology. A POLST is the result of an honest and frank conversation between a doctor and patient and is the result of informed consent. A POLST doesn't replace other advance directives, but it can help define a vague living will.

A study published in the journal *Cancer* found that half of the surveyed doctors don't discuss advance directive planning with terminal patients until all treatments have failed. One difference between POLST directives and living wills is that the doctor actually sits down with the patient and discusses end-of-life care with a POLST. A living will form is given to the patient, and he fills it out at his leisure.

How POLST works depends on the state. If a state doesn't have a POLST program, the form can't be used. A POLST must always be signed by a doctor, but some states require the signature of a nurse or physician's assistant, too.

At this time, fewer than a dozen states have endorsed this program, but many states are beginning to embrace it. To see if your state has POLST laws or is working on developing a program, go to www.polst.org.

The death panel myth

The story of the death panel in the 2010 United States healthcare reform debate started based on POLST directives in Lacrosse, Wisconsin. That state has POLST directives, and more than 90 percent of the people living in that town have a POLST. Hospitals in Lacrosse spend an average of $18,000 on the last two weeks of a patient's life, compared to $64,000 on an average end-of-life span of 39 days at the University of Miami Hospital or 54 days and $66,000 at New York University's Langone Medical Center. The costs are lower because people plan for end-of-life care. Citizens in Lacrosse are angry over the death panel designation. They say that POLST directives are the exact opposite of a death panel because they give the patient choices in care when they can no longer speak for themselves. In other words, POLST forms respect patient autonomy.

Of Sound Mind: Establishing Mental Capacity

Of course, to make an informed decision about end-of-life care, a patient has to be capable of making that decision. Informed consent, the backbone of autonomy, must also be present when planning end-of-life care. Establishing mental capacity can be difficult in some cases, when the patient may be experiencing dementia or the effects of other diseases. It's not ethical to make medical decisions based on a patient's wishes when that patient can't understand what is happening to him.

A patient who isn't capable of making a medical decision may not only refuse care; he may choose care or types of treatments that could actually harm him. The ethical conflict here is between autonomy and beneficence. It's important to understand that capacity can also be questioned if a patient agrees with everything their doctor recommends. It's appropriate for a doctor to assess capacity in a patient at the end of his life to make sure he understands the decisions being made.

In this section, we look at the issue of informed consent when a patient may not have the capacity to decide, and discuss how to check on that capacity. We also examine how substitute decision-makers can be used if a patient can't make decisions about his care.

Understanding informed consent and a patient's ability to give it

A patient can provide informed consent only when he understands what is happening. That is central to the ethical practice of medicine, and healthcare providers have a legal and ethical obligation to understand and embrace this concept. Informed consent is based on a voluntary, uncoerced decision, but it is also based on reasoning and understanding. For more about informed consent, see Chapter 3.

Competency is a legal status that is determined by a judge. When a patient is ruled incompetent, substitute decision makers are appointed for him. So healthcare providers use the word *capacity* instead to judge if informed consent has been given. A patient must have capacity to give informed consent about his care. Capacity is determined by a doctor's assessment and doesn't carry any legal weight.

Just because a patient has dementia or other mental impairment doesn't mean that he can't determine what type of medical procedures he wants and doesn't want. For instance, a patient who can't tell you what year it is may still have the capacity to say they don't want a feeding tube inserted.

There are other factors to consider, too, when considering a patient's capacity to make decisions.

- ✔ Depression can affect decision-making capacity. Many elderly and terminal patients suffer from depression. If the patient has depression, it's important to diagnose and treat it before continuing with any discussions about withdrawing treatment. Not taking this step violates the principle of nonmaleficence.

- ✔ Pain, both physical and emotional, can affect capacity. Researchers have found that atrophy can occur in the prefrontal cortex of people who suffer from chronic pain. This area of the brain controls decision-making ability and lets patients understand consequences of their decisions.

- ✔ Concern about the burdens the illness places on loved ones and caregivers can influence a patient's decisions about end-of-life care. If a patient feels that her family members are unduly stressed about the situation, she may decide not to accept lifesaving treatment. This violates the principle of autonomy.

- ✔ The cost of treatment may be a factor. If medical bills are mounting as a patient approaches the end of life, this worry can cloud decisions a patient makes about her care. Government studies show that 25 percent of Medicare money is spent on patients in their final year of life. Most of that money is spent in the last few months, when benefit to the patient is questionable.

✔ The patient's cultural and religious beliefs should be taken into account. In some cultures, death is seen as a natural part of life, and extending life artificially is objectionable.

Assessing decision-making capacity

Assessing the capacity to make decisions is a critical part of ethical patient care based on the principles of autonomy and nonmaleficence. When decisions are high-risk, such as end-of-life care, you must be sure about the patient's capacity to make decisions.

There are set standards for deciding whether or not a patient has the capacity to make decisions about his care. They are:

✔ The patient can make a choice about treatment and can communicate that choice.

✔ The patient understands the diagnosis, prognosis, recommended care, alternatives to care, and risks and benefits of each.

✔ The patient's decisions are not in conflict with the values and goals he developed throughout his life.

✔ The patient is not suffering from severe mental illness such as depression or psychosis.

✔ The patient uses logical reasoning skills to make a decision about his care.

You can ask questions to determine if a patient has capacity, such as "Tell me how you decided on this treatment" or "Why do you think that angiography is worse than the alternative?" Open-ended questions can be more effective than simple yes-or-no questions. If you are unsure, you can also ask family and friends about the patient's decision to see if the choice is consistent with the patient's belief system.

A person is considered to have capacity unless a doctor decides otherwise. It's just like the legal principle of innocent until proven guilty. Sometimes a patient's lack of capacity is very apparent and obvious and no further testing is needed. But sometimes a provider could have questions about a patient's capacity to understand medical decisions, especially for more serious treatments like chemotherapy or life-sustaining technology.

There are tools available to help you assess capacity. One is the MacArthur Competence Assessment Tool for Treatment (MACCAT-T), an interview guide with a rating system. This tool evaluates

✔ The patient's ability to understand the available treatments

✔ The patient's ability to retain and process information about his care

✔ The patient's ability to reason

✔ The patient's ability to choose a treatment, communicate that choice, and to be consistent with that choice over time

Another commonly used test is the Mini Mental Status Exam (MMSE). This is a brief test of the patient's cognitive function that is used in the doctor's office to provide a quick assessment of capacity.

There is no one threshold or minimum score on a single test that can clearly identify patients who lack capacity. As the risks of a treatment increase, the standard for capacity should also increase. If a patient is found to lack capacity, a substitute decision-maker (SDM) should be brought in (see the next section for more information about SDMs).

Religious and cultural beliefs, along with language barriers, can affect communication, which might depress capacity. See Chapter 7 for more discussion about the impact religious and cultural beliefs can have on informed consent and capacity. And make sure that you don't jump to conclusions about capacity based on appearance, age, disability, or behavior.

In some states, the law requires that a second doctor agree with the diagnosis of incapacity before a surrogate is brought in or if capacity is questioned in decisions about life-sustaining treatment. Capacity can fluctuate depending on health at that moment. For some patients, especially those with dementia or Alzheimer's, you may need to assess capacity more frequently. Capacity is decision specific, so if there is any doubt, an assessment should take place every time an important medical decision needs to be made. To fully respect autonomy, this judgment should be made carefully and cautiously.

It can be difficult to tell a patient that they do not have the capacity to make decisions about their own health. It's important to stress to them that you have their best interests in mind and that by denying capacity you will reduce the possibility of harm. You must still discuss treatments and other medical decisions with an incapacitated patient, and try to get assent from them, which has a lower threshold than informed consent. For more about assent, see Chapter 8.

Substitute decision-makers: When a patient is declared incompetent

If you as a doctor find a patient incapable of making decisions about any type of treatment, no matter how minimally invasive or how vital, you should ask another person to be a substitute decision-maker, or SDM. This person could be a family member, a guardian, an attorney, or a public guardian. If there is more than one SDM, they must agree on any treatment or care decisions.

The SDM gives informed consent in place of the patient. That person or persons is entitled to all of the information that the patient would receive, overturning the issue of confidentiality. Then the SDM tries to reach the same conclusion he believes the patient would make. This is called *substituted judgment*. The principles of beneficence and autonomy should be foremost in making these decisions.

If the substitute decision-maker does not know the patient well, then the best-interests standard will be applied. Using this standard, the substitute, or proxy, thinks of what a reasonable person would want under these particular circumstances. Issues to consider include

- ✔ Freedom from pain
- ✔ Comfort
- ✔ Restoration of physical capability
- ✔ Restoration of mental capability

A substitute decision-maker who does know the patient well will make an educated guess at the patient's point of view. Even if a patient doesn't have capacity, he still may be able to express some beliefs or points of view that should be considered in any decision made about his care.

Relief of Pain and Suffering

One of the primary duties of any healthcare provider is to reduce pain and suffering. At the end of life, many patients fear physical and emotional pain and its accompanying suffering more than dying. The ethical conflict here is how much and what kind of medication healthcare providers should prescribe to relieve pain and suffering. What happens when intention to relieve pain results in the death of the patient?

In this section, we look at palliative care and the ethics of terminal sedation, including the double-effect rule, also called the doctrine of double effect. This ethical rule helps determine how drastic pain relief can be when a patient is suffering.

Understanding palliative care

Palliative care is a concept that provides relief from pain and emphasizes emotional support for dying patients and their families. This concept began with the hospice movement. This type of care supports the principles of beneficence and nonmaleficence, and is used at any stage in disease progression. Relieving pain at the end of life fits right into the principles of beneficence and nonmaleficence.

Palliative care includes

- Control of pain and unpleasant symptoms
- Advance planning, including assistance in forming advance directives and shared decision-making
- Focus on comfort
- Not prolonging the dying process
- Involvement of the family

Walking a fine line: The double-effect rule

Doctors and healthcare providers must figure out how to control pain and symptoms while still providing the best care for the patient. Sometimes the drugs given for pain control can be lethal. The double-effect rule is an ethical principle that affects decisions about death and dying and the medical control of pain and suffering. In a situation where a good action might produce both good and bad effects, the principle of double effect can help resolve the conflict.

There are four conditions of double effect:

- The action must be morally good or morally indifferent. For instance, the administration of morphine, a potentially legal drug, is morally good or neutral.
- The bad effect must not be the means by which the good effect is achieved. In other words, you can't kill the patient in order to relieve suffering.
- The motive must be to achieve only the good effect.
- The good effect must be at least equivalent in importance, or proportionate, to the bad effect. For instance, relieving severe pain is as important morally as the death of the patient at this stage in their life.

For example, if a person is in extreme pain, and a doctor wants to control the pain, he can give the patient a powerful drug such as morphine or another narcotic. Morphine's side effects include sedation and suppression of the drive to breathe. If high enough doses of morphine are needed to control pain, the patient may stop breathing. The intent is to relieve the pain, not to cause the patient's death. If the drug were given to kill the patient, that action would be immoral and unethical. The doctor knows the drug might cause death, but the primary function of the decision to give the patient the drug is to adequately control pain.

Jim's case: Hospice provides care and comfort

Jim was a 48-year-old man who was unexpectedly diagnosed with lung cancer. He had a wife and two children and was in no way ready to die. The cancer had metastasized. He received chemotherapy and radiation, but the cancer continued to spread. It came to the point where no further treatments were available, so Jim and his family decided to involve hospice. The hospice team, including his doctor, the hospice nurse, and the chaplain, visited Jim in his home.

Medications were adjusted to control pain, nausea, and respiratory distress, and increase oral secretions. Jim was very anxious and was helped by the medication and the visits. As he approached death, a hospital bed was brought into the living room because he was bedridden. The family spent his last hours being with him and caring for him with the support of his nurse. He died peacefully at home.

 The action a doctor takes must be in proportion with the situation. The fourth condition of double effect helps to determine proportion. The level of pain and suffering the patient is experiencing must determine the action a provider takes. The more severe the pain and suffering, the more drastic the action can be.

Every state in the United States accepts the double-effect rule as protection for physicians against prosecution. A 1997 U.S. Supreme Court decision that outlawed euthanasia said that "when a doctor provides aggressive palliative care; in some cases, painkilling drugs hasten a patient's death, but the physician's purpose and intent is, or may be, only to ease his patient's pain."

 It's also important that healthcare providers ask the patient if they are experiencing pain symptoms. Patients usually don't complain about these symptoms. Sometimes patients are so sick they have a decreased level of consciousness and are unable to communicate. If a provider doesn't actively ask or observe pain symptoms, there may be undue suffering, violating the principle of non-maleficence. The patient may give clues to suffering, including groaning, restlessness, and agitation.

Easing pain with terminal sedation

Terminal sedation is known as *palliative sedation* or *continuous deep sedation*. The intent is to relieve pain and suffering, not to cure or treat a disease or condition, and it satisfies the principle of beneficence. The principle of non-maleficence is not violated because there is really nothing else that can be done medically to help the patient.

Palliative sedation is usually a series of drugs given to patients whose pain and suffering can't be relieved with opiates. The patient loses consciousness. Some doctors prefer the use of the word "palliative" over "terminal" because the word itself implies care and compassion.

Preserving a patient's dignity: Psychological support

We all know that many medical treatments lead to the loss of dignity, no matter how compassionate the doctor. The end (and the beginning) of life is messy and primal. And pain caused by chronic disease and dying can be emotional, spiritual, and psychological as well as physical.

The five stages of grief, as defined by Elizabeth Kubler-Ross, are denial, anger, bargaining, depression, and acceptance. A dying patient and his family may experience all of these stages. Often, a hospital chaplain, rabbi, or priest can offer emotional and spiritual support to the patient and family.

Psychological support involves active care of the patient, not merely withdrawing or withholding treatment. Believe it or not, there is such a thing as a "good death." Helping a dying patient prepare for death is an important part of medicine and an important ethical role for healthcare providers.

Sometimes a psychologist or psychiatrist can be brought in to assist the primary care doctor. In addition to treating clinical depression, this professional can help ease the transition from life to death for the patient and his family. A spiritual advisor can help, too. Each death is a social experience and affects many people. And remember that everyone grieves differently. Death happens to everyone, but death is a uniquely personal experience.

Terminal sedation is not euthanasia. Actually, it's not easy to end someone's life using pain-relieving drugs. The patient usually does not recover when he has reached this state. It's important to let the families know that this is the end stage of life. The pain is severe because the disease or condition is reaching its zenith.

There are four states that must be met before palliative sedation takes place. They include:

- ✔ Physical symptoms that cannot be managed and are unbearable. They can include severe anxiety because of respiratory problems, terminal agitation, delirium, or extreme pain. At the end of life, some patients literally fight death and can become very distressed and even hurt themselves.

- ✔ A current DNR/DNI order.

- ✔ A diagnosis of an illness or condition that is terminal, usually defined as death occurring within 6 months or less.

- ✔ Imminent expectation of death, within hours or days.

Again, it's important to remember that the sedation itself does not cause death. The underlying illness or condition causes death. The double-effect rule must be considered in this situation. The AMA has endorsed terminal sedation, but doesn't think it should be used when the only distress the patient feels is emotional.

Many hospitals and hospices have clear policies about using terminal sedation. The problem with having specific guidelines is that they can interfere with a doctor's decisions. Every patient and every case is different, and health-care provider's judgment, along with the patient's and family's wishes, should be the primary consideration in this issue. However, terminal sedation should never become routine in any hospital, hospice, or medical practice. No doctor should be complacent about using terminal sedation on any patient.

Organ Donation and Allocation for Transplants

Organ transplantation was a huge advance in modern medicine. Removing an organ from one person and placing it in another has saved thousands of lives, but this process has many ethical considerations.

In the 1960s, when kidney dialysis machines became widely used, the God Committee was formed in Seattle to decide who should receive access to the machines. The members evaluated patients on the basis of age, social worth, income, lifestyle, life expectancy, and contributions to society. So the elderly, the poor, people with different lifestyles, and people who were not active in society were relegated to the bottom of the list.

In response, the government decided to supply kidney dialysis free of charge to anyone who needed it under the End Stage Renal Disease program. Since then, surgeons, doctors, ethicists, and patients have struggled with the issue of who should receive scarce organ donations. Lifestyle and health issues, such as whether the recipient smokes, drinks, takes care of herself, or has other accompanying diseases or health issues, remain factors that many think should be considered.

In 1984, the National Organ Transplant Act went into effect in the United States. It was combined with the federal Task Force on Organ Transplantation in 1987 to create the United Network for Organ Sharing (UNOS). The Network tries to bring fairness in allocation policy into a mishmash of transplant centers, laboratories, and organ-procurement organizations, and is trying to develop the most fair and just system for distributing organs. This is supposed to ensure that donated organs are distributed fairly to waiting patients.

In this section, we look at money and organ transplants. Is it fair for wealthy people to have more access to organ transplants than poorer people just because they can pay for them? If so, what can we do about it? What is the legal standard for organ donation, and what about living donors? We also look at the ethics of paying donors for their organs, including going overseas for organ donation. And we look at the ethical issue of *xenotransplantation*, or transplanting animal organs into people.

Facts about organ donation

More than 100,000 people are waiting for organ transplants in the United States. Organs that can be transplanted include the heart, kidneys, lungs, liver, pancreas, intestine, thymus, and skin. A complicated point system for distributing donated organs has been developed by several organizations. These standards include

✔ Organ type, blood type, and size match

✔ Distance and accessibility from the organ to the patient

✔ Level of urgency and time on the waiting list

✔ Relative health, prognosis, and availability of the patient

At least 5,500 people in the United States die every year while waiting for an organ transplant. And that number is certainly an underestimate.

Legality of organ donation

A person must be over the age of 18 to legally become an organ donor. Parents have the right to donate or refuse to donate a child's organs and tissue. If the parents are deceased or have lost parental rights, they do not have any say over donation.

The National Organ Transplant Act of 1984 made selling or buying of human organs illegal: Organs can only be donated. Some people have signed donor cards, whereas others stipulate donation in living wills. And some families allow their loved ones' organs to be harvested after death.

The family members and healthcare providers must agree on several issues before cadaver donation can take place (for more on each of the following points, see Chapter 12). They are

✔ Realize that the patient is terminal, and his condition is irreversible

✔ Believe it is moral and ethical to stop mechanical life support

✔ Believe that organ donation is a social good and medical necessity

The doctor caring for the patient who may donate organs at death should not ask the family for permission to donate. That should be done by the organ donation committee. The committee members have a better chance of procuring the organs, and there is no conflict of interest because they haven't cared for the patient.

The care of the patient who is on the brink of death and may have viable organs is also an ethical issue. It's better for patients in comas to be kept relatively dry internally, but it's better for organ harvest if the organs are well hydrated. Healthcare providers must be very careful when treating moribund patients. As long as the patient is alive, his interests come first.

Sustaining life for organ harvesting

Most organ donations take place when a person has been on life support for some time and the family has made the decision, after a diagnosis of brain death, to remove that support.

Because the condition of organs begins to deteriorate rapidly after death, the ethical question of when the person is dead and harvesting can begin is difficult. It is decided on a case-by-case basis, following the UDDA and the legal standards of death.

Vital organs like the heart and lungs can quickly become unusable after death, especially in cases of cardiac arrest. But some tissues can still be donated even if other organs are not harvested. Those include skin, corneas, bone, bone marrow, and heart valves.

Is it ethical to for a provider to discuss the possibility of organ donation with his patient's family? The provider usually has a relationship with the patient and the family which could make discussing this option easier. But this request will benefit someone else, not the dying patient, so is the doctor violating non-maleficence for his primary patient by talking about organ donation?

Some ethicists think that a trained organ procurement representative is the best person to bring up the subject of organ donation. The provider probably best serves his patient by being present at the request to answer questions, reassure the family that the patient will not survive, and support the family as they make their decision. And it's important that the provider is not involved with the recipient's care or the harvesting itself.

Notifying a family that their loved one has died should not be done at the same time as a request for organ donation. Family members are under extreme stress and duress at this time and may be unable to make a rational, informed decision.

Looking at living donation

The number of living organ donors has increased as technology and transplant procedures have improved. A live human being can donate a kidney or part of a liver (the liver can regenerate itself), lung, pancreas, or intestine. Living donors must be healthy with no infectious diseases. In 2003, the number of living organ donors surpassed the number of deceased organ donors.

There are problems with living donors. The focus is on the recipient, not the donor. UNOS does not track deaths and serious injury of live donors, which do occur. Ethically, we should take care of people generous enough to give the gift of life. And you must also be aware of pressure put on people to donate organs while alive: Coercion is unethical.

Cost of organ transplants

According to Milliman USA, a healthcare consulting firm, the cost for one year of post-operative care for a heart transplant is almost $500,000, putting them out of reach of poor patients. For liver transplants, the cost is almost $400,000. Some doctors think that financial resources for poor patients should be provided from pools established by governments, drug companies, hospitals, and medical professionals. What makes this problem even more disturbing is that the Journal of American College of Cardiology looked at an organ donation database and found that almost one-fourth of donors would not have been able to receive organs while they were alive because they had no insurance; in other words, they couldn't have paid for the care. They were generous enough to donate their organs to others in death, but couldn't receive them because of money problems while alive. Some ethicists have proposed allowing only those patients who have signed donor cards to be added to the transplant waiting list as potential organ recipients.

Living donation may also violate the principles of beneficence and nonmaleficence. Because living donation is not without risks, it is not often in the best interests of the donor to donate an organ. Of course, it's better for the recipient to get an organ than to die. Doctors must balance the best interests of both patients in this situation.

The financial inequities of transplant eligibility

Wealth plays a role in organ donation and transplantation. Transplants cost a lot of money, both to procure the organ, complete the transplant surgery, and in terms of aftercare, including anti-rejection drugs. Patients either need a lot of money or must have good insurance. Federal law requires that recipients must prove they can pay for all of their treatment before they can even be added to the UNOS wait list. This violates the principle of distributive justice, but unfortunately is a necessary practical consideration. Ethicist Laura Siminoff calls this the *wallet biopsy*.

Some potential recipients use different doctors to get on more than one donor list. This raises their odds of receiving a transplant, but that costs money. The patient must have a relationship with each doctor on each list, and this unfairly distributes organs according to wealth.

The *rule of rescue,* or the preference to save those who appear in the public eye, plays a role here, too. Some wealthy people whose family members need organs will take out ads or appear on mass media to appeal for donations. This unfairly skews attention to those particular patients. Meanwhile, many others die in relative obscurity.

Compensation for donation: The ethical challenges

Organs cannot be bought or sold. The National Organ Transplant Act makes selling or buying organs for profit illegal, whether they come from cadavers or living donors. Unfortunately, because there is such high demand and limited supply of healthy organs, there is a black market for them.

Living donors are on their own, financially and medically, for their care after harvest. This violates the principles of beneficence and nonmaleficence. Donating organs is not free of risk. Some living donors become very sick or die after donation, and many have been forced into bankruptcy because of increased medical costs.

In the United States, several bills are being considered that would offer insurance benefits and medical care to living donors. Such legislation would have to have stringent ethical safeguards to prevent exploitation. Legislators are also considering two new approaches to financial incentives for donation: forward-looking and on-the-spot.

Forward-looking financial incentives include discounting driver's license fees if that person signs a donor card, or paying people to become part of an organ donor registry. Any money given as a result of donations would go to the donor's estate. Some are considering an options market, which would work like a life insurance policy. The donor's family would be paid if his organs were donated after death.

Raj's case: The black market for organs

A black market for organs has developed, especially in poor countries.

Raj was an illiterate farmer in India. He was offered $2,500 to donate one of his kidneys to a wealthy foreigner, who traveled to the country to get the kidney. Raj donated his kidney, but was paid only $1,200. He continued to have chronic flank pain at the site of the injury, making it difficult to work, but he had no way to get help or receive the full payment.

In 2009, an organ ring made up of corrupt medical providers who had harvested Raj's kidney was broken up in New Delhi, India after illegally buying and transplanting 500 kidneys.

On-the-spot approaches would offer some type of incentive to families of patients who are near death and are candidates for donation. The money could be a charitable contribution or used to cover funeral expenses. Or money could be offered to the estate of the deceased donor, in appreciation of their sacrifice. For example, the Ad Hoc Committee to End the Intractable Shortage of Human Organs has recommended a *gift for the gift of life* that would go to the deceased donor's estate. A patient's wishes would still need to be carefully honored above those of the family so this financial incentive would not lead to abuses of the patient's autonomy.

Xenotransplantation, or animal to human transplant

Xenotransplantation is the transplanting of living cells, tissues, or organs from one species to another. This is performed on a limited basis with humans. An example is the use of a porcine (pig) heart valve in valve replacement surgery.

This practice could save thousands of human lives every year. Organs from animals such as baboons or pigs could be treated with human genes so they won't be rejected by the human. But animal rights activists believe it is ethically wrong to sacrifice animals to save human lives. Chapter 16 discusses that animals are considered special populations in research.

Medical and ethical issues related to this subject include disease transmission (xenozoonosis), the lifespan of animal organs, which are shorter than human organs, and alteration to the genetic code. In addition, many religions would have an objection to this practice.

Xenotransplants may relax the barrier between human and animal diseases. If you think that the reaction to mad cow disease was loud, just wait until a disease unique to baboons starts to affect human beings because of a transplant. And because many pathogens are becoming resistant to antibiotics, xenotransplants may exacerbate this problem.

Animal organs are just not designed to last as long as human organs. Pigs, for instance, have a lifespan of only about 15 years. Will the organ transplanted from a pig to a human last that long? Are we sentencing the recipient to a life shorter than he would have lived with a human donor?

Xenotransplantation has the potential to reduce the number of people who die while waiting for organ transplants. The science is at a point where animal tissues, most likely from a pig, can be engineered to reduce the incidence of rejection. Struggling with ethical issues now will help guide researchers through this new frontier.

The case of Baby Fae: Receiving a baboon heart

An important ethical case regarding xenotransplantation is the case of Baby Fae, an infant born in 1984 in California with hypoplastic left heart syndrome. In this condition, the pumping chamber of the heart is underdeveloped, and the infant usually doesn't live beyond two weeks of age.

Baby Fae was diagnosed with this syndrome at Loma Linda Hospital and then sent home with her mother to die. However, a pediatric surgeon at the hospital, Dr. Leonard Bailey, had just been granted permission by the hospital's IRB to perform five xenograft operations. Baby Fae was called back to the hospital, and at five days old, a baboon heart was transplanted to replace her diseased heart. Unfortunately, she soon developed rejection of the transplanted heart and went into kidney failure. She died after living for 21 days.

Many ethical questions were raised about this case. Was this transplant considered treatment, or was it really experimentation? Were the uneducated, uninsured parents offered true informed consent for this procedure? Dr. Bailey felt it was unlikely a small human heart could be obtained for transplant in such a short time, but shouldn't this at least have been attempted? And what about the rights of the baboon?

Part IV

Advancing Medical Knowledge with Ethical Clinical Research

The 5th Wave   By Rich Tennant

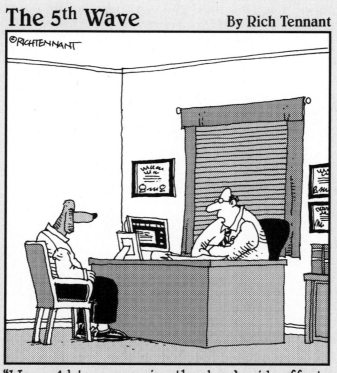

"We could try reversing the drug's side effects with gene therapy, but we don't want to get into trouble with the SPCA."

In this part . . .

Medical research has saved countless lives in the past century. To advance medical treatments, rigorous and ethical clinical studies must be conducted. How can we ensure that these studies provide the most good to the greatest number of patients? How can we protect clinical subjects while they are part of a study?

Ethical clinical studies are important, not only to protect the patients participating in them, but to make sure that medicine and medical advances are trusted and respected. What happens when a trial ends early? How can we prevent problems with medical research in the future?

Chapter 14

Toward Trials without Error: The Evolution of Ethics in Clinical Research

....

In This Chapter

▶ Looking at the history of medical research in America

▶ Understanding the principles of ethical studies

....

Medical research has produced some amazing results. In fact, research in the 19th and 20th centuries has led to medications, vaccinations, treatments, and surgery that have extended the average human lifespan. At the beginning of the 20th century, the average lifespan of a man in the United States was 49 years. At the beginning of the 21st century, the average lifespan of a man in the United States was 77 years.

However, this improvement is not without a dark side, and research is not without controversy. Early studies didn't have appropriate ethical standards, which led to some serious and immoral violations of human rights. Two documents established ethics in modern medical research: The Nuremberg Code and the Declaration of Helsinki. In this chapter, we examine those two documents and look at the guiding ethical principles of medical research, including the most important practice of medical research: informed consent.

An Introduction to Medical Research

Medical research is a valuable tool that has developed many effective drugs and treatments to treat disease and reduce suffering in the past 100 years. Some of the major benefits of research include

✔ Vaccines for measles, polio, and the HPV vaccine

✔ Insulin treatments for diabetes

- ✔ Medications for high blood pressure and high cholesterol
- ✔ Heart interventions such as bypass surgery and defibrillation
- ✔ Improved treatments for HIV and AIDS
- ✔ Increasingly successful treatments for cancer

Whether a patient realizes it or not, many decisions a doctor makes during the course of a clinic visit are based on medical research findings. This is called evidence-based medicine: making medical decisions based on evidence discovered through medical research.

Let's say a patient comes into my office after being hospitalized for congestive heart failure. A new echocardiogram, or ultrasound of the heart, shows that his ejection fraction (indication of the pumping function of his heart) is 25 percent. A normal election fraction is 60 percent. Recent research showed that patients with this fraction should receive an implantable ventricular defibrillator to reduce the risk of sudden death. Using evidence-based medicine, I would refer him to a cardiologist for a defibrillator which may save his life. This is an example of how clinical research guides my everyday practice.

In the following sections, we give you a brief overview of the different types of clinical research and explain why it's critical to get informed consent in clinical trials.

Moving from lab experiments to research on humans

Medical research in the lab at the cellular level and on laboratory animals (called preclinical trials) provides clues to the efficacy of a new treatment. These experiments must prove that the new treatment is effective and will not harm an organism. After this is established, these new treatments are tested on human beings. In the case of a new drug, for example, three phases of clinical trials must be satisfactorily completed before the FDA will approve a drug, and it can be marketed to the public.

There are two types of clinical research: observational and interventional. In observational studies, researchers observe their subjects and measure outcomes. They don't actively manage the experiment. An example of this type of study is the Nurse's Health Study. Researchers studied a large group of women over many years and learned many things about their health. However, observational studies don't provide evidence that is as compelling as interventional studies. Some ethical considerations in observational studies are respect for people, fair distribution of risks and benefits, diversity in the population sample, minimizing risks, and maximizing benefits all need to be considered in observational studies. And the Declaration of Helsinki applies to observational research, too, because these studies use private information for the good of the public.

An interventional study, or a randomized controlled trial, is an experiment on human beings. Investigators give the patients medicine or intervene in some way and then compare the treated patients to a control group that received a placebo, no treatment, or the best current treatment. Statistical tools are then applied to the results to see if there are any differences among the groups and if those results are statistically significant. Interventional studies provide the best evidence that a new treatment will benefit humans. But as you may guess, any experimentation on human beings whether observational or interventional, presents ethical challenges. We explain how to conduct an ethical clinical trial in Chapter 15.

Most medical researchers abide by high ethical standards. They want to treat disease, benefit mankind, and conduct a scientifically sound, medically ethical study. The funding for their research often depends on whether or not their findings are significant, which can motivate them, but can also lead to bias because an entity that pays for a study would like to see results benefiting their product or treatment. For instance, researchers at *The New England Journal of Medicine* found that in some trials of calcium-channel blockers, 96 percent of the favorable studies were sponsored by the manufacturers producing the drug. In contrast, only 37 percent of studies critical of the drug were funded by the drug manufacturers.

Understanding the importance of informed consent in clinical trials

In the early days of modern medicine, many experiments were performed on patients who did not consent to being studied. The populations used in these experiments included people that society judged to be "less worthy", such as people of color, the poor, prisoners of war, and the handicapped. In many cases, these people could not consent to or refuse the intervention, either because they did not know what was happening to them, or they were forced into participation. Subjects were often deceived into thinking they were receiving treatments, rather than simply being subjects of human research.

All of the principles of medical ethics must be considered in clinical research. And these principles are satisfied when patients give *informed consent*. Informed consent means that a research trial must be fully explained to a patient in terms they understand, and they must freely consent to participation. Patients must be informed about the risks and benefits of the intervention, as well as the risks and benefits of receiving the placebo. Informed consent honors patient autonomy. This way the patient is unlikely to be harmed (nonmaleficence) and all of society is more likely to benefit from the research (beneficence). Justice must be addressed, too. Are these trials going to be fairly administered across different gender, age, and racial groups so as many people as possible will benefit from a new treatment? It is also important that study participants must not have unrealistic expectations about the trial. These studies are experiments, not treatments, and no outcome is guaranteed.

Turning Points in Medical Research in America

Randomized, controlled clinical trials are the tools of medical research. But over the years, there have been many significant ethics violations in research. Some trials were performed on subjects who were unaware they were part of a study. The Tuskegee Syphilis Study, described in the following section, is one example.

In this section, we look at the evolution of ethics in medical research in the 20th century. We also examine how the Office for Human Research Protections was established to guide the ethics of clinical medical studies.

The Tuskegee Syphilis Study: The ethics of withholding treatment

The Tuskegee Syphilis Study is held up as the model of an unethical research experiment. It was conducted on African-American men from 1932 to 1972 in the United States and had a major impact on ethics in medical research. Researchers followed a total of 600 African-American men. A control group of 201 men did not have syphilis, and 399 men did have the disease. The study participants were told they were being evaluated for "bad blood," a euphemism that could have meant anything from fatigue to anemia. Even when penicillin, a simple cure for the illness, was available in the 1940s, the afflicted men were not offered treatment for the sake of continuing the study. The study exemplifies racism, physician paternalism, abuse of the vulnerable, and ethical misconduct.

Syphilis is a terrible disease. Untreated, it causes damage to the brain, eyes, heart, liver, bones, and joints. Victims develop paralysis, blindness, and dementia, and eventually die. Men died during the course of this study, but not before passing the disease on to their partners. In some cases, their children contracted congenital syphilis, which causes miscarriage, stillbirth, neonatal death, and birth defects.

The men were the descendents of slaves who lived in extreme poverty in the rural South and were encouraged to participate in the study with offers of free health exams (most African-Americans, at that time, did not receive much medical care), transportation reimbursement, and food. The study even paid for burial costs as the patients began dying, as long as their families consented to autopsies.

The study participants were never given the opportunity to exercise informed consent. They were lied to about the purpose of the study, were not told of risks and benefits, and were denied current and effective medical treatment. Some may have believed that their participation in this study was actually a treatment for the disease.

As mentioned earlier, not one man infected with syphilis in the study was offered any treatment for the disease, even after doctors knew that penicillin would cure syphilis. In fact, the study participants were told that they *were* being treated! The men were never given the option of quitting the project, which is a critical part of informed consent in clinical trials.

The timeline of the study is very long and demonstrates how the basics of medical ethics were ignored over the course of decades.

In 1928, the United States Public Health Service (PHS) and the Rosenwald fund decided to fund a study looking at the health of African-American citizens in southern states. Then the Great Depression began and medical research funding was decimated. The Rosenwald fund backed out of the study.

In 1932, one doctor at the PHS, Taliaferro Clark, tried to rescue the study. He proposed that doctors look at the effects of untreated syphilis on human beings. There was a question in medicine at that time about differences and variations in the effects of diseases based on race. Syphilis was a major health problem at that time, with more than 35 percent of all adults infected with the disease. The Tuskegee Institute in Alabama was chosen as the location for the study. At the time, the Institute was well respected and trusted by the African-American community.

- In 1932, the study began. Patients were examined; those with syphilis were admitted. The PHS prevented other doctors from administering treatment.

- During World War II, some of the study participants were drafted and were found to have syphilis during their draft medical exams. The PHS asked the draft boards to exclude these men from treatment requirements. And the draft boards agreed to this request.

- In 1943, penicillin began to be used to treat syphilis. The patients in the Tuskegee study were excluded from these treatments.

- ✔ In 1972, Peter Buxton, a PHS employee, told J. Heller, a reporter from the Associated Press, about the study. Publicity and the resulting public outcry brought the study to a halt.

- ✔ In 1973, congressional hearings about the study resulted in new regulations about medical experiments on human beings.

- ✔ Also in 1973, a class action lawsuit was brought against the researchers. This lawsuit was settled in 1974 with a $10 million payment. As part of the settlement, all participants were given free lifetime medical care.

- ✔ In 1997, President Clinton formally apologized to all of the study participants and their families. He said the study was "deeply, profoundly, morally wrong." The 11 remaining survivors of the study witnessed the apology at the White House.

The National Center for Bioethics in Research and Health Care was established with a $200,000 federal grant at Tuskegee University in 1997 in response to the civil lawsuit and President Clinton's apology.

The fallout from this study has had wide-reaching implications. In general, African-Americans as a whole have a higher mistrust of the medical community than other populations. A 2005 study done by Oregon State University and the Rand Corporation looked at African-Americans and HIV infection. This study surveyed 500 African-Americans and found that 25 percent believed AIDS was being made in a U.S. government laboratory, and 12 percent of those surveyed felt that AIDS was a form of genocide against black people. A majority of those surveyed thought a cure for AIDS was intentionally being withheld from the poor. These conspiracy theories are viewed as a huge barrier to preventing HIV in the African-American community. Given our history, it is not surprising that African-Americans are more likely to refuse medical care and less likely to participate in clinical trials.

Miss Evers' Boys

The 1997 HBO movie *Miss Evers' Boys* was based on the play by David Feldschuh. The play was written about the Tuskegee Syphilis Study. The tale is told by nurse Eunice Evers, who had a role in the study. She knew that the men she was caring for were not being treated for the disease. Many were her friends. Miss Evers testified before the congressional hearings on the Tuskegee Study. She thought that the study would help improve the lives of African-Americans because this was the first study the government had conducted on that population.

Questioning the honor of being chosen

In my years as a family physician, it has become clear that mistrust of medicine occurs not just in the African-American community, but affects most ethic minorities and the disadvantaged. In the early 1990s, I worked for Indian Health Services in Pine Ridge, South Dakota when the manufacturer of the Hepatitis A Vaccine decided to perform an FDA Phase III clinical trial of the vaccine. Together with the Indian Health Service, the researchers wanted to use the Native Americans who lived in Pine Ridge as subjects. Pine Ridge was chosen because there is a higher rate of Hepatitis A there when compared with the general population. Children ages 3 to 12 were included in the study. The researchers also felt that the Sioux Indians would benefit more from the vaccine after it was approved, so they hoped that patients would want to help with the study. However, some members of the community raised this valid question: "Why are our children being experimented on?" This question made sense given the long history of mistrust that exists between Native Americans and the U.S. government. This issue was picked up by others and the mainstream press. A lawsuit was filed, and the trial stopped in 1992.

The establishment of the Office for Human Research Protections and IRBs

The Office for Human Research Protections (OHRP) was established in 1966. Its job as part of the U.S. Department of Health and Human Services is to monitor medical research as defined in the Public Health Services Act.

The OHRP implements regulations for medical research using human subjects. Any hospital, clinic, or other institution that conducts human subjects research sponsored by the Department of Health and Human Services must establish an institutional review board (IRB) to monitor that institution's human subjects research. The IRB must register with the OHRP.

The OHRP also writes materials and guidelines to help guide institutions involved in medical research. It also provides training for doctors and organizations involved in international research so ethical protections are established in research in other countries.

Nonconsensual research of the 20th century

Before the Declaration of Helsinki was signed in 1964 and the Office for Human Research Protections was established, researchers could perform a medical study without telling their subjects what the researchers were studying, how the condition was being treated, or what the side effects of the treatment might be. Some of the nonconsensual research experiments in the United States included:

- In 1932, a doctor at the Rockefeller Institute for Medical Investigations injected Puerto Rican citizens with cancer cells; at least 13 of these patients died of the disease. This doctor, Cornelius Rhoads, wrote that the Puerto Rican population should be eradicated. During World War II, he exposed American soldiers to radiation to measure the results.

- In 1940, prisoners in Chicago were injected with the live malaria virus in order to evaluate new treatments for the disease. The program was considered essential because of the imminent American involvement in World War II. This study was used by Nazi doctors at the Nuremberg trials to defend their actions in the death camps.

- In September 1950, the United States Army sprayed the serratia bacteria over San Francisco. This was a test to see how vulnerable a city would be to a biological attack. Some people developed drug-resistant bacterial infections, and one man died.

- In New York City in 1966, the United States Army spread the bacteria Bacillus subtilis variant niger through the subway system. Scientists filled light bulbs with this bacteria, which is a harmless variant of anthrax, then dropped them into ventilation grates so a cloud of bacteria spread. Millions of American citizens were unknowingly exposed.

- In Los Angeles in 1990, thousands of Hispanic and African-American babies were injected with an experimental measles vaccine that was not licensed for use at that time. Parents weren't told it was experimental.

- In 1999, the Veteran's Administration West Los Angeles Medical Center had all of its research projects suspended after allegations of research performed without informed consent.

- In 2001, the Federal Office of Human Research Protection (OHRP) suspended Johns Hopkins' research license after they discovered that the hospital failed to tell patients that the drug hexamethonium was experimental and toxic. A patient died after inhaling the drug under doctor's supervision.

- In 2003, three University of Maryland researchers admitted they made up interviews for a research study about AIDS prevention and safe sex to get a $1 million federal grant.

- In 2004, Forest Labs admitted they concealed data of clinical trial evidence that their antidepressant did not benefit children and had severe adverse side effects.

All of these experiments violated patient autonomy because informed consent was not given or even solicited. Many of these studies also violated the principles of beneficence, nonmaleficence, and justice. Before the Declaration of Helsinki and the Office for Human Research Protections were put in place in the mid-1960s, doctors could get away with nonconsensual research. Today, doctors and researchers are subject to swift and harsh disciplinary action.

An institutional review board is a committee established by a medical institution that oversees medical research. The National Research Act of 1974 established IRBs. Studies involving educational tests, existing data, or effectiveness of teaching strategies are exempt from IRB standards. IRBs are also governed by Title 45 Code of Federal Regulations, Part 46 (45 CFR 46) as the primary set of federal regulations regarding the protection of human subjects in research. It defines the laws, criteria for exemption, as well as definition and formulation of IRBs and is also called the Common Rule.

How an IRB is selected is subject to strict regulations. There must be at least five people on the board, of both genders. The members should be familiar with the group being studied and with the research being conducted. They must come from different professions, including at least one scientist and one nonscientist. And the board must have one member who has no association with the medical institution participating in the study.

In addition to following general medical ethics guidelines, the OHRP has established additional guidelines for research using certain populations considered to be vulnerable and in need of increased protection. These guidelines cover:

- **Pregnant women, fetuses, and neonates:** preclinical studies must be conducted on animals to help assess risk, and any risk must be the "least possible." The research must also result in knowledge that can't be obtained in any other way.

- **Prisoners as research subjects:** At least one member of the IRB must be a prisoner to represent that group. The risks must be similar to non-imprisoned volunteers, and the prisoner must be informed that participation in studies will not affect his sentence length or parole possibilities.

- **Children as research subjects:** Parental permission and assent of the child should be obtained. Risk must be only a minor increase over minimal risk, and the study must yield vital information about the condition being studied.

See Chapter 16 for more information about OHRP guidelines as pertaining to children and pregnant women.

Guiding Principles of Ethical Studies

Principles for ethical clinical studies have been well established. All doctors, scientists, and other researchers must follow these principles when conducting any studies on human subjects.

After Nazi atrocities in World War II, the Nuremberg Code was established in 1947. We look at the Code and its five protections for patients in clinical research. Then the Declaration of Helsinki was written by the World Medical Association (WMA) in 1964 and has been revised by the medical community several times. We also examine the Declaration and its effect on medical research studies and the recent acceptance of the Good Clinical Practice Guidance rules in place of the Declaration of Helsinki for guiding research around the world.

Finally, we look at the Belmont Report. This document, written in 1978, establishes the best ethical practices for clinical research in the United States. It is the main reference, along with the Common Rule (45 CFR 46) for IRBs overseeing research projects.

There are eight main guiding principles of ethical clinical studies. Doctors and researchers' primary goal is to protect the life, health, and dignity of all human beings. The principles include these points:

- ✔ Human dignity must be preserved and respected at all times.

- ✔ Risks to human beings must be minimized with established research methods and design. This is in keeping with the principle of nonmaleficence.

- ✔ The benefits of the study must be maximized, following the principle of beneficence.

- ✔ Selection of the study's population must be randomized, so no one particular group of people carries the burden of research and so the benefits reach most of the human population. This follows the principle of justice.

- ✔ All participants must be fully informed of the purpose of the study, the study procedures, risks and benefits of the study, and what alternatives are available to them. They must also freely consent to the study's parameters. Participants must also have the freedom to leave the study whenever they so choose. This satisfies the principle of autonomy.

- ✔ Privacy and confidentiality of the participants must be protected in accordance with autonomy.

- ✔ Participant safety and health must be continuously monitored. If researchers find that the study's risks outweigh the benefits at any point, the study must be discontinued and the results published. And if the study shows that the treatments are vastly superior to the standard of care, the study should be stopped and all participants placed on the study treatment.

- ✔ Any participants who may be especially vulnerable, such as children, pregnant women, prisoners, or the disabled, must be rigorously protected.

The Nuremberg Code: New research standards in the wake of World War II

The Nuremberg Code was the first document in the world to state and preserve the rights of human beings in medical experimentation. It combines the Hippocratic oath and human rights with the focus on the human subject, not the physician performing the experiment.

After Nazi atrocities in World War II were uncovered, the world reacted. The Nuremberg Trials were held from 1946 to 1949 in the Palace of Justice in Nuremberg, Germany. The United States was in charge of the trials. Twelve trials took place. The first, called The Doctor's Trial, or *The United States of America v. Karl Brandt, et al*, was held between December 1946 and August 1947.

The defendants took part in human experiments on concentration camp prisoners, civilians, and prisoners of war. The standard in Germany at the time was of "state before individual," meaning citizens were expected to put the government's interests ahead of their own. Many of the experiments were racially motivated, toward the Nazi goal of "racial and genetic purity." The 23 defendants included Josef Mengele, one of the most notorious war criminals. Twenty of the 23 defendants were medical doctors. The indictment states, in part, that the doctors were accused of

> . . . performing medical experiments, without the subjects' consent, on prisoners of war and civilians of occupied countries, in the course of which experiments the defendants committed murders, brutalities, cruelties, tortures, atrocities, and other inhuman acts.

An example of one of these experiments was the malaria experiment performed on more than 1,000 patients at the Dachau concentration camp. Healthy prisoners were infected by malaria and then experiments were performed on them. More than half of the involuntary participants died as a result of these experiments. Other types of experiments included painful and disfiguring bone, nerve, and muscle transplants, mustard gas experiments that caused terrible burns, experiments in cold water immersion, and different types of forced sterilization.

The doctors were also accused of crimes against humanity and war crimes. Seven of the accused were acquitted. The others were found guilty; seven were hanged and the rest given multiyear prison sentences. The court also rendered a decision on the ethics of human experimentation.

As a result of these trials, Dr. Leo Alexander wrote six points detailing the ethical conduct of medical research. The Nuremberg court accepted those points and added four more. Those points became the Nuremberg Code.

1. The voluntary consent of the human subject is absolutely essential. This means that the person involved should have legal capacity to give consent; should be so situated as to be able to exercise free power of choice, without the intervention of any element of force, fraud, deceit, duress, over-reaching, or other ulterior form of constraint or coercion; and should have sufficient knowledge and comprehension of the elements of the subject matter involved as to enable him/her to make an understanding and enlightened decision.

2. The experiment should be such as to yield fruitful results for the good of society, unprocurable by other methods or means of study, and not random and unnecessary in nature.

3. The experiment should be so designed and based on the results of animal experimentation and a knowledge of the natural history of the disease or other problem under study that the anticipated results will justify the performance of the experiment.

4. The experiment should be so conducted as to avoid all unnecessary physical and mental suffering and injury.

5. No experiment should be conducted where there is a prior reason to believe that death or disabling injury will occur; except, perhaps, in those experiments where the experimental physicians also serve as subjects.

6. The degree of risk to be taken should never exceed that determined by the humanitarian importance of the problem to be solved by the experiment.

7. Proper preparations should be made and adequate facilities provided to protect the experimental subject against even remote possibilities of injury, disability, or death.

8. The experiment should be conducted only by scientifically qualified persons. The highest degree of skill and care should be required through all states of the experiment of those who conduct or engage in the experiment.

9. During the course of the experiment the human subject should be at liberty to bring the experiment to an end if he has reached the physical or mental state where continuation of the experiment seems to him to be impossible.

10. During the course of the experiment the scientist in charge must be prepared to terminate the experiment at any stage, if he has probable cause to believe, in the exercise of good faith, superior skill and careful judgment required of him that a continuation of the experiment is likely to result in injury, disability, or death to the experimental subject.

One of the arguments made by the Nazi doctors' defense attorneys was that there was no standard code regulating medical experiments on human beings. That made the Nuremberg Code a moral and legal necessity.

Research in Nazi Germany

A difficult ethical question that is raised by medical research performed in Nazi Germany is whether information obtained from research performed in an unethical manner on nonconsenting subjects should ever be used. Some Nazi studies have been listed as references in studies performed after the Nuremberg Code was written. For example, prisoners were subjected to severe prolonged submersion in ice water to obtain data about hypothermia.

This information is referenced in some newer studies. Obviously, this data is highly offensive, especially to those in the Jewish community, and to all of us appalled by the mistreatment of so many vulnerable human beings. Is it ever ethical to use results from research obtained in an unethical manner? This is an ongoing debate, but some of this knowledge, also known as fruit from the poisoned tree, has already been used to develop more recent medical research.

The Declaration of Helsinki: A global roadmap for ethical clinical research

The Declaration of Helsinki was codified in 1964 in Helsinki, Finland, by the World Medical Association. The Declaration uses the Nuremberg Code and adds the Declaration of Geneva from 1948, which lists a doctor's ethical duties in clinical research. The document changed the term *human experimentation* to *clinical research*.

The Declaration has been revised and clarified six times, with the last revision completed in 2008. This document is not legally binding, but is morally binding. The Declaration is meant to help officials override national, regional, and local laws, unless those laws hold a higher standard.

The Declaration contains 35 Articles, each stating ethical guidelines in all parts of clinical research. The Articles cover basic principles and operational principles.

Some of the basic principles include

- ✔ There must be respect for the individual, autonomy, and informed consent.
- ✔ The researcher's duty is completely and solely to the patient.
- ✔ The patient's welfare comes before the interests of science and the state.
- ✔ Special attention must be paid to vulnerable patients.

The operational principles state

- Any clinical trial must be based on science and a complete knowledge of medicine.

- The trial must have a reasonable likelihood that it will be beneficial to the group being studied.

- Only trained researchers should conduct the trial.

- Only approved methods and protocols should be used in the trial.

- The trial should be ended if the patients are being harmed.

- The trial should be as transparent and public as possible.

- The research should compare the best known treatments against the experimental treatments in most cases. In some cases, a placebo can be used.

- The patients should receive care after the trial has ended.

Good Clinical Practice Guidelines: Replacing the Declaration of Helsinki

In 2008, the FDA replaced the Declaration of Helsinki with Good Clinical Practice Guidelines. Under these new guidelines, drug companies can now conduct trials outside the United States where regulations and ethical considerations are not as strict. For instance, in some countries, patients who do not receive the experimental treatment (the control group) can be given a placebo instead of the best current treatment. These guidelines apply to any clinical trials on drugs, treatments, procedures, or equipment conducted on human beings outside the United States. Good Clinical Practice Guidelines do include protection of human rights of any subject involved in a research trial. They also include standards on how clinical trials are conducted and monitored, and the assurance of safety and efficacy of newly developed treatments. It's just that these guidelines are more relaxed than the guidelines for research done in the United States put forth by the Belmont Report and the Common Rule.

As a result, many drug manufacturers are moving clinical trials for their new products offshore because the ethical standards are lower than in the United States. Under the new guidelines, the authors of clinical studies conducted outside of the United States no longer have to

- Reveal funding sources or other conflicts of interest.

- Publicly reveal the design and scope of the trials.

- Submit an investigative new drug application (IND) to the FDA before beginning a trial, which makes the trials impossible to monitor.

- Consider the health concerns of the country hosting the trial.

- Restrict use of placebos. Patients only have to receive standard care established in that foreign country.

✔ Give treatment to patients after the trial is completed.

✔ Publish negative results of the trial.

The Good Clinical Practice Guidelines document was developed by the International Conference on Harmonisation (ICH), a committee with international interests that defines ethical standards in medicine. The FDA's switch to use these guidelines in place of the Declaration of Helsinki was opposed by patient advocates, consumer groups, and public interest groups, and supported by drug companies. Some ethicists believe that the new guidelines may reduce ethical standards for international clinical research trials.

The use of placebos instead of the best current treatment is problematic because it means that those who receive the placebo are not receiving treatment, which is a violation of the principle of nonmaleficence. Many drug companies prefer using a placebo because it is easier to prove the new treatment is better than nothing at all rather than proving the new treatment is better than the best current treatment. Comparison trials, or trials of a new drug against an older drug, are more difficult and costly than a trial against a placebo.

There's another problem with testing drugs in other countries and then selling them around the world. The drugs are tested in countries with a lower standard of care and then are used in countries with a higher standard of care. That is unethical because the standard of care should be the same for all patients around the world In poorer countries, after a drug proves beneficial in a study, the participants in the study and others in their country do not have access to this drug because they cannot afford it. Some ethicists argue that this violates the principle of justice, and that a drug that is proven beneficial should be provided without cost to the study participants.

There has always been a dichotomy between medical research studies conducted in rich countries versus poor countries. In countries where there is no standard of care or that standard is poor, the patients may not be as protected using Good Clinical Practice standards. Some ethicists want the Obama administration to force the FDA to return to the Declaration of Helsinki as the research standard both within and outside of the United States.

Pfizer fined for unethical sales practices

In 2009, the large drug manufacturer Pfizer was fined $2.3 billion in criminal and civil fines by the U.S. government over sales practices for Bextra, Lyrica, Geodon, and Zyvox. The firm marketed the drugs for off-label uses; in other words, uses not approved by the FDA. That sounds like a lot of money, but it was only three month's worth of profit. Although doctors can prescribe drugs for off-label uses, drug manufacturers can't. The government investigation found other ethical problems with the company, too, including kickbacks to doctors. The felony charges were actually levied against a Pfizer subsidiary, Pharmacia & Upjohn, so that Pfizer could keep accepting government funds for research.

The Belmont Report: Best ethical practices in U.S. research

In 1974, the United States Department of Health, Education, and Welfare (now the Department of Health and Human Services) created the National Commission for the Protection of Human Subjects of Biomedical and Behavioral Research. This Commission laid out the ethical standards for biomedical and behavioral research on human beings. This took place at the Smithsonian Institute's Belmont Conference Center, so the report became the Belmont Report. As mentioned previously, the Belmont Report is an essential reference for IRBs and lays out guidelines to follow when evaluating potential research studies.

The Report consists of three parts: boundaries between medical practice and medical research, a list of the best basic ethical principles in medicine and research, and applications of these principles.

The boundaries between practice and research must be distinct. The practice of medicine is to diagnose and treat patients using accepted methods that have a high rate of success. On the other hand, research is used to test a hypothesis and develop or expand knowledge. Any innovation, which is defined as a treatment that is significantly different from established practice, must be first tested in a clinical trial before it is used in medical practice.

The ethical principles are introduced in Chapter 1 and were laid out in the Belmont Report. The first principle, autonomy, is expressed in respect for persons. Any patient who consents to a clinical trial must either be free and uncoerced, capable of consenting, or protected because of diminished capacity.

Two other principles, nonmaleficence and beneficence, are elaborated on in the report. The study must first of all, do no harm or minimize harm (nonmaleficence), and maximize benefit. Beneficence demands that patients in a clinical trial are treated with kindness and compassion

Another principle is justice. The burdens of research and the benefits of new treatments developed from that research must be as equitably distributed as possible among different groups of people.

These principles are applied in the requirements of informed consent and clear communication. Information about the study must be supplied in a manner and style the patients can understand. Patients must freely volunteer and not be coerced in any way. The purpose of the study, the study procedures, any risks and benefits, and alternatives to the study must be clearly laid out, and the patients selected for participation in the study must be randomly selected. All of this is evaluated by the IRB before a research study is given approval to proceed.

Chapter 15

Beyond Guinea Pigs: Anatomy of an Ethical Clinical Trial

*W*hen you were a kid, did you ever put baking soda in a bottle and add vinegar to make a mini volcano? That was a simple science experiment with no ethical dilemmas (unless your mom needed the vinegar for something). But things are different with clinical trials; they are experiments on human beings. Before a trial can proceed, researchers must decide what type of drug or treatment they want to study, what they want to measure, and who can participate. They also need to set parameters, study the potential risks and benefits, and communicate this information to participants. Every study must have a *protocol,* or a detailed plan set up to answer questions about the new treatment and to protect the health of patients participating in the trial.

In this chapter, we look at how an ethical clinical trial is set up, how participants are told of risks and benefits, and the importance of full disclosure. We also look at the role of the institutional review board (IRB), how to set up a valid trial, and how to end a trial early if there are problems.

All the principles of medical ethics are involved. Patient autonomy is critical such that a patient needs to give true informed consent to participate in the trial. Beneficence demands that there be a likelihood of some benefit to trial participants and to the larger community through scientific discovery. The principle of nonmaleficence applies in that the risks involved in participating must be less than the likely benefits of the study results to society. And with justice, the trials must be fairly set up and balanced, with diverse participants drawn from as large a pool as possible.

Elements of a Valid Trial: Leveling the Playing Field Ethically

If researchers are trying to figure out which treatment is more effective, it's ethical to use patients in a clinical trial. There are many reasons why a clinical trial should be valid and ethical. Good science is the only way to move medicine forward. Patients aren't going to trust medicine unless trials really show a clear benefit associated with new treatments and medications. And unless a trial is valid and ethical, much harm can come to the human subjects in the trial and to patients who use these new treatments in the future.

A trial's results will be considered valid only if the trial is fair and balanced, and it is conducted in an ethical manner. A double-blind, placebo-controlled, randomized trial designed to yield statistically significant results is the best way to determine the effectiveness of any new drug or treatment. In this section, we look more closely at the elements and design of a clinical trial, including blinding, randomization, using placebos properly, avoiding harm, and giving reasonable care to the control group.

Collective clinical equipoise: Asking whether a trial is needed

For a trial to be justified, researchers as a group must be genuinely uncertain if one treatment is better than another. This is called *equipoise*, or the uncertainty principle, or the condition of being balanced. When there is genuine uncertainty in the medical community as a whole about whether the study treatment or standard of care is the best treatment, a trial can proceed until enough statistically significant results have been obtained to show that one treatment is better than the other.

If the medical community knows that one treatment is better than another, they are ethically obligated to give the better treatment to patients. If they don't know, a clinical trial should be conducted to determine beneficence for their patients.

Equipoise has a basis in the principle of justice and the pursuit of knowledge. Participants in any clinical trial should be representative of the larger population that could be helped by this drug or treatment. The burdens and benefits of scientific research should be fairly distributed.

There's a second factor in clinical equipoise. For a trial to be considered effective, equipoise should be disturbed at the end of a randomized controlled trial (RCT) (see the later sections "Preventing bias with study blinds and randomization" and "Choosing ethical controls"). There should be a clear benefit showed by the treatment, or no benefit shown.

There is some ethical debate about equipoise being used as a principle for clinical research. Some ethicists point out that researchers often have a hunch that a certain treatment is better and, therefore, want to test it in a trial. This is not equipoise, but it is still ethical. Others who support the principle of equipoise point out that if researchers think a treatment is superior to other treatments, it should be offered to all patients instead of only those in the treatment group of a study. They argue that research should only be done when physicians truly do not know which treatment is better (equipoise).

Understanding basic trial design

Clinical trials are conducted in four phases. The first phase tests the new treatment in a small group to find the best way of administering the treatment and check for safety and toxicity. For instance, researchers will test for the highest level of dosage that is tolerated without causing harm. Phase II adds more people and tests the treatment for effectiveness and best dosage. Phase III looks at the overall risk-benefit ratio of the new treatment and looks for side effects. And Phase IV is an aftermarket study that looks at possible long-term side effects and more risk-benefit ratios, as well as unauthorized uses of the drug for treating other diseases.

In Phases I and II, when the drug is being tested for safety and to determine dosage, there is usually no benefit to the participants; these trials are nontherapeutic. The participants all receive the experimental treatment. Phases III and IV are where the subject might benefit, but because the trial is randomized, the subject isn't guaranteed to receive the experimental treatment. This must be stressed to the participants.

According to the National Institutes of Health, there are six kinds of clinical trials:

- ✔ Prevention trials look for ways to prevent disease.
- ✔ Screening trials try to find the best way to detect disease.
- ✔ Diagnostic trials look for the best way to diagnose conditions.
- ✔ Treatment trials test experimental treatments or drugs.
- ✔ Quality of life trials try to find ways to improve the quality of life for people with a disease.
- ✔ Compassionate use trials offer experimental treatment to people who have run out of treatment options.

Choosing ethical controls

Clinical trials have different *arms*, which are groups of patients who are receiving different treatments. These arms represent the group of patients receiving the experimental treatment and groups of patients who receive either no treatment at all or the *best available treatment.* A trial can be *placebo-controlled,* which means the control group gets sugar pills or other medically inert drugs, or *active-controlled,* which means that the control group gets an active treatment, usually the best available. These arms must be balanced for a valid trial.

Placebos aren't used in many trials because there are usually best available treatments for most diseases. And if a patient who is ill receives a placebo instead of conventional treatment, his health will be adversely affected, which violates the principles of nonmaleficence and beneficence. Those who oppose the use of placebos do so from the deontological point of view; that it is always unethical to deceive patients, even if they have been forewarned. Those who support the use of placebos do so from the consequentialist and utilitarian points of view: that the best clinical results come from the use of placebos, and the greater good is served.

Placebo controls can be used if

 ✔ There is no standard treatment for that particular disease or condition.

 ✔ Doctors and researchers have determined that the standard treatment is no better than a placebo.

 ✔ Standard treatment(s) results may be questionable because new evidence about the treatment or the disease has been unearthed.

 ✔ Effective standard treatments do exist, but aren't available because of limited supply or cost that puts it out of reach of most patients.

Most ethicists agree that using placebos in clinical practice is unethical *if* there is a standard treatment for the disease. This type of practice undermines the doctor-patient relationship by violating trust and truthfulness.

Preventing bias with blind studies and randomization

Blind experiments and randomization are two of the essential tools of a legitimate scientific experiment. The concept of justice requires that trials have some blinding and randomization.

Assigning people to experimental or control groups

Randomization is an essential tool in clinical trials. In a *randomized trial,* participants are put into a large group as long as they fit certain criteria, but then they're selected at random. Assignment to the control group and the group that receives the treatment is done at random, but each group should be closely balanced with respect to race, gender, economic status, geographic location, and other factors. If these factors aren't balanced, these simple differences rather than the difference in therapies may account for the difference in outcome.

Positive thinking

The *placebo response* or *placebo effect* is well documented in scientific studies. Studies have shown that about 30 percent of patients will feel better after taking a placebo. The mind is a powerful tool, and some patients can believe they are getting better because they think they're receiving a new medical treatment. The brain can release endorphins after the patient receives a placebo. The response varies from person to person. No one understands why some placebos work because the biological mechanisms are complex.

The placebo effect comes into play in everyday clinical practice, whether a physician realizes it or not. A provider can use the placebo effect to treat patients more effectively. If a patient comes into your office with migraine headaches, for example, there are a number of medications that could be prescribed. Because we know that placebos work at least 30 percent of the time, you can be confident that your choice of medication will work at least that often. As I discuss a new medication with a patient, I describe how it works and convey confidence that the therapy will be effective. If the patient also feels confident in the therapy, he will be more likely to be compliant with the treatment, and the outcome is more likely to be successful. This is not deceiving the patient; it is simply engaging the patient's mind and body more actively in the treatment and increasing the chance of success.

Randomization helps researchers achieve certain goals:

- Offers more robust results due to equal sizes of the control and placebo groups
- Allows each patient an equal chance of receiving the treatment
- Eliminates selection bias
- Reduces the probability of accidental bias

Randomizing is the gold standard in clinical trials. And most researchers believe that when researchers are in equipoise, offering random assignments is the ethical response.

Keeping assignments under wraps

A *blind* experiment is one where the researchers and subjects don't know some of the information about the trial. The word comes from the idea of blindfolding someone. Single-blind experiments are where the subjects don't know what type of treatment or drug they are receiving, and double-blind experiments are where neither the subjects nor the researchers know who gets what treatment. This helps prevent bias, which can skew findings and result in false positives or false negatives.

Some experiments involving blind studies can violate the principle of non-maleficence. In trials studying drugs or behaviors, it's fairly easy to conceal which group gets the placebo or standard care. But if researchers are conducting a trial that uses surgery or other invasive technique, blinding becomes more difficult. If, for instance, doctors who wanted to study the effectiveness of arthroscopic knee surgery for knee arthritis put patients under sedation and made small skin incisions around the knee to make it look like surgery occurred in the placebo group. In this case, sedation and small incisions did carry some risk to the patient. But the study concluded that this type of surgery did not help knee arthritis, thus preventing thousands of unnecessary knee surgeries. Some ethicists argue that this sham surgery is never ethical because of potential harm to the patient. Other ethicists allow for sham surgery with tight restrictions. To be ethical, studies such as this that evaluate more invasive procedures must be small, offer significant benefit to patients, there must be no other way to test the treatment, and the trial must be constantly overviewed by the IRB. (For more on the IRB, see the later section "The Institutional Review Board: Ethical Gatekeepers of Clinical Research.")

Because the best studies are set up so no one knows who's receiving the experimental treatment and who's getting the placebo or alternative treatment, someone on the IRB must be able to break the code in case of an emergency. The patients participating in the trial should wear some type of identification so that if they do need emergency treatment, the attending physician knows about the research and can contact someone for more information.

Some studies require a data and safety monitoring board (DSMB) if they are particularly complex or risky. The DSMB's functions include

✔ Specifying the type of data collected and presented

✔ Examining the data by group without knowing which group is receiving the tested treatment

✔ Breaking the code and unblinding the study

✔ Monitoring the safety of patients more easily than the IRB because they have more access to information

Minimizing any risk of harm

It's just not possible to avoid all harm in life, let alone in medicine or clinical trials. You can go huddle under your bed in fear, but you're going to miss your life. But when performing ethical experimenting on human beings, the risk of harm must be minimized. The risk of harm must also be much less than the hypothesized benefit to society of the new drug or treatment.

Of course, sick patients who participate in trials must be protected against harm. But some ethicists think that healthy participants in these trials must be even more protected simply because they won't benefit from the results of the trial, at least not yet. As much data as possible should be collected from standard of care procedures before the trial to minimize risk. And trained medical personnel should be available 24/7 to respond to emergencies.

The Institute of Medicine commissioned a committee to recommend a framework to minimize harm in clinical trials. Their recommendations are

- ✔ All clinical trials should be overseen by protection programs specifically tailored to minimize risk of harm.

- ✔ The leaders of the trial and the protection programs should be made known to the public and commit to the highest ethical standards.

- ✔ Whoever makes the decisions about protocol development should be highly trained in medical ethics.

- ✔ Participants in the trials should have some say in protocol development.

- ✔ IRB reviews before approval should look carefully at conflict of interest.

- ✔ The IRB itself should be called an *ethics review board* and reshaped to focus on minimizing harm and adhering to ethical principles.

- ✔ When participants are harmed, they should be compensated for injuries.

The Institutional Review Board: Ethical Gatekeepers of Clinical Research

Institutional review boards (IRBs) are the watchdogs of clinical research. The members of these boards must make sure that the trials meet the highest ethical standards possible. The safety of participants must be at the top of the list, and scientific integrity must be maintained.

In this section, we look at the role of IRBs in clinical trials and how they evaluate a trial and give researchers permission to proceed. As we discuss in Chapter 14, an IRB must be composed of at least five people from different professions, including one nonscientist and one member from the community who has no association with the trial, its sponsors, or the institution running the trial. The members must have enough education and knowledge in medicine to make an informed decision about the ethics of the trial and necessary safeguards.

In the United States, IRBs are governed by the National Research Act of 1974 and are themselves regulated by the Office for Human Research Protections (OHRP), under the Department of Health and Human Services. IRBs are usually outsourced by the company or institution running the trial.

Every single trial must be reviewed individually by an institutional review board. Risks and benefits are different for every trial. Knowledge of risks gained through laboratory or animal research may or may not apply to risks and benefits in human trials. If there is no indication of risk in animal trials, that doesn't mean no risk exists in human beings.

Looking at the role of the IRB

The Belmont Report, as discussed in Chapter 14, is the guiding document for institutional review boards. Beneficence, justice, nonmaleficence, and respect for autonomy all play a role in reviewing and approving clinical trials.

The IRB must make sure that risks to patients are minimized, that unnecessary risk is eliminated, and that procedures used in the trial are scientifically sound. The board scrutinizes the research protocol and informed consent forms, analyzes the risk-benefit ratio to make sure that it is acceptable, and looks at the qualifications of investigators.

The board not only reviews and approves the research before it begins, but it also must review the research as the trial proceeds. The reviews must be done at least once per year, every year that the trial is in progress. A trial with minimal risk can be monitored less frequently than a trial which has more than minimal risk.

The IRB identifies the risks of harm present in the research that are separate from risks of the usual therapies used to treat the disease or condition. There are several types of harm that can come to trial participants. These are

- Physical harms, including discomfort and injury that may be mild or serious. Patients have died while participating in clinical trials.
- Psychological harm, including mood alteration from drugs, or feelings of guilt, stress, or depression.
- Social harm, which is defined as invasion of privacy and confidentiality breaches that could end in stigma or embarrassment.
- Economic or financial harms, which could be the result of employment loss or future ineligibility for insurance.

And at the annual review, the IRB must be sure that the informed consent forms are clear and thorough, will be been discussed with each potential participant, will be documented and recorded, and will be properly reviewed. In some long trials, informed consent may need to be explained to patients again, especially if new data is discovered during the process. (For more on informed consent in clinical trials, see the later section "Recruiting Study Participants.")

Evaluating and green-lighting a clinical trial

Before a trial can begin, the IRB must examine all of its facets, evaluate the risk-benefit ratio, and determine that the trial has scientific merit. Several factors must be met for a clinical trial to get the go-ahead to begin:

- ✔ An informed consent form must be approved for patients who are voluntarily participating in the trial.
- ✔ The research must be scientifically sound.
- ✔ The risk-benefit ratio for trial participants must be favorable.
- ✔ The selection of patients must be randomized to eliminate bias.
- ✔ Privacy and confidentiality safeguards must be in place.

The size of the trial is also an important consideration. Trials that are too large expose too many patients to risk. Trials that are too small don't yield statistically significant information. If more people take part in a trial, that trial is said to have more *statistical power*.

The IRB is also responsible for making sure that the participants are drawn from a large pool, so the risks of research are spread evenly across the population that may benefit from the newly approved treatment or drug. Then the principle of justice is satisfied. The National Commission of IRBs has recommended that, to be as fair as possible, trials should use adults before they use children, competent patients before incompetent, and noninstitutionalized patients before institutionalized patients. Other burdens of research, such as discomfort and embarrassment, should be minimized.

After everything has been reviewed and the board is satisfied, the trial can begin. If the trial is testing a new drug, device, or treatment, a government agency will review the data before the trial begins. And the FDA can audit trial documentation after it ends.

And finally, researchers have to remember that IRB approval is temporary. Approval of a clinical trial can be withdrawn at any point in the trial if the board thinks the risks and harm are too high. The ratio of risk to benefit can change at any time during a clinical trial. Research can be modified or brought to a halt if the IRB demands it.

Recruiting Study Participants

Say you're a researcher, and you have a good idea for a new type of blood pressure medication. You develop the drug, test it in laboratory experiments and cellular research, and then the drug is tested on animals (see Chapter 16). It looks promising, so you want to start a trial on human beings. How do you recruit trial participants?

In this section, we look at the ethics of asking patients to participate in a trial. And we look at the importance of informed consent in clinical trials and the importance of full disclosure.

Deciding to ask patients to participate

One of the first steps in any research protocol is to determine who to study. When researchers decide the parameters of inclusion and exclusion, these parameters must be strictly followed so the study is not compromised. Some criteria may include age, how long the patient has had that particular illness, previous treatments, and overall health of the participants.

It's difficult to balance beneficence with nonmaleficence, or maximizing benefit and minimizing risk, when asking patients to participate in a clinical trial. Participating in a trial can expose your patients to significant risk. For example, if a patient receives a placebo instead of the experimental drug, the risk is their condition will get worse because they aren't receiving treatment. There are some cases when a placebo can ethically be used, such as if researchers think the standard medication may not be very effective or has side effects that limits patient compliance. In these cases, omission of the treatment must not increase mortality or cause significant long-term harm to the patient in the event they receive the placebo. And many patients who enter trials do so because there are no more treatments for their condition, or the available treatments no longer work.

The ethical justification for participation in clinical trials is that risk is minimized to the best of the researcher's ability, and that the most people possible benefit from this research. Doctors have a duty to promote scientific knowledge and the advancement of medicine. By participating in a trial, patients will not only help themselves, but they will help future patients by testing new and hopefully better treatments. Patients who participate in clinical trials receive excellent medical care, usually more care, more often than they would receive if they did not participate.

So should you recommend a clinical trial for your patients who qualify? Some ethicists feel it is never the treating physician's role to recommend that a patient consider a clinical trial because it is never better for the patient as pure treatment would be. Other physicians, especially oncologists, recommend clinical trials for their patients, especially when no other options are available. These trials may provide the potential for benefit to the patient, will further cancer research, and have little potential for harm. As is often the case, this question should be considered on a case-by-case basis. Consider your patient's condition, their desire to participate and the specific clinical trial, and recommend it if the potential benefit seems likely to outweigh any possible harm.

Laying out all the risks and benefits with informed consent

Informed consent, of course, is an important part of any medical practice, but it's especially important in clinical trials. Although prospective subjects are asked to sign an informed consent form, informed consent is a *process* a patient goes through, not just a form that is explained to them and signed. Patients must understand that they aren't receiving treatment for their illness; they're being studied to see if a new medication or treatment is effective against their illness. Since many of the patients who participate in trials are at an advanced stage of their disease, they must understand that a trial isn't necessarily going to cure their disease or prolong their life. They also must be aware of possible side effects before they agree to participate.

Knowing what goes on informed consent forms

These are the important components of informed consent forms in trials:

✔ The form must include what the purpose of the study is, what procedures will be undertaken, what the researchers hope to see happen, what treatments are being tested, and why the participants are being invited to participate in the study.

✔ All of the risks and benefits of the study should be reviewed.

✔ The consent form must be easy to read and understand, and must contain all relevant information about the study. Many IRBs say that consent forms should be written at the level of an eighth-grade education. Culture and language should be considered when writing the consent form. A translator or interpreter should be used when necessary.

✔ Patients should be told that clinical trials aren't considered treatment for their disease, but that they are helping develop future treatments. If patients think that the trial will offer them therapeutic hope, this is called *therapeutic misconception*.

✔ The researchers must point out all alternatives treatments to the patient's condition so they understand that participation in the trial is simply a way to test treatments.

✔ There must be a statement telling patients that they can leave a study whenever they want to.

✔ There must be no coercion involved, including the use of study names or acronyms that might offer misleading hope to a distressed patient, such as HOPE, MIRACLE, or SAVED.

✔ Confidentiality must be stressed, and participants must be told how their participation will remain confidential. Full confidentiality can't be guaranteed, so the statement "every effort will be made to keep your information confidential" is usually added.

✔ Patients can be paid to participate in some clinical trials, but the National Institutes of Health discourages this practice. There are some exceptions to this general standard. Participants can be paid for transportation costs or missed work opportunities. All payment methods and accounting methods must be completely transparent.

✔ Participants should have easy access to study contacts if they have questions, develop problems, or have concerns about their participation.

✔ The doctors and researchers involved in the study must not have any financial ties to the outcome of the trial.

✔ A statement that informed consent is *not* a contract. A patient participating in a clinical trial can leave at any time, for any reason.

Telling your patient what to expect

Describing placebos, blind studies, and randomization to patients is difficult. Patients must understand these terms and how these factors will apply to them as they participate in the trial. It's your responsibility to explain all the risks and benefits of a clinical trial so your patients can make a rational, informed decision about whether or not to participate.

Some study participants enroll because they think the trial may benefit them. It's important to let them know that it might, but that there are no guarantees. And others enter trials altruistically, hoping to add to scientific knowledge and medicine that will benefit others.

A patient's trust in you has to be considered in informed consent. If you have a patient's trust, your recommendation that they enter a clinical trial will probably carry more weight than it should. You must always emphasize the difference between therapy and research, and that participation is optional. Because you have more power than the patient in this relationship, be careful to stress that you are asking your patient to participate, not telling her or recommending that she do so. Patients must be told if the part of a trial in which they are participating is therapeutic or nontherapeutic. And, of course, the patient's emotional state has to be taken into consideration. After a serious diagnosis, offering a patient an experimental treatment through a trial may give them false hope.

Finally, it's important to remember that the process of informed consent should continue throughout the trial. Researchers should always be available and able to explain the purpose of the study and explain risks and benefits, as well as hear concerns and questions from participants. For example, if a patient is recruited into a study as they enter the hospital, their distress about their condition and their physical and emotional state may negatively affect their ability to give informed consent. It is important to follow up with these patients when they have stabilized to review the study and confirm informed consent.

Full disclosure: Explaining financial and institutional conflicts of interest

The National Institutes of Health and the Food and Drug Administration started the Clinical Trials Data Bank in 2000 (http://clinicaltrials.gov). This bank maintains information about clinical trials that shows the *sponsors* (those who fund the research) of the trials and publishes all results. This data bank was established to promote transparency in clinical trials after several studies found that negative results were being dismissed, and positive results stressed in some trials.

Because many clinical trials are sponsored by industry, and those industries want to keep results of such trials, especially negative results, as quiet as possible, a call for full disclosure about clinical trials, made by the editors of *The New England Journal of Medicine*, went out in the United States. Clinical trials are expensive and time-consuming. Most trials are conducted by large corporations, research hospitals, and the government. Scientists can sign funding agreements with companies to produce a drug even before a clinical trial has ended.

Some press has indicated that scientists receiving funding from pharmaceutical companies have not disclosed some negative side effects, and many scientists must sign nondisclosure agreements before their projects are funded. Ethicists think that patients should be told of researcher's financial and institutional ties before the study begins, and that this information should be included in informed consent forms.

If doctors are paid to enroll patients in clinical trials, this information must be reported to patients as part of informed consent. Other conflicts of interest include bonuses to the investigators and stock options from the sponsor as a reward for a successful trial. Any type of monetary gain could influence the outcome of a trial. In reality, all research and trials do have some built-in conflict of interest because the researchers hope that the new treatment will be effective.

Knowing what to disclose

These are the financial and institutional ties that should be disclosed before a clinical trial begins:

- ✔ It should be clear how the researchers are compensated for their time and effort.

- ✔ Information should be presented detailing if the researchers have a proprietary interest in the treatment. This includes patents, funding agreements, copyrights, or licensing agreements with corporations.

- ✔ Equity interest of more than $50,000 in the company producing the drug or treatment should be disclosed.

- ✔ Clinical researchers or members of their immediate family shouldn't have a direct interest in the product or treatment being studied.

- ✔ Payments to the researchers by study sponsors, whether the sponsors are corporations or institutions, should be disclosed.

- ✔ Institutions and corporations should not be allowed to review the data or conclusions before results are published.

- ✔ Whether or not the institution conducting the trial is being paid for participation should also be disclosed.

- ✔ The coordinators of the trials should understand financial and institutional ties and be able to clearly explain them to potential participants.

Noting whether the study's integrity may be at risk

In 2004, the *New England Journal of Medicine* published data from a five-year Conflict of Interest Notification Study conducted by the National Heart, Lung, and Blood Institute. The study developed disclosure statements about conflict of interest to use in informed consent documents. The study author agreed with the National Human Research Protections Advisory Committee that there are two types of disclosure: when a financial interest doesn't present a risk to the study's integrity, and when there is question about risk or integrity because of financial interest.

In the first case, a general financial disclosure form is sufficient. But in the second case, a specialized disclosure must be developed, including prompting questions from potential participants.

Risk of bias because of financial or institutional ties is subjective. Each IRB should use a separate algorithm to discover if these ties pose a risk to patients or the study's soundness. Then the type of financial and institutional disclosure form should be decided upon by the IRB and the researchers.

A 2003 survey from the University of Michigan found that when potential trial participants were told that the research was funded by a company or institution, they would be more willing to participate. But if they were told that a researcher had a financial interest in the treatment, they were less willing to sign up. Most patients surveyed wanted to know about potential conflicts of interest.

Ending a Trial Early

A trial may be ended early for two reasons:

- ✔ If a trial shows early negative effects, the IRB must be informed and the trial may be ended. No scientist or researcher should ever try to hide negative results about any research; that act violates all the principles of medical ethics.

- ✔ A trial may also be ended early because the results are so positive or promising. If it looks like a treatment or drug is more effective than the standard of care treatment against a condition or disease, researchers are obligated to end the trial and make the therapy more widely available.

In this section, we look at a researcher's obligation to patients, the implications of ending a research trial early, and when preliminary results should and should not be publicized.

Remembering obligations to patients

Any healthcare provider or medical researcher's first obligation, of course, is to her patients. The four principles of medical ethics (see Chapter 1) are designed with patients in mind. And remembering the physician's obligations to patients is the reason for undertaking the trial in the first place. Patient obligation must also be a primary reason a trial is ended early.

It's important to remember that the more participants are involved in a study and the longer a study lasts, more statistically significant information will be collected. A 2010 international study published in *The Journal of the American Medical Association* looked at almost 100 trials that were ended early and compared them with 400 similar trials that were completed. The study found that in the trials that ended early, researchers gave too much weight to early evidence. The data showing that the treatment was promising was at a random high, which meant that if the trial had continued, less positive results may have accrued. As results begin to come in, false positives or negatives can start to appear.

The problem is that ending a trial early due to positive results can sometimes benefit everyone except the patient. Researchers, pharmaceutical companies, journals, and funding bodies will receive benefits in the form of critical acclaim and money from new treatments. But if patients are given a treatment that has not been adequately tested, no benefit, or even harm to many patients, can result. This could be seen as a financial conflict of interest.

The Women's Health Initiative study

A recent example of an important trial that was ended early because of negative results was the Women's Health Initiative. This study, which was initiated by the NIH in 1991, studied hormone replacement therapy (HRT). Healthy postmenopausal women in the treatment group were given HRT in the form of estrogen (Premarin) and progesterone (Provera). The control group received a placebo. The study was ended early in 2002 because of increased risk of breast cancer, heart attack, stroke, and pulmonary embolism in the treatment group. Although the increased risks were slight, they were statistically significant. The study was ended to protect the women in the HRT wing and to publicize the information on these risks. Since the study ended, fewer women are using HRT, and the incidence of breast cancer has actually declined.

Clinical trials should be ended early only with a very good reason, such as significant harm to participants. A trial may be ended early because

- ✔ Unexpected harmful side effects are found.
- ✔ Not enough patients sign up for the trial to make a statistically significant group size.
- ✔ Early results reveal no benefit or very marginal benefit.
- ✔ The treatment presents unreasonable and significant risk to patients.
- ✔ The trial's sponsor may be unable to manufacture the drug or have determined that market potential is insufficient.

When a trial ends early, participants need to be notified as soon as possible. They should be told why the trial is ending, about any safety considerations or concerns, about available after-care, and be given a timetable for after care. Patients must be monitored after any trial, but especially after a trial that has ended early, for positive or negative reasons. If the trial was studying a drug, for instance, should the patients be weaned off the drug and monitored for side effects during withdrawal? Even if a study's funding source is cut off, the patients still need to be given adequate medical care.

Looking at implications for research

Ending a trial early can have a negative effect on further medical research. If a trial shows very promising results, other scientists will be less likely to investigate the treatment or drug. There isn't a point to conducting expensive and time-consuming research on a treatment that has already been proven effective, even if it hasn't been through a full trial.

Researchers will also likely not research treatments or drugs that show adverse effects because of the principle of nonmaleficence. But if a drug that did show promise is marketed and then starts causing problems, doing additional research on that product is ethical, as long as strict precautionary measures are in place and the IRB reviews the trial closely.

In 2007, the United States gave the FDA new powers for oversight of drug safety, including requiring after-market clinical trials. For instance, the cholesterol drug Vytorin was marketed as an improvement over traditional cholesterol-lowering drugs. But an after-market study found that it was no more effective than cheaper generic drugs. The study that showed clinical benefit, which was nicknamed ENHANCE, may have been flawed. Congress is investigating whether researchers withheld negative results.

When conducting clinical research, it's ethical to design the best study, protect participants, and tell the truth. Science in general and medicine in particular are hurt by poorly conducted trials. Medical mistakes get a lot of press, and unethical trials hurt future research. Patients will be less likely to sign up for trials if they don't trust researchers. And patients in general will be harmed by improperly tested treatments.

Publicizing preliminary results

Preliminary results are usually not publicized unless there is clear and convincing evidence that the treatment or drug is extremely beneficial. After Phases I and II, results are used to determine whether the trial can continue. When Phase III is complete, researchers look for medical significance. If it is present, the trial is publicized.

Publicizing preliminary results is called *science by press conference* and this practice is ethically questionable. Most researchers think that studies should be finished and reviewed by peers or experts in the field before the new knowledge is released to the general public. Releasing results can also depend on the disease or condition in question. For instance, at the insistence of AIDS activists, new research about treatments and cures is generally released more quickly than treatments for other diseases. And when scientists were investigating the SARS (severe acute respiratory syndrome) outbreak, they notified the media quickly, rather than publishing results in journals.

If a disease is fast moving and life threatening, it is tempting to release results of promising studies. But researchers and doctors must temper their eagerness with caution and pragmatism. Offering false hope before studies are completed is not ethical.

Pfizer drops the drug Mylotarg

In 2010, Pfizer ended a trial of Mylotarg, a drug that researchers thought would increase the lifespan of elderly patients with acute myeloid leukemia. In fact, the drug was put on the accelerated approval program because the drug showed promise early. But researchers found that more patients were dying on the combination of Mylotarg and chemo together than on chemo alone. This drug will not be available to new patients.

Chapter 16

Research in Special Populations

C linical research is essential to the practice of medicine. We examined some of the ethical issues involved in research in Chapters 14 and 15. Now we take this a bit further and look at research in special populations.

It's interesting to note that clinical practice *is* experimental, even with established drugs and treatments, because doctors and healthcare providers are always looking for new reactions to medications, both positive and negative, and trying to learn something new. In fact, many new surgical treatments were developed by surgeons and doctors making changes in methods out of necessity.

Special populations are those patients for whom obtaining informed consent is problematic because they either lack mental capacity to understand or because they lack freedom in some way. These groups are also called *vulnerable subjects* because they are unable to protect their own interests. That includes animals, prisoners, children, people with mental health issues and diseases, and pregnant women.

In this chapter, we look at the ethics of research in these vulnerable groups. We explore the responsibility of the researchers and institutional review boards (IRBs). We try to understand why animals are used in scientific research, how to ensure that they are treated in an ethical and moral manner, and why some people are opposed to using animals this way.

We look at psychiatric research and the issue of capacity. We also look at why research on children and pregnant women is pursued more cautiously, and the ethics behind this research, including the issue of direct benefit and the lure of a potential cure or treatment for those who have lost hope.

Animal Research

Most drugs and treatments are first tested in the laboratory using cells and tissue. Animal testing is usually the next step. When a drug is first developed, researchers aren't sure what, if any, side effects it will have. It is considered more ethical to experiment first on animals and then on human beings. In fact, using human beings as a first step in research would violate the Declaration of Helsinki and federal law in most countries.

Of course, the animals used in research still must be treated in an ethical manner. Some people believe that animal testing is unnecessary and immoral. In fact, in the past several groups have stormed research facilities, freeing the animals and destroying the projects.

Through animal research, medicine has developed

- ✔ Immunizations for polio, diphtheria, mumps, and hepatitis
- ✔ Biomedical advances in cancer research, including bone marrow transplants
- ✔ Pacemakers
- ✔ Artificial joints
- ✔ Development of insulin and antibiotics
- ✔ Organ transplants
- ✔ Treatments for glaucoma

The American Medical Association (AMA), the American College of Surgeons, the American Veterinary Medical Association, and the Association of American Medical Colleges all recognize that animal research is needed. The important ethical point is that animals used in medical research must be respected and protected.

In this section, we look at the ethics of using animals in medical research. We try to explain why animals are used and talk about the standards set to ensure that animals are treated in an ethical manner.

Understanding why animals are used

Before drugs and treatments can be used in human beings, they must be tested. Tests are run in the laboratory on cells and by using computer models. But proponents of animal research point out that testing on isolated cells is very different from testing on a whole body system. If reactions to the drug, efficacy, and safety were tested first in human beings instead of animals, many deaths would result.

Animals have been used in medical research since the 17th century. The first experiments were quite cruel, such as vivisection, which is the dissection of animals while they are still alive. Most scientists at the time didn't think that animals could even feel pain, let alone learn or remember. The philosopher Descartes proposed the theory that animals were more like machines.

We now know that is wrong. Animals do feel pain, suffer, remember, and learn. My cat Muffin once stepped on a threshold we were painting. We had to scrub the paint off her paw with turpentine and then wash it many times with soap and water, much to her distress. For the next few months, every time she approached that threshold she would jump over it rather than step on it. She remembered her suffering caused by that threshold every time she approached it, and modified her behavior by avoiding it.

Cell function and even organ function is similar in all mammals and in all vertebrates. When a system works, it is replicated in other species. Our skin is similar to pig's skin, so research on pigs developed skin grafts for burn patients. Our eyes are similar to the eyes of the rabbit, so animal research on rabbits led to successful corneal transplants.

Computer model studies of cells and even organs, can give research scientists an idea of how a drug or treatment will affect a whole organism. But even results from computer models can't predict what will happen when that drug or treatment is used on a mammal. Will a medication to treat glaucoma raise blood pressure? Computer models can't predict this. And data used in computer models comes from animal studies.

As with human subjects research, the gain from animal research must be significant enough to justify the pain and suffering caused by the research. Animals shouldn't be used in research for frivolous reasons, such as the testing of cosmetics.

Animal research advocates point out that advances in veterinary medicine have come from research performed on animals. Research on HIV in animals led to the vaccine for feline leukemia. And research on diseases such as diabetes and heart disease has led to new treatments for dogs and cats.

Ethical treatment of research animals

In the 1970s and 1980s, fringe groups such as the Animal Liberation Front raided labs and destroyed research materials. Although these groups did damage, they also exposed how badly many research animals were treated and highlighted the need for change.

Practicing invasive medical procedures on animals

On rare occasions, animals are used not just in research, but in doctor's training. Minnesota's Medical School started a class to train rural doctors in skills they will need when staffing emergency rooms and taking calls in small towns.

The class includes a 2-day classroom course focused on different scenarios and then a skills lab. When I took the class in 1999, the benchmark lab taught many critical skills including emergency intubation of adults and children, emergency tracheotomy, chest tube insertion for chest trauma, inserting central IV lines in children and adults, and emergency thoracotomy. We practiced the pediatric skills on a rabbit and the adult skills on a sheep.

The animals involved were paralyzed and sedated with general anesthesia. After the skills were learned and the lab completed the animals were humanely euthanized. The animals were treated in a compassionate manner during the entire process. I was grateful that I had a chance to learn these skills in the lab before I had to use them in an emergency on a human being.

Several laws have been passed in the United States regarding the ethical treatment of animals in medical research. The Animal Welfare Act of 1966 sets the minimum standard of conditions in research labs. And the Health Research Extension Act of 1985 expanded the Animal Welfare Act and added the requirement to provide veterinary medical and nursing care for animals both before and after research. That law also established animal care committees to oversee publicly funded research. The Guide for the Care and Use of Laboratory Animals is the source for regulation of animal welfare in medical research.

Medical research using animals follows basic guidelines called The Three Rs: reduce, replace, and refine. In other words, researchers must reduce the number of higher species used in experiments, such as primates, horses, dogs, and cats, and reduce the number of animals used in any experiment. Animals should be replaced with other research methods and models when possible. And scientists should refine experiments and tests so the research parameters are humane.

More than 90 percent of all laboratory animals are rats and mice bred specifically for research. Other animals used in research include guinea pigs, dogs, cats, pigs, sheep, leeches, squid, and fruit flies. The laws only apply to warm-blooded vertebrates.

Because animals are sentient beings and cannot give informed consent, special procedures to protect them must be followed. These include

✔ A veterinarian should be on staff to monitor the animals' health and comfort and provide medical support.

✔ The research should be designed with the greatest good in mind.

✔ The fewest number of the most appropriate species are used in research; this should be justified statistically. Other models, including in vitro and computer models, should be used first. And experiments should not be unnecessarily duplicated.

✔ The living conditions should be appropriate and correct for the animal's comfort and health. Some regulations require environmental enrichment, which can include playing and petting the animals and providing toys and exercise.

✔ Personnel conducting this research should be trained and experienced.

✔ Animals must experience the least amount of distress possible, and pain must be avoided or minimized.

✔ If the research causes pain that is more than slight or momentary, the animal should receive sedation or analgesia.

✔ Animals that suffer chronic pain that can't be relieved should be painlessly euthanized as soon as possible.

✔ If problems are encountered or exceptions to these rules made, a review group should be consulted for proper protocol. The animals should be given care after the procedure.

Yes, animals suffer and feel pain and fear. These facts give them the moral status of sentient or feeling beings, but do not give them the moral status of human beings who can make ethical decisions. Some ethicists use this standard to judge if a test should be performed first on a human being or an animal: if you had to evacuate a burning building, would you rescue a human being or an animal? If you answered "human being," then animals are not in the same class as humans to you.

Animal Liberation

The author Pete Singer wrote the book *Animal Liberation* in 1975, considered the primary guide for opponents of animal research. In it, he coined the term *speciesism*, or devaluing life because it is in the form of another species. Singer wrote that speciesism was as indefensible as racism. He rejects the thesis that if suffering must exist, it's better for beings with lesser moral status to suffer. Opponents of Singer's philosophy point out that we have to draw a line somewhere. If it's immoral to cause suffering in a rat, how about insects or an amoeba? The line in medical research must be drawn somewhere, so it is drawn between humans and animals.

When I (co-author Linda) was studying at Rush Presbyterian-St. Luke's Medical Center in Chicago, I took part in an experiment to study mitochondria. We performed what I now consider a frivolous and possibly unethical experiment. A mouse was sedated and then a portion of its liver cut out to be examined with an electron microscope. No medical benefit emerged from this experiment; it was a learning experience for the students. This lesson could probably have been learned without sacrificing an animal.

Psychiatric Research and Consent

The American Psychiatric Association (APA) has special ethical guidelines for research. The same basic principles and ethical guidelines in other forms of medical research are followed, but more guidelines are needed in this specialty. The APA has added annotations to the AMA Code of Medical Ethics.

Research on people suffering from mental illness can cause serious harm. There are five areas to consider:

- ✔ **Respect for a person's rights and dignity.** There is a history of mistreatment of psychiatric patients in medical research, so these patients need to be treated with special care.

- ✔ **Weighing risks and benefits.** Psychiatric patients often are already distressed or have a distorted view of the world. Very sensitive questions are usually asked, which could trigger stress, anxiety, or depression. A study must combine great benefit with minimal risk.

- ✔ **Informed consent.** Competence and capacity come into question in psychiatric patients. If the researcher is also the patient's primary doctor, this may create undue pressure on the patient to comply with the study. An ethics committee should decide if those patients should participate in any of that particular doctor's studies. Extra effort should be made so the patients understand the risks and benefits of entering into the study. Informed consent in these cases should be checked as the study progresses as well as at the beginning.

- ✔ **Confidentiality and privacy.** Most psychiatric research is sensitive, and questions asked are very personal. Subjects in these studies may be more vulnerable to identification than in non-psychiatric studies, so composites of patients should be used when reporting results. And if information regarding a threat to the safety of others comes out in a study, the researchers are obligated to report it.

- ✔ **Conflicts of interest.** Ethics committees must require all doctors and researchers involved in the study to disclose conflicts of interest, such as financial interest in the outcome. Using their own patients is usually forbidden, and the design of the study must include care and treatment of subjects both before and after the study.

In this section, we look at how researchers assess decision-making ability in psychiatric patients, as well as protecting the patient by evaluating the risks and benefits of the study.

Assessing decision-making ability in psychiatric patients

The patients who are most needed in research studies are often those who are the least likely to be able to give informed consent. Patients who suffer from schizophrenia, dementia, and psychotic depression may not be able to understand a study or make a rational decision to participate. This means there is a potential for skewed results. For example, if a certain group is more easily coerced into participation in a study (such as depressed, apathetic patients) this may mean the study is not as applicable to the general population. And if patients with severe mental illness aren't included in studies because they can't give informed consent, then the study results are less likely to apply to them even though they may be most in need of the treatment.

Coercion in these cases can be real or may be perceived by the patient. Because bonds and emotions can develop between the patient and the psychiatrist, a patient may want to participate in the study to please their healthcare provider. And some patients might understand the risks involved, but not care about them because of an illness like clinical depression.

Involuntary patients are those patients who are involuntarily committed to a psychiatric institution. They pose a very ethically challenging question: can they give informed consent? There are mental health laws in place to protect patients in these situations. Involuntary patients must be told that they can refuse to take part in the study, and an ethics committee should evaluate and reevaluate informed consent in these cases.

Researchers must develop informed consent forms and capacity protocols specifically for psychiatric research. Some researchers have a sliding-scale approach to assess capacity. In other words, as the risks of the study increase, the patient's capacity to understand and consent must also increase. In the more extreme cases, a patient should at least be capable of choosing a proxy to decide for him. An independent patient's advocate can be an important part of any psychiatric research study because they may be more capable of logical reasoning and their judgment wouldn't be skewed by the disease itself.

When a patient has been ruled legally incompetent, or has been judged to lack capacity, doctors must conduct an *explicit assessment* of capacity. This involves:

- ✔ Researchers must decide if the study involves more than *minimal risk*.
- ✔ If there is more than minimal risk, researchers must develop a special protocol to handle patients with diminished capacity.

✔ A standard cognitive test can be used to determine capacity, such as the Mini-Mental State Examination. More testing of the patient's understanding of the study should be conducted during the study.

✔ Doctors should use an independent panel to evaluate capacity.

✔ An IRB should mandate repetition of consent during the study so patients are asked more than once if they understand the trial.

Institutionalized patients or those who are under the day-to-day care of providers need to be treated with great care. In some cases, assent (simple consent) instead of informed consent can be enough to enroll these patients in a study, as long as they are functional, and only if the study poses minimal risk.

The patients must always be able to leave the study at any time. When there is any doubt about capacity, researchers should always contact the ethics committee or the Office for Human Research Protections (OHRP), a part of the U.S. Department of Health and Human Services.

Protecting the patient: Risk versus benefit

When creating any psychiatric study, the likelihood of benefit to the subjects from the study and others with similar conditions should be stressed. The United States has formed a National Bioethics Advisory Commission (NBAC) that oversees research in patients with mental illness.

The type of psychiatric research that is most controversial is placebo trials, followed by studies that discontinue needed medications, and then testing with medications that can induce psychiatric symptoms. These types of studies must produce evidence of clear-cut medical benefits prior to the study being conducted, and the maximum in safeguards must be instituted. The National Institute of Mental Health (NIMH) has established the Human Subjects Research Workgroup to intimately examine these high risk studies.

As in all medical research situations, the risks and benefits must be balanced. Any study with high risk should result in great benefits. And informed consent is more important in high-risk studies. More controls should be built into those studies.

Pregnancy and Pediatrics

Pregnant women, fetuses, and children are special populations who must be protected in medical research. Research on these groups is necessary, but great and direct benefit must result, and risks must be minimized.

In this section, we look at the risks and benefits of research in pregnancy, as well as research on children. The issue of the *mature minor* comes into focus again as we decide if children or their surrogates should give informed consent or at least have input into the research participation. (See Chapter 8 for more details about mature minors.)

Understanding research with pregnant women

The prescribing of thalidomide to pregnant women in the late 1950s prompted the government to start thinking about changing the FDA's research recommendations. More than 10,000 babies were born with deformed or missing limbs because thalidomide was prescribed for morning sickness without being tested on pregnant women.

In 1977, the agency excluded women of childbearing potential from research. Now there is a lack of scientific data on the effect of many drugs on women and pregnant women. In 1988, the FDA called for safety and efficacy profiles on treatments for women and pregnant women. And in 1993, that agency eliminated the restriction on women of childbearing age participating in research.

Excluding women from research trials violates the principle of justice, because excluding women from studies deprives them as a whole from benefiting from discoveries in research.

When conducting research on pregnant women, preclinical studies must be performed first, including research on pregnant animals and women who are not pregnant. The fetus cannot give consent to participating in a study, and the pregnant woman is vulnerable because the fetus may be harmed. This is one time that the father has a say in what happens to the unborn child. Consent of the mother and the father should be obtained before a pregnant woman is enrolled in a clinical study. Of course, if the father is unavailable, incompetent, or the pregnancy happened because of rape or incest, he is not involved in the study.

Informed consent for pregnant women is more complicated than informed consent for other research participants. These factors must be considered:

- ✔ The researchers are acting in the best interests of the fetus and the woman.
- ✔ The study will not increase pain or suffering on the part of the mother or the fetus.
- ✔ The woman should consider her own interests in this study and not dismiss them because of potential benefit to the fetus.

✔ Informed consent during labor and delivery may be difficult or impossible to achieve, so women ideally shouldn't be recruited during that time. But sometimes research during this time may be necessary, so "emergency exceptions from informed consent" could be used. In this case, the standard is what a reasonable and competent patient would agree to.

✔ The parents understand the study's focus and trust the doctor who tells them about the study and explains the risks and benefits. The balance of information should be that enough information about risk is presented without causing anxiety, and enough information about possible benefit is presented so hopes aren't unrealistically raised.

✔ Both parents should be able to ask questions and take the time to decide whether or not to participate.

Many studies about pregnant women and fetuses are conducted using *active surveillance*, also called *delayed surgical intervention* or *watchful waiting*. Doctor visits are carefully monitored and medications given according to established protocol. In 2009, the New York Department of Health conducted this type of research on pregnant women admitted to the hospital with H1N1 infections.

Why risk may outweigh the benefits

Pregnancy changes a woman's body in many ways. These changes alter the way the body uses, reacts to, and processes drugs. So this research is essential to help prevent tragedies like the thalidomide disaster.

Pregnant women can be included in clinical trials and studies if that is the only way that a woman with a life-threatening condition can receive treatments that are still experimental. There must be a direct benefit from the research to the woman and the fetus: this is different from ordinary clinical research standards.

Some necessary studies are conducted on the health issues that arise during pregnancy, such as maternal diabetes or hypertension. But pregnant women aren't included in more general medical studies simply because of the risk to themselves and the fetus.

The pregnant woman's needs are considered more pressing than the fetuses' in many of these studies. The exception is if the benefit to the woman is small and the risk to the fetus is high. In those cases, doctors think the risks outweigh the benefits and the study should not be conducted.

Some clinical studies may inadvertently include pregnant women. In the United States, regulations require researchers to tell women who may participate in a study that there may be risks to the embryo or fetus if the woman becomes pregnant during the course of the study. Some studies specifically exclude pregnant women, require a pregnancy test before a woman can be enrolled in the study, and require women (as well as men, sometimes) to practice birth control while the study is in progress.

When considering the risks and benefits of pregnancy research, doctors must consider:

- ✔ Have studies been conducted on this treatment with nonpregnant human beings and pregnant animals first?
- ✔ Is the risk to the fetus minimal?
- ✔ Is the risk to the mother and fetus kept to the least possible?
- ✔ Will the mother be informed of any risk to the fetus as well as herself?

The National Academy of Sciences has proposed that research on pregnant women be conducted in three instances: when a condition arises that threatens the pregnancy, when preexisting conditions may affect the pregnancy, and when conditions arise that affect the pregnancy outcome, such as preterm labor.

No fetuses in utero can be studied unless the research is designed to meet the specific needs of that particular fetus and the risk is minimal. And researchers must be sure that the knowledge they want to gain from this research cannot be learned in any other way.

Research on children: Surrogate consent

Children present a special case in medical research. When is it ethical to test unproven drugs or other medical treatments on children? The problems inherent in this type of research include children's inability to give informed consent and the understandable motives of parents who want to see their children cured. And children are especially vulnerable because they are growing quickly and may be more sensitive to drugs and other treatments.

Children don't respond to medications the way adults do. Estimating a dose based on body weight, for instance, can lead to overdose or other complications. So research on children is necessary. The NIH now requires investigators to include children in research or provide good reasons why using children is inappropriate, such as when the condition being studied does not occur in children. In fact, current policies require that drugs that are used in substantial numbers of children be tested on children for safety and efficacy. This ensures proper labeling of medications and highest safety standards.

The American Academy of Pediatrics produced a document in 1995 stating the ethical principles that should guide pediatric research. They are

---

Timothy's case: A teen's decision on participating in a clinical trial

Timothy was a 13-year-old boy who had fought leukemia since the age of 10. He was initially treated with chemotherapy, and then underwent bone marrow transplant. His disease was in remission for a year, and then reoccurred. His doctors had no further proven treatment to offer, so he was considered for a clinical trial of a new chemotherapy agent.

There were significant possible side effects of this medication, including vomiting, diarrhea, shortness of breath due to lung scarring, and possible damage to his heart. His parents were anxious to proceed with the new drug in an effort to save his life. However, Timothy knew the drug was unlikely to be of benefit and had significant side effects. He had come to terms with dying and wanted to live the rest of his life without the side effects. After long discussions with his parents and his oncologist, everyone honored his wishes and withdrew him from the trial.

✔ Studies should be conducted with adults before children, if feasible.

✔ There must be sound reasons why the clinical research must be performed with children, such as treatments for cancer that only affect children, or for calculating dosage of drugs specifically for children.

✔ The level of risk to the child has to be carefully assessed and weighed against the potential benefit to that particular child as well as other children in the same or similar condition.

✔ Any research proposal that may involve more than minimal risk to the child and no personal benefit requires special review by an IRB or other board.

✔ Informed consent, informed permission of the parents, and their close involvement in the research must be obtained whenever children are involved in a clinical trial. Consent of any child considered a mature minor should be obtained as well, and children should give assent.

Parents are heavily involved in medical research on children. They give *informed permission* to their child participating in a clinical trial. But the children themselves must be considered. Many researchers think that after the age of 7, children should be involved in discussions about clinical participation, and if the child does not want to participate, that refusal should be respected. The older child who has a role in decision-making is considered a *mature minor*. But even mature minors need special consideration because their brains are not fully developed and they do not have the full intellectual capacity and reasoning ability of adults.

Some trials are randomized, with one group getting the experimental treatment and another getting the best known current treatment. By being involved in the study, a child may miss out on the best current treatment if he or she receives the experimental drug. The parents and the patient must be informed about this fact. And as with other types of research, a child must be allowed to withdraw from the trial at any time.

Experimental treatments may be the only hope for some children with terminal illnesses. This raises an ethical dilemma for the doctors and the parents, who may be desperate for any treatment to save the child. It must be emphasized that research is not the same as therapy and there are no guarantees that the child will benefit from the research or improve at all. Much medical research with children simply provides hope for future generations rather than extending the life of the children in the study.

But so many of the improvements in survival of these terminal conditions are due to the willingness of children and their families to take part in clinical research. We owe a great debt to them.

Chapter 17

It's All in the Genes: The Ethics of Stem Cell and Genetic Research

*O*f all the topics in medicine, stem cell research and cloning have received the most media attention. These medical advances seem like the stuff of science fiction, yet researchers think treatments using these methods aren't far away. In 2008, scientists used adult stem cells to rebuild a woman's trachea, and within days it was indistinguishable from the rest of the tissues in her body.

So what's all the fuss, and why the controversy? Why do some people oppose this type of research that has so much potential to help heal and treat disease? The most useful stem cells are derived from a *blastocyst,* a fertilized human egg which has just begun growing. In this chapter, we look at the controversy over stem cell research, focusing on stem cells from embryos and contrasting them with adult stem cells. We also look at the risks and benefits of genetic testing, including genome sequencing, gene therapy, and who owns your DNA. Finally, we address the ethics of cloning.

Understanding Stem Cell Research

Stem cells are very basic human cells that can develop into many different types of cells, tissues, and organs. For instance, stem cells can become heart tissue or skin or cartilage to rebuild a trachea.

These cells are called *pluripotent,* literally meaning multiple potential. They can differentiate into any of the three main types of cells in the human body:

the *endoderm,* which becomes the GI tract and lungs; the *mesoderm,* which becomes muscle, bone, and blood; and the *ectoderm,* which becomes the skin and central nervous system. The only organs pluripotent stem cells can't become are the placenta and umbilical cord. *Totipotent* stem cells can become all the cells in the body, including the placenta and umbilical cord. And *multipotent* stem cells, or adult stem cells, are limited in their ability to become different organs. For example, bone marrow stem cells are multipotent because they can become blood cells, but not other cells such as kidney cells.

Scientists are hopeful about embryonic stem cells because they can literally develop into any tissue. For instance, researchers think that some day, instead of relying on cadavers for organ donation, we'll be able to grow someone a new heart or kidney using their own DNA. Not only will this solve the problem of organ scarcity, but it will also eliminate *host-and-transfer disease,* in which the body attacks the new organ because it has different DNA and is seen by the immune system as an intruder.

Stem cells can be naturally pluripotent or can be artificially induced into that state. In the latter case, there is hope that adult stem cells, usually harvested from skin, bone marrow, or the brain, may be used in stem cell research. This would eliminate the ethical issue of destroying an embryo to obtain the cells.

In this section, we look at the ethical debate about embryonic stem cell lines. We also look at who will benefit from stem cell research and what kinds of diseases and conditions that treatment from this research might cure. And we look at the promise and problems of adult stem cells.

Who will benefit? The case for stem cell research

There is the potential for thousands, if not millions, of people to benefit from the cures and treatments that may come from stem cell research. Some people say that every single human being will benefit from the research. Some stem cell treatments are already available. Bone marrow transplants that are used in the treatment of leukemia use adult stem cells.

These are the kinds of diseases and conditions that scientists hope stem cell research may be able to treat or cure

- ✔ Spinal cord injuries
- ✔ Parkinson's Disease
- ✔ Huntington Disease
- ✔ Cancer
- ✔ Blindness and deafness

- ✔ ALS
- ✔ Muscular dystrophy
- ✔ Strokes
- ✔ Burns
- ✔ Organ transplants
- ✔ Diabetes
- ✔ Heart disease
- ✔ Osteoarthritis and rheumatoid arthritis

Scientists are using adult stem cells to create better drugs to treat diseases. This type of research is progressing quickly, and may help treat some of these diseases before a cure is found. New treatments for Parkinson's disease and diabetes using stem cell research show promising results. Scientists are also learning more about how cells work, including how they go off-track and develop into birth defects, cancer, and other diseases. This research can also help improve drug development. If new drugs can be tested on stem cells, it may speed up the clinical trial process and make those drugs safer.

Most of these treatments, of course, are years in the future. But some of them may become reality within 10 to 20 years. Clinical trials using stem cell treatments for some of these diseases are now being conducted.

The ethical debate over embryonic stem cell lines

In 1998, scientists learned how to grow embryonic stem cells in the lab. Of course, the issue of using embryonic stem cells in research is just as contentious as abortion, discussed in Chapter 11. As you might expect, opponents of stem cell research are against embryonic stem cell research because it destroys an embryo, which is considered destruction of a human life. Stem cell proponents support this research because it may improve or save many lives, and they don't consider a blastocyst to be a complete human being.

Some people think that destroying an embryo, even to potentially create a way to improve and even save thousands of people's lives, is unethical. And others think that *not* using these cells to help human beings live better lives is unethical. And still others believe, according to their definition of personhood, that an embryo isn't a human life until it's implanted in the womb, so using them for research is acceptable.

One of the main ethical arguments of opponents to stem cell research is that the potential good that may come from stem cell research at this point is largely theoretical, or in the future, whereas the harm that is coming to embryos is happening now. So the good that comes from stem cell research is a theoretical good rather than a tangible good, and this is ethically not worth the destruction of human embryos.

The moral question is: What is the harm, and how can we balance it? Destroying embryos does end life. But disease also destroys lives. For proponents of stem cell research, embryos do not have the same moral status as full persons, the ones who will benefit from stem cell research. So it follows that the potential to prevent pain, suffering, and death of many full persons through the advancement of this research outweighs the harm coming to a blastocyst. And to those who say that the good that may come from this research is theoretical, we won't know until we try. Much medical research is theoretical, especially when a branch of science, such as stem cell research, is new.

Creating stem cell lines: Do you have to destroy an embryo?

Because of legal restrictions, the benefits of stem cell research so far have been seen with adult stem cells. However, the stem cells that show the most promise — and generate the most controversy — are derived from blastocysts. (Actually, they should be called *blastocyst stem cells,* not *embryonic stem cells.*) *Blastocysts* are the stage in human development between a fertilized egg and an embryo. They exist about five days after fertilization. A blastocyst is a hollow ball of 50 to 100 cells, with an inner and outer layer. Blastocysts do not have the *primitive streak* that becomes the spine, and they have no heart, lungs, brain, or any specialized tissues. The development of the primitive streak is important because some believe this point distinguishes a blastocyst from an embryo.

Embryonic stem cell lines are created from cells removed from the blastocyst's inner layer, the part that would become an embryo and then the fetus in a normal pregnancy. The cells keep replicating without changing their basic state as long as they are properly cultured in the lab. They do not differentiate until they receive a signal from a *growth factor,* usually a special protein. These cells must be able to divide over a long time to demonstrate potency before they can be used in research.

Not all cells from every blastocyst divide and become a stem cell line. It can take up to 100 cells to get one that will be used to create a stem cell line. To become a line, millions of cells must be successfully replicated from that one original cell. The cells must be free from defects, viruses, or any problem with DNA.

Other possibilities may allow research using embryonic stem cells without destroying actual blastocysts. Unfortunately, there are problems with many of these methods.

> ✔ The Parthenote method uses unfertilized eggs and triggers them into acting as if they are fertilized, so they produce all 46 chromosomes in a blastocyst. Unfortunately, these eggs usually have a poor or faulty genetic structure, which means they are too flawed to use.

✔ Amniotic stem cells are found in the amniotic fluid in the womb. These cells can be used without destroying embryos. Scientists think that these cells are not pluripotent, but they can form *embryoid bodies,* which are disorganized aggregates of cells, just like embryonic stem cells can, which is a good sign.

✔ The Morula method uses a fertilized egg that has developed into eight cells. Just one cell is removed and then that cell is replicated. The remaining cells in the morula can develop into a healthy embryo. Morula cells are *totipotent,* meaning they can develop into any tissue or organ, including the placenta. This technique is used when evaluating embryos for pre-implantation genetic diagnosis, but deriving a line from a single embryonic cell doesn't work yet.

✔ Somatic cell nuclear transfer (SCNT) is a method where the nucleus is removed from an egg, which is then labeled *enucleated.* A nucleus from another cell is added to the egg, which begins to replicate.

✔ Alternate nuclear transfer (ANT) method uses an embryo that doesn't have a gene regulating development. Those embryos usually turn into *teratomas,* which are tumors made up of all three germ layers. Again, problems with this method include defective cells and difficulties with genetic manipulation.

Using unwanted embryos

Hundreds of thousands of frozen embryos created in the IVF procedure are stored in clinics. These embryos, if not implanted into a uterus, are frozen for long periods of time, then donated or thrown away. Some researchers think it would be better to use some of the cells from these embryos to help find cures for diseases rather than discard them as medical waste. And many of those embryos will never be implanted because they aren't rigorous enough to develop into a fetus. Those embryos have three fates: thrown away, frozen indefinitely, or used in research.

Intention is a critical ethical principle in this debate. Proponents of stem cell research argue that if the intention for using unwanted embryos is to improve someone else's life, you are taking a bad situation and turning it into something good. When someone dies and donates their organs, accepting that organ doesn't mean you approve of their death. Receiving the polio vaccine, which was developed using fetal tissue, doesn't mean you approve of that research. And if some blastocysts created for IVF can't develop into a human being, using their cells to help treat disease is making the best of what some think is a bad situation.

This is consequentialist ethics, which argues that we should do everything we can to reduce suffering, or achieve the best possible consequences, especially because the embryos are going to be destroyed anyway. This position could also be defined as a utilitarian position, or getting the greatest amount of good for the greatest number of people.

Snowflake infants

Some pro-life advocates are calling frozen embryos *snowflake infants*. There are more than 400,000 embryos frozen in IVF and research labs, and that number is increasing. Embryos that are not implanted by a couple can be donated to other couples, discarded, or donated to be used in research.

The Snowflakes Embryo Adoption Program began in 1997. Fewer than 200 babies have been born through this program. Many parents are uncomfortable with the thought of their biological children being raised by another parent, so many back out of the donation at the last moment. And many of these embryos were not used by the original couple because they have genetic problems or weren't healthy enough to be implanted.

There is only about a 10 percent chance that these frozen embryos (that have been frozen five years or less) are healthy enough to ever be implanted and become a baby.

The parents of these embryos often face emotional and psychological difficulties when deciding what to do with them. And infertility groups are nervous that laws designating the embryos as human beings may restrict fertility treatments. Some fertility clinics have lost track of the parents of these embryos. Some scientists think it's only a matter of time before the status of these embryos is challenged in court, which raises the ethical issues of autonomy and privacy. If embryos aren't in a woman's body, who do they belong to?

Those who oppose stem cell research see it differently. They feel the embryo is a full person and has a full right to life. Because they have a right to life, they shouldn't be killed even for a good cause, or a potential good. Any good that might come from an immoral act is, therefore, itself immoral. Opponents argue that similar to the research done in Nazi concentration camps, research that is done in an immoral way is never justified. We do use data from Nazi experiments, but many are morally opposed to this.

Looking at funding and regulations on stem cell research

In 2003, President Bush restricted stem cell research funded by federal money to embryonic stem cell lines that existed before August 9, 2001. President Obama lifted that ban; however, he couldn't lift a legislative ban that forbids researchers from using federal money to create new lines using destroyed embryos. That amendment is attached to every National Institutes of Health (NIH) funding bill that passes through Congress. But federal funds can now be used to perform research on new lines created using private funding.

Confused yet? So are many people. Scientists think that the newer lines, produced using private money, are healthier and stronger than the lines created before August 9, 2001. They need the best possible lines with the strongest cells to do their research. Those lines created before 2001 were

✔ Cultured using cow serum and mouse cells, making them unsuitable for human use because they may carry animal viruses.

✔ Not grown in consistent, approved environments, making them difficult to verify for FDA clinical trial approval.

✔ Needing constant care in the lab to keep them healthy and replicating. Newer stem cell lines are more resilient.

✔ Aging at a rapid rate, making them unreliable.

✔ Not from diverse populations. Diversity in stem cell lines is crucial for developing treatments that will help the most people. One of the problems with the earlier developed stem cell lines is that almost all of the embryos used to develop those lines came from wealthy white parents.

For now, research in the United States on embryonic stem cell lines is publicly funded. But that could, and probably will, change with each national election. The problem with restrictions on public funding of this research is that all scientific research is very expensive, so federal funds are important. Not many private companies have the funds or want to spend the money to sustain research of this type from the very beginning. Stopping and starting federal funding is frustrating to scientists.

What about the courts and the government? The court system regards frozen embryos as property, but property that has a moral status. They are not viewed as human beings. The FDA has decided that embryos are biological tissue. The state of Louisiana has stated that embryos are *juridical persons*, a designation that was used to describe slaves: not totally human, but holding some rights. That means that embryos cannot be thrown away.

The laws are different in other countries. In England, frozen embryos are discarded after five years. In Italy and Germany, freezing embryos is forbidden by law. Every embryo created must be implanted.

The National Institutes of Health has issued specific guidelines pertaining to stem cell research. Detailed and extensive informed consent forms, approval of protocol by an IRB, and free and uncoerced donation of the blastocysts are all part of the guidelines. See www.stemcells.nih.gov for more information.

Focusing on adult stem cells

Adult stem cells are also called *tissue stem cells* because they are found in all tissue of every body, including fetuses. Every type of cell in your body needs stem cells to replace them as they age. Adult stem cells tend to hide in the body and are present in only very small numbers, so they are difficult to find. There are skin tissue stem cells, intestinal tissue skin cells, liver tissue stem cells, and so on.

Scientists have learned how to change adult stem cells, from umbilical cord blood, bone marrow, brain, neural stem, muscle, and T-cells, into *multipotent cells*. Multipotent cells don't have the capacity of pluripotent cells. Multipotent cells can only become a few different types of tissue. Scientists have just created pluripotent stem cells from adult stem cells, but they have to use a treatment made from embryonic stem cells to induce pluripotency.

The research on adult stem cells is less controversial simply because no embryos are used to start these lines. Some people claim that because scientists know how to use adult stem cells, embryonic stem cell research is no longer needed. But that isn't true.

The problem is that adult stem cells, although promising, may not have as much promise as embryonic stem cells. Embryonic stem cells divide more rapidly, are more resilient, have more *plasticity* (or ability to potentially treat more diseases), have longer lives, and will not contain the damage or abnormalities that can be found in some adult stem cells. In fact, some adult stem cells treatments have caused tumors, meaning they are *tumorigenic*. Genetically altering adult stem cells could also trigger cancer-causing genes in those cells. And these risks may exist with embryonic stem cells as well. The true potential and the possible risks of embryonic stem cells will not be known until much more research with these cells is done.

It's true that some very successful therapies have been developed using adult stem cells but not embryonic stem cells. That could be because restrictions placed on federal funding for embryonic stem cell research stifled it. And embryonic stem cells have been isolated for use only since 1998. Adult stem cells have been used for decades, so they have been more extensively studied.

It's also important to remember that even though there are thousands of clinical trials going on right now using treatments derived from adult stem cells, they are focused mainly on cancer. Adult stem cells have been successfully used to treat only two diseases: cancer and heart disease.

Scientists think that we need as many stem cells from as many different sources as possible to do the best research, and different kinds of stem cells will be needed to treat different diseases. We need embryonic stem cells and adult stem cells. We need stem cells from every culture and genetic background. Proponents of stem cell research feel that putting limits on this research will limit treatments and cures in the future. If we had limited funding for bone marrow transplants or heart transplants, for instance, many people would not be alive today.

Genetic Testing: Looking for Problems in DNA

If someone gave you a crystal ball that showed your future, would you look at it? If someone offered you a book detailing parts of your future life, would you read it? Those are simple examples of what genetic testing can do.

Genetic testing is performed by taking samples of your body's cells, growing them in the lab, and then looking at your DNA to find defects and problems. This type of testing can be done on blastocysts, fetuses, children, and adults. We can test embryos before they are implanted in IVF treatments, and children and adults for later onset diseases. Currently, doctors can test for about 400 different genetic diseases using this technology.

Whereas genetic testing offers promise and hope, it can also be a minefield full of potential problems and issues. Who should be offered this type of testing? Who should be tested? What about counseling for those who are tested? Should children be tested without their parent's consent? And what about keeping this information private?

Should there even be genetic testing for those diseases that have no treatment or cure? What happens if someone has a test but can't afford the medication to help alleviate symptoms? If someone wants to be tested, can insurance companies deny them insurance or raise their rates based on the results?

In this section, we look at the reality, limitations, and expectations of genetic testing. The risks versus the benefits of genetic testing need to be clearly spelled out to anyone who wants to be tested, including the impact this information may have on their insurability and employability. And the need for genetic and psychological counseling must be discussed.

Knowing what we can and can't change

Before anyone is tested for a genetic disease, it's important to tell them what, if anything, can be done to help them if they have the gene that causes the disease. Some genetic centers offer tests only for diseases that have established, proven treatments. What is the point of testing for a disease with no cure or treatment? Telling a patient they have a disease that will only get worse, with no hope for a cure, can violate the principle of nonmaleficence because it may cause significant anxiety and suffering.

Some diseases, such as Huntington's Disease, have no treatment and no cure. And if you have the gene, your chance of developing the disease is 100 percent. Many people who are at risk for Huntington's choose not to be tested because if they have the gene, there's nothing they can do about it except wait for the inevitable and dread the future. On the other hand, even if someone has an untreatable disease, this knowledge may affect their life decisions, especially when it comes to having children. Some people do take the test.

On the other hand, some tests can prompt action. Women who have the BRC1 and BRC2 genes, for example, have a greatly increased risk of developing breast and ovarian cancer. They can have therapeutic mastectomies (removal of the breast before cancer develops) and prophylactic oophorectomies (removal of the ovaries before cancer develops) so they won't develop those diseases. Or they can have more frequent screening tests to detect those cancers early. It's also important to remember that having the gene does not result in a 100 percent chance of developing the cancer. Women without the gene will get these cancers, too.

At the same time, everyone has to realize that the answers to all diseases do not lie in our genes. Mutations can arise spontaneously, and environmental factors play a big role in disease development.

Weighing the risks and benefits

The physical risks of genetic testing differ depending on the age of the patient. For blastocysts and fetuses, the risk entails damaging the blastocyst or fetus or causing a miscarriage. For children and adults, testing entails a blood draw, and the risks are really nonexistent. Emotional, psychological, and financial risks, however, can be severe. These risks can all violate the principles of nonmaleficence, beneficence, and justice.

Considering tests before birth

Amniocentesis, chorionic villi sampling (CVS), and genetic testing done in utero bring up ethical questions as well. These tests have risks for the mother and increase the risk of miscarriage. Should they be ordered if the results put the pregnancy at risk, but are unlikely to change the pregnancy's outcome? If it's unlikely that the results will affect a couple's decisions about the pregnancy (termination or a higher level of prenatal care), some ethicists say it's a waste of valuable medical resources, violating the principle of justice. And risking a miscarriage if the pregnancy won't be voluntarily terminated violates the principle of nonmaleficence. But others think that women need time to prepare for the birth of a child with medical problems, which satisfies the principle of beneficence.

The case of Jessica: Prenatal genetic testing

Jessica was a 27-year-old single mother whose first infant had Down syndrome. She became pregnant for a second time and requested genetic testing to determine if this fetus was at risk. She was referred to a perinatologist and saw a genetic counselor. She agreed to proceed with CVS, knowing the risks. She wasn't sure if she would terminate the pregnancy if the fetus had Down syndrome, but she was very worried and hoped to be reassured. Fortunately, the genetic test came back normal and her mind was eased.

Pre-implantation genetic testing has become almost routine in in vitro fertilization (IVF), which is discussed in Chapter 10. Pre-implantation genetic diagnosis (PGD) can be performed on blastocysts and even eggs before they are fertilized. Embryos can be tested for

- ✔ Sickle cell disease
- ✔ Cystic fibrosis
- ✔ Tay Sach's Disease
- ✔ Huntington's Disease
- ✔ Klinefelter's syndrome
- ✔ BRCA1 and BRCA2, the genes that increase the risk of breast cancer
- ✔ Fragile X syndrome
- ✔ Hemophilia
- ✔ Duchenne and spinal muscular dystrophy

In PGD, blastocysts created in the lab have one cell removed when at the 8-cell stage. This cell is cultured and analyzed for genetic problems. A procedure called comparative genomic hybridization (CGH) analyzes cells from an older blastocyst when it has about 100 cells. More than one cell can be removed for testing, which makes test results more accurate.

The doctor selects embryos that are healthy and implants them in the uterus. There are problems with false positive (1 in 6) and false negative (1 in 50) results. Not all cells in all embryos are perfectly consistent. Any embryos that do transplant successfully should be tested again for abnormalities with amniocentesis or CVS around 11 weeks gestation.

Huntington's pre-implantation ethics

Parents who have Huntington's Disease in their family, but who don't know if they themselves have the disease, often use pre-implantation genetic diagnosis (PGD) to choose healthy embryos to implant. That way the disease is not passed on to their children. But what happens when the parents don't want to know if they have the gene? If all of the embryos have the gene, none can be transferred, and the parent will know he or she has the gene. Ethicists think that in this case, exclusion testing should be offered instead. This test links chromosomes with special markers and matches them to the affected grandparent. That way, embryos that have that entire chromosome from the affected grandparent, but not necessarily the specific gene for Huntington's, can be eliminated before implantation.

Weighing emotional risks for children and adults

The emotional risks for genetic testing are high. Tests for late-onset diseases, like Huntington's Disease and cancer, can lead to a life filled with dread, waiting for symptoms. Is it better to know if you carry a certain gene, or better to be blissfully ignorant?

Surprisingly, those who are tested for serious genetic defects and found they *didn't* have the gene can also have emotional problems. Survivor's guilt or decisions made that can't be undone (such as choosing not to have children because you thought you were at risk) can be emotionally devastating.

Some companies are offering home-based genetic tests, which have real risks associated with them. The problem is that the standards surrounding the testing are not known, so accuracy can be an issue. Also because these companies never see the patient face-to-face, sending results of a genetic disease in the mail can be devastating. And these patients aren't given automatic access to necessary counseling. This failure to provide needed psychological care is unethical because it violates nonmaleficence.

And what about children born into a family with a history of genetic disease? Should they be tested before they can consent to a test? Many ethicists think that parents should not test their children for later-onset genetic disease because that removes autonomy and choices from the future adult. If you are tested for a disease and you know the result, you have no chance to decline the test.

Of course, if the test is for an early onset disease, it's to the child's benefit that the test be performed. Babies born with Phenylketonuria, or PKU, can't metabolize the amino acid phenylalanine. This protein builds up in the body and retards brain development, leading to brain damage and seizures. If the infant is tested, found to have the gene, and immediately placed on a special diet, the baby can grow and develop normally. The test for PKU isn't expensive, but the special formula and lifetime restricted diet can be. This test, and a few other genetic tests, are now part of state mandatory newborn screening done soon after birth.

Counting costs of genetic tests

Cost is also an issue; genetic testing isn't cheap. Even home genetic tests can cost $1,000. But denying a genetic test to someone based on cost violates the principles of nonmaleficence and justice.

Insurance can be a concern as well. An example of a genetic disease that people are tested for is hemochromatosis. This is an autosomal recessive gene, meaning a patient needs two copies of the gene, one from each parent, to express the disease. If someone has two copies of this gene they inappropriately store iron in their liver and heart, leading to severe damage. Symptoms don't show up until late in the disease progress, so genetic testing determines if a patient has the disease or if family members are at risk. Phlebotomy, or blood removal, can prevent these late complications. But insurance often doesn't pay for the expensive tests, and until recently, patients were uninsurable if they are diagnosed with this disease.

And what about patients who take a test, find they have a gene that may cause disease, but can't afford treatment? This issue relates to universal healthcare, discussed in Chapter 6. Many people in the United States cannot obtain life-saving medical treatments because they can't afford medical care.

Considering privacy

Of course, privacy is important. Thanks to the 2010 Health Insurance Reform Act, insurance companies will no longer be able to refuse insurance to people with preexisting conditions, including genetic predispositions to disease. But there was nothing in that bill to control costs these companies can charge higher-risk patients. And keeping genetic information totally private can be difficult.

What about genetic information a patient discovers that may affect other members of his family? We discuss the joint account model for genetic information in Chapter 3. Ethicists think that doctors can breach confidentiality about genetic information when certain factors are met. They include

- Can you persuade your patient to share this information?
- Will withholding this information from relatives cause serious harm?
- Will telling the relatives about the genetic condition prevent harm?
- Will you tell the relatives *only* about the genetic information?
- Does the risk of harm to other people outweigh the harm of violating confidentiality?

Offering emotional counseling for patients

Emotional counseling should always be included with any genetic testing. The risk of suicide can be fairly high for some people and some genetic diseases. The counseling should be offered both before the tests and after. And this work should be done by doctors or counselors who have been trained in the specialty of genetic counseling.

Unless you keep up with this field, it's difficult to accurately counsel a patient about genetic testing. Knowing the symptoms and progression of different genetic diseases, as well as the probabilities of passing them on, is critical. The medical jargon can be difficult to translate so laypeople can understand it, and technology is progressing at a rapid pace.

There are certain steps to genetic counseling to make sure the patient receives the best care, that their autonomy is respected, and that harm to the patient and his family is minimized. Genetic counselors should

- ✔ Take a complete family history of the patient.
- ✔ Get more detailed information on medical history or other patient data, such as symptoms and physical signs.
- ✔ Educate the patient about the test, the possible results, and follow up, as well as about the disease for which they are being tested.
- ✔ Discuss options available to the patient.
- ✔ Make sure the patient understands all the risks and benefits of the test.
- ✔ Set up a plan for action after a test if the results are positive, or offer more counseling if the results are negative.

Pre-test counseling should assess the emotional stability of the patient. Questions such as "What will you do if you find out you do have this gene?" should be asked and the answers carefully noted. Many people can handle the results of a test, but some are more fragile and need more help.

Researchers have found that if a patient is very anxious and distressed before a genetic test they are more susceptible to psychological problems after a test. Of course, the difference between distress and emotional problems that cause functional impairment is impossible to predict.

Family dynamics also play a big part in genetic testing and should be investigated during counseling. Genetic testing can have a huge impact on the family, especially if the gene in question is likely to be present in other family members.

Pre-test education and informed consent must be part of the counseling. Counselors should stress risks and benefits of every test, what to do if a test is positive, and how to make a plan for the future.

Genome Sequencing: Mapping DNA

In 2003, the Human Genome Project was completed. Scientists mapped out the entire human genome sequence. Well, really only about 92 percent of the genome was actually mapped, because 8 percent of our genes are in a genetically inactive state called heterochromatin.

More than 3 billion pairs of DNA make up the genes of a human being, using four nucleic acids: adenine, thymine, cytosine, and guanine, also known as ATCG. And the differences among people are created by several million of those pairs: about 0.3 percent. And only about 2 to 5 percent of our genes actually code proteins, the building blocks of life.

The genome project is exciting because it may unlock the mystery of disease and let medicine be individualized. Scientists hope that someday medications can be tailored to each individual patient based on his or her genes. This would provide better outcomes and reduce adverse reactions.

The ethical principles of beneficence, nonmaleficence, autonomy, and justice play a part in this critical issue. Learning about our genetic code benefits us all in many ways. But are there ways that it can lead to harm? For example, testing someone for a gene that will cause a disease for which there is no cure may violate the principles of nonmaleficence and beneficence if that person is devastated by such news. These tests are expensive and can only be afforded by some people, which may violate the principle of justice. And what about patient autonomy? Can a company actually own a patent to a defect in your genes?

In this section, we look at the ethics of genome sequencing. Are your genes your own, or can they belong to someone else? And who gets to see your genes? Who can use the genome? Is it public property, or will private companies be able to patent our genes? Ethical issues are raised by these *intellectual property laws,* which restrict research because a company can patent a gene. This is in contrast to the rights of research scientists to use all available information from the genome in the lab and in clinical trials.

Gene patents: Deciding who owns what

Your genes are your own. That seems simple and straightforward, right? Well, no. Companies that have literally unraveled human genes and deciphered what the information means are patenting their work.

The companies defend this practice, saying that they don't hold a patent on a private person's genes, but they hold patents on specific isolated and purified nucleic acids. This is called the *patent thicket*, describing a thicket that scientists must fight through to get patented information. Information about more than 20 percent of the genes in our bodies are owned by private companies.

Scientists get genetic material from two sources: they are collected from patients who consent to the retrieval, or from a tissue bank of samples taken from patients who have given informed consent. So even though the material comes from individuals, corporations can own the material. Cooperative tissue and blood banks are set up to avoid trampling on patent issues.

For a gene to be patented, scientists must meet several standards set by a patent office. The patents issued so far for genetic research are from the United States Patent and Trademark Office, the European Patent Office, and the Japanese Patent Office. A patent is issued only for research that

- ✔ Identifies novel or newly discovered gene sequences
- ✔ Specifies the product of that gene sequence
- ✔ Shows, in detail, how that product is used in the body
- ✔ Proves that the sequence can be used to make that product in the lab

As mutations in genes are discovered, tests to find those genes are developed. Those tests are always patented by the company that owns the disease gene patent. Companies own this patent for 20 years.

A basic premise of science is that studies progress quickly when scientists have free and complete access to study results. But money plays a part, too. If a company can't make money from its research, there is no incentive to do that research in the first place. Although applying for a patent is inexpensive, the research that goes into the discovery for that patent runs into the millions of dollars.

Companies know that patents can help spur research. If someone owns a patent on a particular discovery, scientists won't waste time duplicating that work and research will expand into new areas. As long as you can afford the information protected by a patent, you can use it. Companies don't have to guard discoveries because they can charge for access.

There's one big difference between a patent on genes and a patent on a new kind of cell phone. Many argue that a product of nature can't be patented, and discovering or even purifying it doesn't change its fundamental nature. In fact, in March 2010, U.S. District Court Judge Robert Sweet ruled in a case regarding breast cancer genes BRCA1 and BRCA2 that the U.S. Patent and Trademark Office never should have granted these gene patents in the first place because the genes are a "law of nature." No one can have a patent on rain or the wind or dolphins. Still, companies have been applying for patents based on their discoveries. There has to be a way to protect researcher's investments and rights while still allowing the public access to this important information.

Looking at ethical problems with patents

Ethicists who are against patenting our genes state the *universal heritage* argument. They think that because our genes belong to everyone, the research on our genes should belong to everyone.

Researchers are worried that intellectual property rights and restrictions may affect breakthroughs in genome research. The National Academy of Sciences has issued a statement saying that Congress should write legislation to let researchers work on patented products relating to the genome without being afraid of patent infringement liability. This is especially important as it relates to public health.

Patents on genes have already slowed research on treatments for some diseases and have raised costs on genetic tests. The cost for some genetic tests, such as the gene for the BRCA1 breast cancer gene, have tripled in the past few years.

There are conflicting studies about whether or not gene patents are stifling research. One study published by the National Academy of Sciences found that only 5 percent of scientists even check for patents related to their research. And because research in this area is exploding, there is little real-world evidence that patents are limiting research. But, almost half of geneticists' requests for data relating to their research have been denied based on patent privacy.

A bill was introduced in Congress to limit patent protection in genetic research. The Genomic Research and Accessibility Act was introduced in 2007, but it never became law after languishing in committee for two years.

And scientists are finding that filing for patents is becoming more common than writing journal articles to tell the world about genetic discoveries. This reduces accessible information in medical literature.

The Ethical, Legal, and Social Implications (ELSI) Research Program (www. ornl.gov/hgmis/research/elsi.shtml) was started in 1990 as part of the Human Genome Project. This program identifies ethical and social challenges in gene therapy, including intellectual property issues, the conduct of genetic research, and implications to society of unraveling the mystery of our genes. The program establishes high standards to protect human subjects, ensures that clinical trials are valid, and evaluates new tests and treatments as they are developed.

Deciding who can use the human genome

All of the information generated by the Humane Genome Project is in a free public database called GenBank (`www.ncbi.nlm.nih.gov/genbank`). Anyone with Internet access can access this information. But patented information is kept private until someone pays to see it. Researchers feel that they deserve credit and compensation for their ideas and their work. But in some ways, that violates the principles of justice and beneficence by adding monetary cost to medical research that could save and improve lives, thereby limiting its use.

When a gene responsible for the presentation of a disease is mapped, scientists hope they will then understand the pathology of the disease from its genetic sequence. Scientists have already cloned the genes that are responsible for Duchenne muscular dystrophy, cystic fibrosis, and retinoblastoma. Blood tests can now screen for the presence of those genes. It is only right that people at risk for genetic diseases have access to tests that will tell them if they have that particular gene.

The genome is continually changing. And most of our DNA doesn't seem to have a specific use that we understand: this is called *non-coding DNA* and probably has a regulatory function. Tests and treatments developed from the human genome are going to be important tools in medicine, but will not be the only tools.

Gene Therapy: Changing the Code

Gene therapy, or using a specific gene inserted into a medical treatment, is moving from the realm of science fiction into our current reality. DNA or RNA is inserted into cells to change the genetic code. A specific gene can be inserted into a host patient's DNA using retroviruses, adenoviruses, or liposomes. Gene therapy is accomplished by adding genes to cells, turning off genes so they cannot be expressed, repairing a faulty gene, killing diseased cells, or improving the immune system so it will kill faulty or diseased cells.

Currently, gene therapy is used to treat bone marrow or blood diseases. Another type of gene therapy, which is controversial, is called *germ-line gene therapy,* where a gene is inserted into or removed from eggs and sperm, so certain traits are passed on to children or removed from the line. Basic gene therapy is approved by the National Institutes of Health, whereas germ-line gene therapy is not.

In this section, we look at the risks and benefits of gene therapy. We also look at cost and access issues, which are only going to increase as this therapy becomes available because companies are patenting genes, which increases legal fees and arbitrary pricing.

Weighing the risks and benefits of gene therapy

Genomics, or the study of the genome, must be pursued to minimize risks and maximize benefits of gene therapy . Most gene therapy, at this point, involves *somatic gene therapy*, or inserting DNA into cells that will not be involved in reproduction because they will not be present in the sperm or egg. These therapies are in the clinical trial or experimental stage. In this section, we discuss the possible benefits of gene therapy as well as safety concerns.

Looking at the promise of gene therapy treatments

The benefits of gene therapy could be limitless. They include

- ✔ Potentially stopping a disease at the very beginning
- ✔ Providing individualized treatments for diseases
- ✔ Eliminating cancer cells without chemotherapy or radiation
- ✔ Stopping the expression of dominant and recessive genes in offspring

At this time, most gene therapy treatments are being used to manage disease or develop better treatments, not to prevent or cure them. For instance, there is a gene therapy that can lessen the effects of Parkinson's disease. This treatment involves giving patients an infusion of genes that create a critical enzyme that controls neurotransmitters, and it has worked in clinical trials.

Adenosine deaminase deficiency (ADA) was the first disease that received an approval for gene therapy treatment. This disease manifests from a defect in just one gene, which makes gene manipulation easier. And the amount of adenosine deaminase in the body can fluctuate naturally, which means it doesn't have to be tightly regulated.

A genetic disease, linked to the X chromosome, called severe combined immunodeficiency, or SCID, is also in trials for therapy. This is the Bubble Boy disease, where children with this gene do not have an immune system. They must live in a completely sterile environment until they get a bone marrow transplant. Infants have been treated with gene therapy for this disease and they have developed their own immune systems.

Still, gene therapy is quite expensive. Some ethicists worry that this expensive therapy may be available only to the wealthy, which would violate the ethical principle of justice, especially distributive justice.

Considering safety issues

Doctors are concerned about the safety risks in gene therapy. The issues scientists are facing include effectively delivering the DNA to the cells, controlling the distribution of the new DNA, and making sure the new genes aren't overexpressed, or become too active, which could cause problems from too much of that specific protein, causing inflammation or even cancer. And most of the diseases gene therapy could treat are the result of mutations in multiple genes. Doctors can only treat diseases that are the expression of a single gene.

How safe does this therapy have to be before we can begin clinical trials? The risks of gene therapy include

- ✔ The insertion of the genetic material into the wrong gene
- ✔ The virus used to transmit the DNA may affect other cells
- ✔ The immune system could treat the healthy DNA as a foreign object and respond with host-and-graft disease
- ✔ The immune system may be over stimulated
- ✔ The gene may over-reproduce, causing other diseases

In fact, some patients in clinical trials for gene therapy have died. In 1999, Jesse Gelsinger, an 18-year-old patient who was in a trial to cure a nonfatal metabolic disorder, died from an immune system reaction that caused kidney and liver failure. This case is discussed further in Chapter 19. Two children in France developed leukemia while being treated with gene therapy for X-SCID. That case prompted the FDA to put a hold on trials using retroviral vectors. And in 2007, Jolee Mohr died after inclusion in a clinical trial for gene therapy against arthritis. That trial was just to test the safety of the new treatment, and would not have benefited Ms. Mohr. Her husband has stated that she didn't understand this fact despite a signed consent form, but her primary physician disagrees.

Gene therapy has the potential to help many people and remove the risk of disease, but we don't know what problems this tinkering with the genetic code might cause years down the line. One tiny error could create huge problems. And the children conceived using the gene-line therapy method can't choose to accept or refuse this type of treatment.

Designer genes: Going beyond therapy

Although everyone can understand that gene therapy to treat a disease such as cancer is ethical, not all opportunities that this therapy presents are obviously beneficial to all. There's a big difference between repairing a defect and simply improving physical characteristics. What conditions should be treated with this therapy? Should someone receive expensive gene therapy treatments because they think they're too short? What about athletes using gene therapy to build muscle or strength? Society will have to be careful that so-called normal individuals aren't diminished if this type of therapy becomes more common.

As we begin to manipulate germ-line genes, are we wandering into eugenics? It is clearly ethically wrong to create "a master race," as was promoted in the eugenics movement in Nazi Germany. But could we, perhaps, create a new line of human beings who have exceptional skills in certain areas? And will that redefine what "normal" is? If a large group of people have genetically enhanced IQs, will that cause discrimination or problems for people with "normal" intelligence? This raises some difficult ethical issues. The focus of genetic manipulation should be to learn about disease and figure out ways to treat it to benefit patients (beneficence). It is important that we monitor this research ethically so that it does not cross over into making some people superior to others based on certain genetic characteristics.

Ethicists are also worried about germ-line gene therapy. Making deliberate changes in the genes of future children removes some of their autonomy. If parents want to design children with certain characteristics, such as height or intelligence in math or science, that will remove some lifestyle choices from those children. Are we placing an undue burden on genetically altered children? Where are we going to draw the line? These are questions that will need to be answered in the future.

Cloning: Making Copies

In the movie *Attack of the Clones,* an exceptional army is cloned from a single bounty hunter. The scary scenes in that movie, which was made in 2002, inflamed public fears about human cloning. But if you have ever grown a plant from a cutting, you have cloned something. *Cloning* means making an exact genetic reproduction of a plant or animal. Understandably, many ethical issues swirl around this technology.

In this section, we look at the ethics of cloning as an option for reproduction. We also look at the possibility of cloning organs, also known as *therapeutic cloning,* and its implications. And we look at the ethical cases for and against cloning.

There are three different kinds of cloning: DNA cloning, reproductive cloning, and therapeutic cloning.

- ✔ In DNA cloning, a fragment of DNA is transferred to a virus or bacteria and is then replicated. This technology has been in practice since the 1970s.
- ✔ Reproductive cloning creates an exact copy of a plant or animal.
- ✔ Therapeutic cloning uses stem cells to create organs and tissues.

These last two types of cloning will be looked at now in more detail. Both reproductive and therapeutic cloning use *somatic cell nuclear transfer* (SCNT). This is a method where the nucleus is removed from an egg, which is then labeled *enucleated.* A nucleus from another cell is added to the egg, which begins to replicate.

Cloning as a reproductive option

In Scotland in 1996, Dolly the sheep was the first mammal to be cloned. Dolly was a direct copy, or clone, of the sheep that donated the nucleus. An enucleated cell with a donated nucleus was inserted into an unfertilized egg, and then the egg was stimulated to divide into a blastocyst with electric stimulation. The blastocyst was then inserted into a uterus of a sheep and Dolly was eventually born. This type of cloning is very difficult to accomplish successfully. And the clones have had many health problems. Dolly, for instance, aged much more rapidly than normal and eventually died at the age of six of a lung disease common in much older sheep.

Scientists have successfully cloned other animals, including cats, cows, goats, and mice, although less than 10 percent of cloned embryos actually result in the birth of a healthy offspring. And some of these cloned animals, similar to Dolly, have significant health problems. So why are animals being cloned? Some researchers think that cloned animals could provide an unlimited food source in the future, and others believe that cloning animals will help develop new treatments for diseases, both for animals and human beings.

Many ethicists think that that reproductive cloning introduces unacceptable medical risk into medical research. The process is very inefficient and difficult, and we don't know the long-term effects of this process. There has been very limited success in cloning animals, so cloning humans seems unlikely. It's morally objectionable to clone a human being who might have serious genetic flaws just for the sake or science of learning. Cloning entire mammals has been very problematic, but animals can be euthanized when they are suffering. Human beings cannot.

Even if we do eventually clone humans, we aren't creating a Xeroxed copy of another person because factors other than genetics play a role in a person's development. Even identical twins, who are technically clones, are different because of their environment and life experiences. But ethicists worry about the psychological harm that may affect cloned human beings. Knowing that you are an exact genetic copy of another person may have a big effect on psychological health. The principle of nonmaleficence to both animals and humans seems to be at risk as we proceed with reproductive cloning.

Growing tissues with therapeutic cloning

Therapeutic cloning, or cloning stem cells to create tissues for transplant or disease treatment, does not result in a human being. This is the type of cloning that most scientists are pursuing. It's important to note that scientists don't intend to clone a person and then harvest his organs for transplant. The organ in question would be grown in the lab from stem cells and the patient's cells. This is also accomplished by somatic cell nuclear transfer.

In therapeutic cloning, a nucleus of a desired organ cell, say a liver cell, is inserted into an enucleated embryonic stem cell. These cells are then grown in tissue culture to the point where they may regenerate an entire organ such as a liver.

Few people argue that developing an ability to clone specific organs would be a bad thing. This technology would reduce a tremendous amount of suffering in the world. It could help alleviate some of the dilemma associated with the huge shortages of organs available for transplantation. Some believe that it is unethical to stop this research that has so much potential.

Of course, because this type of cloning involves the destruction of embryos, some people will have moral objections to it. The ethical case against cloning involves some of the same ethical issues surrounding abortion. To make a clone, embryos must be destroyed to get at the stem cells needed to grow the organ or tissue you're trying to replicate. If you believe that a human life or personhood, with all its moral rights, begins at conception, you would be opposed to cloning because therapeutic cloning destroys an embryo and reproductive cloning recreates a human being.

In fact, that is one of the ethical cases against cloning. If a fertilized egg is a complete human being with a totally unique DNA, infused with a soul, what about the moral status of an exact copy of that egg? These questions about personhood don't get any easier! And again, we find ourselves in the ethical dilemma of weighing the harm to an embryo versus the potential medical benefits that likely could be derived from research on cloning.

Cloning likely will be a part of medicine's future. We may be able to alleviate a lot of suffering with this technique, and with controls in place regarding ethical research, there is potential for great good. Banning all forms of cloning would be like banning all organ transplants. It isn't wise to cut off a whole branch of medicine because of ethical concerns that not all people share. Using biotechnology to improve life seems to be a moral imperative in medicine.

So as the cases for and against cloning continue to be fought, and the political climate swirling around this issue continues, scientists are still involved in stem cell research, gene therapy, and cloning. The fact that so many people are concerned about the ethics of these issues makes it less likely that science will cross an ethical line into ethically unacceptable behavior. It's important that we continue to struggle with ethical issues surrounding cloning, and develop acceptable ethical as well as scientific guidelines as we move forward.

Part V
The Part of Tens

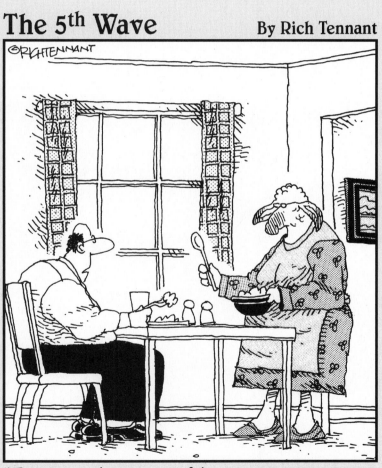

"Exactly what type of hormone replacement therapy <u>are</u> you taking?"

In this part . . .

In this final section, we look at some important ethical cases, including ten issues to review with your patients, ten landmark ethical cases that helped shape medical ethics principles, and some issues that will (we think!) be important in the future.

Chapter 18

Ten Ethical Issues to Address with Your Patients

Medical ethics may seem like a challenging class in medical school, or a topic that occasionally makes the evening news. But after you become involved in patient care, ethics becomes a part of your everyday practice. Here are some of the most important issues to talk about with your patients. The more honest and open the communication between you and your patients, the better the outcomes will be. Talk is not only cheap; it's invaluable!

Confidentiality in the Patient Visit

It's critical that your patients know their medical information is kept confidential. The primary ethical issue here is nonmaleficence, or do no harm. It could be very harmful if someone's medical information were to become public. You can certainly imagine a situation where a person might be denied employment because of a medical condition, or when medical information may be used against someone in divorce proceedings.

When a patient trusts a provider with very personal information, the patient-physician relationship is greatly strengthened. Patients will be more likely to disclose information that will help you care for them and maximize their health when they trust you. It's important to reassure a patient that everything talked about during their visit will remain confidential. (See Chapter 3 for more on the patient-provider relationship.)

The widespread use of computerized medical records has made the business of confidentiality more challenging. Instead of walking to the medical records department and fishing through lateral files for paper charts, you can access any record with a few clicks of the mouse.

Many hospitals and clinics have a zero-tolerance policy regarding breaches in confidentiality. That means if you inappropriately access a patient's record, you will be fired. When you go into a record, always ask yourself, "Am I directly involved in the medical care of this patient?" If the answer is yes, then ask "Is this the reason I am accessing this information?" Never access the chart of a family member or personal acquaintance without the filed written consent of this person.

Informed Consent

Informed consent is part of every patient encounter. A patient must be instructed on the risks and benefits of evaluations or tests, treatments, or medications prescribed, and procedures or surgeries performed. The primary ethical principle here is autonomy. Patients can make the best decisions about their healthcare when they are well-informed.

For more significant office procedures such as biopsies, hospital procedures such as blood transfusions and surgeries, or transfer from one medical facility to another, a written consent form is used. This must be reviewed with and signed by the patient. But for most other interventions, the informed consent is verbal or even implied.

Informed consent is simply good communication. For example, when a young woman comes in for her first pelvic exam and Pap smear, as her doctor, I take time to explain the procedure to her while she is seated and fully dressed. I show her the speculum, the cytobrush, the spatula, and the Pap smear vial, and explain how they are used. I explain that the pathologist will look at the cells obtained as a screening test for cervical cancer.

I am sometimes surprised at the misunderstandings about pap smears. Some women think pap smears screen for uterine cancer or sexually transmitted diseases. The truth needs to be conveyed to the patient. It's important that women understand how their regular pap smear is done and what information is revealed. This takes a little time, but is clearly in the best interest of the patient.

Integration of Religious and Cultural Beliefs into Patient Care

One of the great joys of practicing medicine is getting to know people with a diversity of cultural and religious practices — many of them integral to their very being. It's important that as a provider, you understand these beliefs and how they affect your patient's health. The ethical principle of benefi-cence is the focus here. It's a great benefit to the patient that he is under-stood as a whole person. In this setting, healing is more likely to occur.

So how do you find out about a patient's cultural or religious views? Often, important information is shared by the patient in a visit. A Muslim woman may request to see only a female provider based on her faith. A Native American man may share that he has already seen a traditional healer for his problem, and only wants advice from you. An elderly Lutheran woman of Scandinavian descent may be at peace when facing death because of her deeply entrenched Christian faith.

But what if a patient doesn't share information that may be important for you to know for the best care? Sometimes an interpreter or family member can help you learn important background information about the patient's culture or religion. And you may want to ask the patient outright, "Are there any cul-tural or religious beliefs or practices that are important to you as you think about your health?" (See Chapter 7 for more on cultural and religious beliefs.)

An excellent book that explores the importance of considering a patient's cultural and religious practices is *The Spirit Catches You and You Fall Down* by Anne Fadiman. The book tells the story of a young Hmong boy with a sei-zure disorder, and how cultural misunderstandings between his family and his medical providers ultimately led to tragedy. It's recommended reading for anyone going into the field of medicine.

The Ethics of Clinical Research

There is great reverence for clinical research within the medical profession. We all know that great advances in medicine have come and will come from medical research. However, as we reviewed in Chapter 14, the quest for medical knowledge has sometimes led to unethical treatment of patients.

As a provider, whether you are a researcher or a physician with patients involved in trials, you must make sure the patient clearly understands the study in which he is participating and the safeguards in place to shield him from harm. The ethical principles here are autonomy and nonmaleficence.

If you have a patient participating in a clinical trial, it's important for you to understand as much about the research as possible. What blood tests or other screening tests are being done to monitor your patient? What possible side effects might occur from a study drug? What benefits are afforded the patient for participating in the trial?

For instance, a primary care patient with breast cancer could be in a study where she is receiving a standard treatment such as tamoxifen plus a study drug or a placebo. If this patient develops a new symptom such as severe dry mouth, you may want to confer with the oncologist administering the study. You need to know how to manage your patient's symptoms, and make the researchers aware of this possible side effect. By staying in communication with your patients in clinical trials, you can advocate for the patient and for advancement of medicine.

Help for the Uninsured

For those who enter the medical profession, the first statement of the Declaration of Geneva reads, "I solemnly pledge to consecrate my life to the service of humanity." This document goes on to state that nothing, neither race, creed, or social standing, can come between the doctor and his duty to his patients. As providers, we're committed to caring for all people with compassion, to the best of our ability. It's one of the things you can be most proud of as a member of the medical profession. This is the principle of justice.

There are many people who are uninsured or underinsured in the United States. Many people are burdened or even bankrupted by medical bills. It's critical that you give all patients the best care possible, regardless of their economic status. However, it's also helpful to understand your patient's financial situation, if they're willing to talk about it. The goal is to try to not add to the problems he's experiencing by ordering more expensive tests or medications than necessary.

Patients need to understand the costs of visits and procedures before they're ordered. Tests can sometimes be effectively delayed and the patient given time to recover. For example, a patient with low back pain doesn't immediately need an MRI (which costs around $1,500). Research has shown that anti-inflammatories, ice, and back exercises are the most effective treatment for lower back pain, and that imaging is usually not needed until more conservative management hasn't improved the condition after 4 to 6 weeks.

Another way to help an uninsured patient is to choose equally effective generic medications over new brand name medications, especially for a condition such as hypertension. This can result in great savings. A patient can also be directed to free clinics, local programs, and government programs to help with their medical expenses. The disadvantaged patient needs you as an ally. It's a great honor and responsibility to help patients any way you can.

Screening for Genetic Diseases

The field of medicine is characterized by constant striving for more knowledge and information. But is it always best to know as much as you can about yourself and your health? Is there some information that it may be better *not* to know?

Genetic testing, for adults and pregnant women, can give the patient information to help guide medical and personal decisions. This is the principle of beneficence. But sometimes harm can come from too much information. It's important that your patients understand the ethical issues associated with genetic screening.

For example, a young woman comes to you for help. Her mother has Huntington's disease, which is a progressive, incurable disease that leads to chorea (involuntary movements) and dementia. The gene that causes this disease is autosomal dominant, which means there's a 50 percent chance this woman carries the gene and will develop the disease.

If she is tested and has the gene, it may affect her life in a negative way. She may be uninsurable. She may choose never to marry or have children. She may suffer from anxiety or depression as she awaits her fate. But, on the positive side, this information could allow her to prevent transmission of the gene to her children through IVF and genetic testing of embryos before transfer. It may help her better prepare for her future.

And, of course, there is a 50 percent chance that the test will be negative. The woman could be free of the gene and this devastating disease. This information could lift a great burden of fear and worry that she may be carrying. It's important that your patient understand all of the risks and benefits of the test before you begin.

Ethical Dilemmas in Infertility

Infertility is one of the most difficult situations a couple can face. It's a journey of emotional extremes. A couple becomes hopeful and joyful when they think they are pregnant; then a negative pregnancy test dashes those hopes and triggers a period of grief. The couple builds up the courage to try again and then the cycle repeats. This path may lead to more advanced technologies such as IVF (see Chapter 11). There are a number of ethical issues associated with these technologies, and it's helpful to the patient and her partner if they understand them before proceeding. The ethical issues here are beneficence and autonomy.

As a couple undergoes IVF, multiple embryos are created. Some are implanted and some stored for future use. If multiple embryos implant at once, selective reduction of one or more of the embryos may be recommended to improve the chances for the rest to survive. For someone who tried so hard to get pregnant, it may be difficult to face losing an embryo.

Obviously, the patient's feelings on abortion are important. And what if there are extra stored embryos that are no longer needed? What happens to them? These are just a few of the ethical issues that a patient facing infertility may struggle with. Your role during this difficult time is to discuss issues, listen with compassion, and help your patient make decisions.

Minimize Suffering in Terminal Conditions

One of your most important roles is to relieve suffering, especially when an illness is terminal. We may think that the more pain is relieved, the better. But there's a balance to reach, and this is the crux of the ethical dilemma. As a patient's pain is controlled, more beneficence is achieved. But, medications to relieve pain, primarily narcotics, can cause sedation, respiratory depression, and even death. Overuse of these medications can reduce autonomy by sedating the patient so he can't make decisions.

If you have a patient with significant pain because of a terminal condition, it's important to discover how he feels about this balance. Some patients want to use as much medication as possible to control pain and other symptoms, even if it means they are heavily sedated. Others prefer minimal medications so they can be more alert to make decisions and spend meaningful time with family.

It's important to remember that there's a difference between pain and suffering. Pain is the physical perception of discomfort. Suffering is a broader phenomenon, defined as an individual's emotional experience associated with harm or threat of harm. There are many things besides medication that can relieve suffering.

Treating a patient's anxiety or depression can be very helpful. Providing spiritual support with a pastor or chaplain can relieve suffering. Other treatment modalities to control pain, such as meditation, music therapy, biofeedback, and acupuncture, have been proven to relieve suffering.

And finally, simply being present for your patient during his illness is the most important thing you can do as a provider. See him regularly, return phone calls promptly, and keep in touch with other members of the care team to coordinate care. When a person has someone with whom to share a burden, that burden is considerably lessened.

The Living Will Discussion

End-of-life issues are difficult to discuss with patients. Very few patients are interested in deciding if they would like CPR, tube feedings, or terminal sedation at the end of life, especially when they are living healthy, active lives. However, all patients should be encouraged to complete a healthcare directive or living will, especially those who are elderly, those who have serious or terminal medical conditions, or those facing major surgery.

The healthcare directive is the champion of the ethical principle of autonomy. This document allows a patient to state their wishes for end-of-life care (see Chapter 13 for more details). If the patient is unable to speak for herself, the healthcare directive speaks for her, allowing her wishes to be fulfilled. This document is legally binding and can't be changed or overruled by family members or even medical professionals who may prefer a different course of action.

Here's a common scenario you may face as a medical professional. A patient comes in for an unrelated office visit or just stops by the front desk. He pulls a crumpled stack of papers from his pocket and says, "Here it is, Doc. My living will. Just file it on my medical chart." It's tempting to just write FILE on the papers, sign and date them, and send them on to records to be entered on the patient's chart. But this is a great opportunity to get to know your patient and his wishes. Encourage him to make an appointment to go over the living will with you. Ask him to bring his closest family member or friend. His wishes are more likely to be carried out in the future if they are discussed and clarified with you and his loved ones.

Honor the Patient-Provider Relationship

The medical profession is historically a profession of honor and noble traditions, according to the Declaration of Geneva. There is great honor in the tradition of treating illness and of scientific advancement. But truly, the most important moment in medicine is when a physician and a patient connect in the context of a healing encounter.

It's a great privilege to intimately share in another person's most important life moments: the birth of a child, the diagnosis of a serious illness, a miraculous recovery, and the moment of death. It's also a great honor to simply hear about a patient's summer garden or the birth of a grandchild. There's something sacred about connecting with another person, whether it's in a lifesaving moment of CPR or simply seeing them for an annual exam.

As discussed in this book, there are many challenging moments in medicine as well. Difficult decisions must be made, and often in a timely fashion. Remember that excellent care of the patient is always your highest priority. Think about the ethical principles of beneficence, nonmaleficence, autonomy, and justice, and how they might apply in each individual situation.

Turn to colleagues for help and support, and don't be afraid to admit mistakes. Remember that you won't always be able to offer a treatment or cure, but you can always offer your ongoing support and compassion for a patient during difficult times.

Chapter 19

Ten High-Profile Medical Ethics Cases

Medical ethics cases are often in the news. You may have heard of some of these cases because many were widely publicized. Examining these issues is an important way to advance the field of medical ethics In fact, some ethics experts feel that the only way to advance our knowledge and understanding in medical ethics is through difficult cases, or *case-based* ethics. The publicity about these cases also helps to educate the public.

In this chapter, we look at ten high-profile medical ethics cases from the past 30 years or so. Each addresses a different ethical issue, including advance directives, surrogacy, end-of-life questions, life-saving treatment for children, and gene therapy.

Terri Schiavo: The Right to Die

There are a number of important cases about the ethics of withdrawing life support. The most recent and newsworthy is Terri Schiavo in 2005. She was a woman in a persistent vegetative state (PVS).

In 1990, Terri Schiavo, a 26-year-old, collapsed from cardiac arrest, perhaps caused by eating disorders. Her brain was deprived of oxygen, which caused severe anoxic brain injury. At first, her husband wanted everything done for her and even trained as a respiratory therapist to take care of her. After 15 years, her husband wanted her feeding tube removed, stating that Terri wouldn't want to continue living in this condition. Terri's parents disagreed with this plan and wanted her kept alive no matter what. They accused Mr. Schiavo of abuse and tried to have him removed as legal guardian.

A nationwide furor exploded. Right-to-life advocates supported Terri's parents. The ACLU supported Mr. Schiavo. Doctors testified in the case on both sides. Some of these doctors seemed to be promoting untested therapies for brain injury and seeking fame. Politicians soon were involved, and the U.S. Congress subpoenaed Michael and Terri Schiavo to testify in their debate on this case. The Florida legislature passed Terri's Law, giving the governor authority to intervene. This law was soon declared unconstitutional. And of course, the news media provided 24-hour coverage of the drama.

Finally, a judge ordered that the feeding tube could be removed on March 18, 2005. Terri received palliative care and died 13 days later, not of starvation, as has been claimed, but from dehydration. An autopsy established that her brain had hydrocephalus ex vacuo, or was almost completely liquefied and that she couldn't see, hear, think, feel, or interact, with no chance of recovery. There was also no evidence that she had ever been abused.

This case highlights both the need for advance directives and an understanding of who can decide when a person in a PVS lives or dies. Because Ms. Schiavo didn't have an advance directive, but had apparently told her husband she didn't want to be kept alive with artificial means, the doctors had only his word about her wishes. Her husband was appointed her legal guardian, with the right to make any decisions about her health. Ethics committees and the courts were heavily involved in the case, with the ultimate decision in favor of Mr. Schiavo and Terri's perceived wishes for her life.

Daniel Hauser: A Child's Right to Refuse Lifesaving Treatment

The concept of *mature minor* is gaining importance. A mature minor is a person who is below the statutory majority age of 18, is still dependent on parents, but can make reasoned judgments. This concept raises some difficult medical issues. In Minnesota in 2009, a 13-year-old boy named Daniel Hauser developed Hodgkin's lymphoma, a very treatable type of cancer. His parents didn't want to give him traditional medical treatment, in spite of a 90 percent cure rate for this type of cancer. His religion was against medical treatment, and his family preferred to use natural therapies such as vitamins and herbs. He received one course of chemotherapy in the spring, and the mass in his chest shrank after the treatment. The chemo made him sick, and he refused to undergo a second round of treatment.

The doctors took the case to court; a judge ordered that Daniel was medically neglected and must resume treatment. The county was given custody of the boy. In May, Daniel and his mother disappeared rather than undergo treatment, and an order was issued for their arrest. After a week on the run, Daniel and his mother, Colleen, returned and agreed to comply with the judge's order. While Daniel was on the run, the tumor in his chest grew and began to interfere with his breathing. His mother was treating him with ionized water and herbs during this time. After returning to Minnesota, he completed treatment, and in May 2010 was declared free of cancer.

So what about autonomy in this case? Does a 13-year-old have the right to refuse lifesaving medical treatment? That is the age that minors can be considered mature enough to participate in their medical treatment. Was Daniel able to make reasonable judgments, and should his autonomy to decide against treatment have been honored? There are several relevant issues in this case. Daniel was homeschooled and couldn't read. The judge found that the boy couldn't understand the severity of his medical condition and because he thought that herbs and vitamins could cure him, he wasn't capable of making a reasoned decision about his care.

The judge ruled that the state had a compelling interest in the life and welfare of Daniel and that his parents didn't have the right to refuse treatment for him. And because Daniel didn't have the knowledge to give informed consent, he couldn't ethically refuse treatment.

Angela Carder: Maternal versus Fetal Rights

Some of the most difficult ethics cases in medicine involve pregnancies when the rights of the mother are at odds with the best interests of the fetus. Angela Carder was a young woman who was diagnosed with sarcoma, an often-fatal form of cancer, at age 13. She survived treatment, and the cancer went into remission. She grew up, married, and became pregnant. Unfortunately, her cancer reoccurred during the pregnancy and metastasized to her lungs. She became gravely ill. At 25 weeks gestation, the hospital recommended that she undergo Caesarean section to save the fetus. She and her husband opposed this. Angela was so gravely ill at this point, it was felt she would not survive the surgery.

The hospital's administrators went to court and had a lawyer assigned to Angela's fetus. A neonatologist testified that the fetus had a 60 percent chance of survival. Angela's husband testified that she clearly did not want the surgery performed. Before the surgery, Angela had stated she didn't want it done. At the time of the court case, she was so ill that she couldn't testify. The court didn't interview Angela's long-term cancer doctor.

Although by the time of the surgery she was too sick to communicate, the court ordered the Caesarian; none of the obstetricians familiar with the case would perform it. Eventually, another doctor agreed to perform the surgery. The Caesarean was performed, the fetus died, and Angela died two days later.

Her estate sued the hospital, and in 1990 the U.S. Court of Appeals ruled that the lower court mistakenly favored the state's interest in potential life over

Angela Carder's right to autonomy, upholding the pregnant woman's right to autonomy. Some attorneys who have studied the case felt that the judges thought that because Ms. Carder was "almost dead," the rights of her fetus outweighed her rights. How much should the rights of a fetus, a potential person, infringe on a mother's autonomy?

Sister Margaret Mary McBride: Religion in Conflict with Medicine

Sister Margaret Mary McBride was an administrator and member of the ethics committee at St. Joseph's Hospital and Medical Center, a Catholic hospital in Phoenix, Arizona. In November 2009, she was presented with a case of a pregnant women, a mother of four, who was suffering from pulmonary hypertension in the 11th week of gestation. Sister McBride agreed with the patient, her family, and her doctors that the only way to save the mother's life was to perform an abortion.

Sister McBride was relying on the *double effect rule*, that the main goal was to save the mother's life, and that the abortion, while regrettable, was a secondary effect of the surgery. Without the abortion, both mother and baby would likely have died. The abortion was performed, and the mother survived. Because of her role, Bishop Thomas Olmsted excommunicated Sister McBride from the Catholic Church.

More than one in six hospitals in the United States are Catholic hospitals. This is the relevant question: How much should hospitals be allowed to let religious teachings about ethics dictate medical care? What about patient autonomy and justice? Even among Catholic theologians and physicians there was disagreement about the bishop's decision and ongoing discussion about what this means for patients in church-affiliated hospitals.

Baby Manji: An Unclear Identity

Surrogate arrangements in pregnancy can raise many difficult ethical issues. In 2008, a baby girl named Manji was born through a surrogate arrangement in India. The surrogate mother received a new house, a lump sum payment, and living expenses. The couple who started the process, the Yamahas, lived in Japan but traveled to India for this process. Unfortunately, they divorced the month before the baby was born. Manji was conceived from a donor egg and Mr. Yamaha's sperm and then implanted into another woman's womb.

Technically, this child had three mothers: the surrogate mother, the egg donor, and Mrs. Yamaha. But after the divorce, Mrs. Yamaha did not want to raise the baby. The issues were this: Who was Manji's legal mother? What was her nationality? A birth certificate in India requires the names of father and mother. With no birth certificate, the state of India wouldn't issue a passport for the baby. And India doesn't allow single fathers to adopt infants.

Then a social welfare agency called Satya got into the act. The agency filed a petition against the clinic, saying the clinic was trafficking in infants and selling them to foreigners. The agency also claimed that Mr. Yamaha should not have custody of his biological daughter because India lacked proper surrogacy laws.

In the end, a court issued a birth certificate for Manji that was actually an identity certificate, which didn't mention a mother's name or the baby's nationality. This document let officials issue a humanitarian visa to the baby. The baby's paternal grandmother was given custody. Many issues with this case are still unresolved. In surrogacy, there are at least four involved parties (including the baby), and all of these parties want their autonomy honored, especially when disagreements arise. It's difficult to decide whose rights are most important. When surrogates are paid for their work, questions about coercion and justice are raised. And what about fertility tourism? Are women in poor countries being exploited by this issue with the lure of money?

Louise Brown: The First Test Tube Baby

Louise Brown was the first baby to be born after being conceived by in vitro fertilization. She was the original *test tube baby,* and her case raises ethical issues with clinical research and fertility treatments. She was born in Oldham, England, on July 25, 1978. Her parents, Lesley and John Brown, had tried to conceive for nine years, but had been unable to because of a blockage in Lesley's Fallopian tubes.

Drs. Patrick Steptoe and Robert Edwards had been working for a decade on in vitro pregnancy. They recruited infertile women for their experiments and harvested their eggs. The eggs were fertilized in a petri dish and then implanted in the uterus. Lesley Brown was their 102nd patient. With the correct hormonal balance, the pregnancy was a success.

The couple was told that the in vitro fertilization (IVF) procedure was experimental, but doctors didn't tell them that no child had ever been born alive as a result of this procedure. Looking back, this is a breach of the couple's autonomy because of lack of informed consent. However, the pregnancy went well, and Louise was born a healthy baby by Cesarean section. She is now married and has a son of her own.

Since Louise's birth, many advancements have been made in IVF, which has led to issues about the creation and storage of embryos. What value and rights do these embryos have? How should they be disposed of? Should certain embryos be selected because of their genetic makeup — even for trivial matters such as gender or eye color? These questions remain unanswered.

Jesse Gelsinger: The Risks of Gene Therapy

Gene therapy is a medical treatment in which a disease-causing gene is replaced with a healthy one. All of our cells have genes, so this is a monumental process. There have been several clinical trials of this therapy, with many issues and problems.

Jesse Gelsinger was an 18-year-old man who had an X-linked genetic liver disease called ornithine transcarbamlyase deficiency that was the result of a mutation. His disease had been well controlled with diet and medication, although the disease would eventually kill him. Jesse had the opportunity to participate in a clinical trial of gene therapy for this disease and decided to enroll. His decision was based on the altruistic attitude of advancing science and helping others with the disease. He had health conditions that should have excluded him from the trial, and he wasn't informed of serious treatment side effects that had already been noted.

When he was injected with adenoviruses carrying a healthy gene in a Stage 1 trial, his body responded with a massive immune response that led to organ failure. He died, and the trial was discontinued. It was revealed that the principle investigator in the trial was an investor in the company that had sponsored the trial — a clear conflict of interest.

Some doctors and researchers think gene therapy trials should have stricter protocols and be followed more closely by Institutional Review Boards and regulators. A few scientists think there should be a moratorium on gene therapy until more lab and cell research has been done. There's also a concern that gene therapy may be used to enhance human beings cosmetically, or improve IQ or mental acuity rather than treating disease. Informed consent and ethical clinical trials are the issues here. Patients must be told of all of the risks and benefits of a trial, and must understand that trials are not therapy. Researchers must report adverse effects immediately.

Nadya Suleman: Too Much Fertility

The case of Nadya Suleman (a.k.a. Octomon) raised ethical questions about infertility. In 2009, Ms. Suleman gave birth to eight babies at once. The six boys and two girls joined six siblings (all under the age of 8) for a total of 14 children. The single mother had used fertility treatments to achieve her multiple pregnancies, and had 11 embryos implanted, resulting in eight babies.

Ethical questions immediately bounced around the country. Carrying that many babies at once poses a real risk to the health of the mother, not to mention the babies. Should Ms. Suleman's doctors have allowed her to undergo fertility treatments, let alone in vitro fertility treatments, when there were questions about her financial stability? Ms. Suleman lived with her parents, who had just declared bankruptcy. Should finances play a part in determining who has children? Who is going to pay for the neonatal care?

There are no laws regulating assisted reproduction in the United States, although since this event, both California and Georgia have introduced legislation regulating fertility clinics. The proposed laws would limit the number of embryos implanted in each round of treatment. The American Society for Reproductive Medicine (ASRM) has guidelines that state a woman under age 35 should be implanted with no more than two embryos at one time.

Although patient autonomy is important, there are other ethical considerations. Isn't risking the health and lives of so many fetuses violating the principle of nonmaleficence? What about scarce medical resources and justice? The cost of neonatal intensive care can run into the millions of dollars. What about the lives of the children Ms. Suleman already had? Is their quality of life going to suffer because she has so many children to take care of?

The fertility doctor or doctors bear some of the responsibility in this case. Transplanting that many embryos at one time can lead directly to difficult ethical issues. Will the mother agree to selective reduction, if necessary? Who will pay for intensive care, if necessary? And who will take care of the children if something happens to the mother during pregnancy or labor?

Ms. Suleman's fertility doctor, Dr. Michael Kamrava, is under investigation for over-implanting several other patients. In 2009, the ASRM expelled the doctor. In January 2010, the California Medical Board filed a complaint of gross negligence against the "octodoc."

Glen Mills: Autonomy versus Protecting Society

Some high-profile HIV cases have made news, most notably Glen Mills, a New Zealand man who was incarcerated after he knowingly had unprotected sex with at least a dozen men and women whom he contacted on the Internet. Doctors believed he was deliberately spreading the disease and should be restrained for public safety reasons.

Healthcare providers were aware that Mr. Mills, who was diagnosed with HIV in 2007, was having unprotected sex, but couldn't inform authorities about it because of ethical considerations and privacy laws. However, it became clear that he was intentionally infecting others, and his doctor's duty to report harm to others overcame the patient's right to privacy and confidentiality. In 2009, he was charged with reckless endangerment and remanded into custody. He died in jail in November 2009 before his trial began. In 2010, an

Indiana man, Tony Perkins, was arrested and accused of knowingly infecting as many as 100 women with AIDS. Mr. Perkins was informed of his *duty to warn* in 2008 by state health officials, but he ignored the message.

The issues of autonomy, nonmaleficence, and justice are important in these cases. Concerns about public safety and public health can override confidentiality and patient autonomy when a person is a clear danger to the health and welfare of others. These cases are not always so clear. What about the pregnant mother who is abusing drugs? What about the father who spanks his children and leaves bruises? When should a person's autonomy be restricted to protect the lives of others?

Baby Jane Doe: Treatment of Impaired Babies

When babies are born with severe defects, difficult ethical decisions must be made about treatment. An early and notable case is Baby Jane Doe. She was born to parents Linda and Dan in New York in 1983. At birth, she had spina bifida, hydrocephalus (fluid on the brain), a damaged kidney, and microcephaly (small head).

The pediatric neurologist who first examined her issued a grim prognosis. He said she would either die soon or she should have immediately surgery, but would be paralyzed, retarded, and vulnerable to bowel and bladder infections. Given this poor outlook, the parents elected to forgo surgery and continue with *comfort care.*

The story broke in the national media and a right-to-life lawyer filed a suit to force treatment. The courts eventually decided that if there were two medically reasonable options for treatment of an infant, the decision should be left to the parents. In the meantime, doctors discovered that the initial prognosis was too negative, if not outright incorrect. Baby Jane's head was actually a normal size, and doctors thought she would be able to walk with braces. The parents decided to go ahead with the surgery. In 1998, when Baby Jane was 15 years old, she was living with her parents and attending school for the disabled.

Many ethical issues come into play when treating impaired infants. Should disabled children be allowed to die just because they don't fit into their parents' plans? Are there different degrees of defects? Are some defects more acceptable than others? How does one predict an impaired infant's future quality of life, and how does this affect the parents? Whose autonomy takes precedence? Is there a time when letting an impaired infant die is the most compassionate treatment? With the increase in premature births, these ethical questions must be faced more often.

Chapter 20

Almost Ten Ethical Issues for the Future

In This Chapter

▶ Creating new life and organs

▶ Deciding who receives treatment

*I*n this chapter we look through a telescope at the future. Given how far medicine has advanced in the past 50 years, we may have difficulty imagining what new medicines, treatments, or cures await us in the future, and what ethical issues they will generate. But we're going to try!

Cloning

Scientists once thought that cloning mammals was impossible. Then in 1996, the Roslin Institute in Scotland cloned a lamb named Dolly. Although Dolly lived a short and sickly life, she showed that cloning is a real possibility. The field holds a lot of promise for treatments and even cures, but there are huge ethical issues surrounding it. Should human beings be cloned? Many people feel that re-creating exact genetic copies of people is unethical. Cloning involves creating embryos that may be defective or that will have to be destroyed, which raises ethical issues.

But what if we can literally grow a new heart or kidneys for someone? Just think of the thousands of lives that could be saved if we didn't have to rely on cadaver donation for organ transplant. The amount of suffering that could be alleviated is tremendous. Strict oversight on cloning research and tough ethical guidelines will need to be put in place for this research to advance.

Designer Babies and Future Elites

Pre-implantation genetic testing before in vitro fertilization (IVF) lets would-be parents avoid passing on diseases to their children. Most people feel that's a good thing. But how far are we going to go with this testing? If we can avoid passing on the gene for cystic fibrosis, for instance, can we also choose hair color and intelligence? There's an ethical difference between medical treatment and genetic enhancement; one improves lives, but enhancement could result in devaluing "normal" human beings.

Sex selection is another issue when we "design" babies. Abortion because of gender is already a huge issue in some parts of the world, usually favoring male infants. Many people think this practice is unethical and immoral because favoring one sex over another is discriminatory. What if we discover a gene that favors homosexuality? Or a gene that controls physical coordination? We are going to have to set limits on acceptable tweaking of traits and genes.

Rationing of Medical Care

In the summer of 2009, there was a huge ruckus in the United States about proposed healthcare reform. Wild accusations flew around, and discussions got very heated. Many people were upset at the thought of changes in their healthcare. But with tens of millions of Americans uninsured and the cost of healthcare spiraling out of control, something had to be done. Reform was passed, and the heavens didn't fall. Another thing that didn't happen was a clear and calm discussion of healthcare rationing. This is something we can hope for in the future.

As we discussed in Chapter 6, every service on earth is rationed. What we have to decide is *how* medical care is going to be rationed. Are we going to keep rationing by cost? Will only the wealthy have good healthcare? Or are we going to see to it that as many people as possible receive a decent minimum of care? Using other countries' models will be helpful as we pursue healthcare reform. Controlling the cost of insurance and care is going to be important, not only to our health, but also to our country's economic future.

Who Owns Your Genes?

When the Human Genome Project was completed in 2003, scientists were overjoyed. For the first time in history, all of the genes in human DNA were identified. This could open the door to medical treatments tailored specifically to each patient, lead to cures, and improve diagnostics.

Of course, ethical questions were also raised. And what happens if information in our genes becomes public? In 2008, President Bush signed the Genetic

Information Nondiscrimination Act (GINA), which protects Americans against discrimination from insurance companies and employers based on what's in *our* genes. Is that going to work in practice?

Can a company patent a gene? Aren't our genes our personal property? This issue hasn't been addressed with legislation. Companies have tried to patent genes, but in March 2010, a judge struck down patents on two genes linked to breast and ovarian cancer. The argument was that genes are products of nature and can't be patented, and that these patents stifle research. The company argued that work on DNA turns it into something else and makes it patentable. We'll see what happens.

The Doctor Is Online

The Internet has changed society. You can order books online, chat with someone on the other side of the world, and learn about anything with the touch of a button. You can even have an online doctor's visit. In fact, more and more healthcare organizations offer e-visits, and patients in small towns use telemedicine to visit with specialists from larger hospitals. But is an important part of the provider-patient relationship lost when it is done by computer? The American Academy of Family Physicians has written guidelines for *e-checkups,* most notably that the patient must have seen the doctor in real life before accessing this service. And can we be sure that these online encounters are secure? The doctor's visit is based on confidentiality and autonomy. We must ensure that safeguards continue to be at the forefront as computer technology advances.

Pandemic Influenza Outbreak

Infectious disease experts predict that a more virulent influenza outbreak will spread across the globe and take thousands of lives in our future. This will raise many ethical dilemmas. How do we decide which patients should get some of the limited supply of medication to treat the disease? Should infected patients be quarantined? And how should the vaccine be distributed as it becomes available? Medical and ethics experts are already devising policies for this situation so we are prepared, but more work needs to be done.

Future Clinical Trials

The Belmont Report and Declaration of Helsinki were written years ago to prevent unethical clinical trials. But even today, some researchers and companies sponsoring research are violating ethical standards. Researchers face a great deal of pressure to publish meaningful findings and to develop new treatments. Sometimes this great pressure leads to unethical behavior. As clinical trials reach into new areas of medicine, ethical standards for Institutional Review Boards (IRBs) are going to be more specific and over-arching. Unethical clinic trial practices undermine the advancement of medicine. Patients lose trust in doctors and medications when ethical standards are violated. Most important, patients are hurt by these violations. Federal legislation may be needed to strengthen IRB oversight and responsibility. If abuses continue, the way research trials are designed may have to change.

Artificial Wombs

And you thought test tube babies were the stuff of science fiction! What happens when a workable artificial womb is created? This technological advance could help women who have had hysterectomies or other uterine abnormalities have children. But it also raises questions about cloning and *snowflake babies*. Will some people demand that currently stored and frozen embryos be grown in artificial wombs as a principle of the pro-life cause? And what about the attachment that a mother develops toward a baby growing inside her body? Isn't that important?

In 2002, scientists cultured endometrial cells from a uterus and engineered them to form a uterus. Embryos were implanted in this uterus, and they started to grow. The experiment had to be discontinued after six days to comply with current IVF legislation. So the future may be upon us. But legal and ethical issues will have to be addressed before this technology moves forward.

The Global Spread of AIDS

One of the primary goals of global bioethics must be to stop the spread of HIV around the globe. This starts now and will extend into the future. Americans first heard of AIDS in 1981. Twenty-five years later in 2006, 25 million people around the world had died of HIV. Prevention tactics raise ethical questions, especially because the disease is spread primarily through sex.

Does attempting to restrict infected patients' sexual practices limit patient autonomy? Do needle exchange programs for IV drug users encourage drug abuse? Now that we have expensive drugs that slow progression of HIV, who should have access to them? In 2010, it's estimated that 14 million children in Africa are AIDS orphans. This problem must be addressed now and well into the future.

Index

• K •